[redacted]

# ILLNESS BEHAVIOR

## *A Multidisciplinary Model*

# ILLNESS BEHAVIOR

## *A Multidisciplinary Model*

Edited by

Sean McHugh

and

T. Michael Vallis

*University of Toronto*
*Toronto, Canada*

PLENUM PRESS • NEW YORK AND LONDON

Library of Congress Cataloging in Publication Data

International Conference on Illness Behavior (2nd: 1985: Toronto, Ont.)
Illness behavior.

"Proceedings of the Second International Conference on Illness Behavior, held August 14–16, 1985, in Toronto, Canada"—T.p. verso.
Includes bibliographies and index.
1. Sick—Psychology—Congresses. 2. Medical personnel and patient—Congresses. I. McHugh, Sean. II. Vallis, T. Michael. III. Title. [DNLM: 1. Attitude to Health—congresses. 2. Behavior—congresses. 3. Sick Role—congresses. W3 IN181P 2nd 1985i/WM 178 I61 1985i]
R726.5.I585 1985 616′.001′9 87-2530
ISBN 0-306-42486-X



Proceedings of the Second International Conference on Illness Behavior,
held August 14–16, 1985, in Toronto, Canada


A Division of Plenum Publishing Corporation
233 Spring Street, New York, N.Y. 10013



Printed in the United States of America

## PREFACE

In August, 1985, the 2nd International Conference on Illness Behaviour was held in Toronto, Ontario, Canada. The first International Conference took place one year previous in Adelaide, South Australia, Australia. This book is based on the proceedings of the second conference.

The purpose behind this conference was to facilitate the development of a single integrated model to account for illness experience and presentation. A major focus of the conference was to outline methodological issues related to current behaviour research. A multidisciplinary approach was emphasized because of the bias that collaborative efforts are likely to be the most successful in achieving greater understanding of illness behaviour.

Significant advances in our knowledge are occurring in all areas of the biological and social sciences, albeit more slowly in the latter areas. Marked specialization in each of these areas has lead to greater difficulty in integrating new knowledge with that of other areas and the development of a meaningful cohesive model to which all can relate. Thus there is a major need for forums such as that provided by this conference.

The traditional biomedical model is frequently criticized by both the public and members of the health and social science professions for a multitude of perceived inadequacies. This might be construed as indicating the time for a paradigm shift in medical treatment. Kuhn (1962) has written, from the philosophy of science, about the evolution of theoretical models proposed to account for given phenomena. Models are initially accepted and widely endorsed with enthusiastic support. This is followed by the emergence of critical data pinpointing model inconsistencies. This, in turn leads to disfavour and replacement with newer models. We would argue that current knowledge should force the rejection of the traditional biomedical model but the complexities required of a replacement model impedes this transition such that Biomedicine supported by technological advance, is itself experiencing a re-emergence. Most health and social science workers are in favour of a replacement model (i.e., biopsychosocial model) but are stymied by its complexity and the lack of specification as to how to translate it into workable terms. The fact that Biomedicine is a "cultural" system, with numerous economic and political factors promoting its maintenance also impedes change.

The organization of this book requires little explanation. It is not all encompassing as neither conference time nor book space permitted addressing all areas of significance. For example, the area of social supports is a major factor in deciding help-seeking behaviour but is addressed only indirectly and not according to its significance. Presumably, future conferences on illness behaviour may deal with the limitations of previous meetings or go on to newer subject areas (e.g., self-care and lay referral; defining the nature and role of unconscious thought processes in illness experience).

Our attempt to integrate the contributions to this text and the current state of knowledge of each of the related disciplines is outlined schematically (Figure 3, p.11) and is analogous to Leigh and Reiser's attempt to focus inquiry into specific dimensions (see PEG, p.62). The multiplicity of variables and their interactions is obvious. We believe the model shows that, despite different scientific backgrounds, it is possible to relate the various interest areas in a meaningful fashion. Further, it emphasizes the importance of continually trying to define the relationships/contributions of each of the component parts of the model if we are to make the biopsychosocial model more workable in practical terms for daily useage.

The contributions of the conference participants deserve mention and thanks including several whose texts are not included herein (Dr. A. Detsky, University of Toronto; Dr. D. Meichenbaum, University of Waterloo; Dr. V. Neufeld, McMaster University; Dr. J. Ware, Rand Corporation). A special mention is deserved for Drs. Arthur Kleinman and David Mechanic who provided much advice and encouragement in the planning of the 2nd International Conference. Lastly, Miss Ginger Paul and Mr. Steven Lico warrant a special thanks for their careful work in the preparation of this book.

Sean McHugh
and
Michael Vallis

REFERENCE

Kuhn, T. S. (1962). The structure of scientific revolutions. Chicago: University of Chicago Press.

CONTENTS

# PART I INTRODUCTORY ISSUES

# ILLNESS BEHAVIOUR: OPERATIONALIZATION OF THE BIOPSYCHOSOCIAL MODEL

Sean McHugh and Michael Vallis

Departments of Medicine and Psychiatry
University of Toronto

The management of illness behaviour has become a major area of interest, as well as a significant challenge, for the health and social sciences. Despite the amount of attention paid to illness behaviour, it is an area which is poorly understood and many (including patients, health care providers, social scientists, and health care systems analysts) might argue, is not effectively managed. In this chapter, the essential components of an illness behaviour model will be outlined, drawing upon the concepts of the various health and social sciences. This model is intended to facilitate effective and integrative management of the myriad of factors relevant to illness behaviour.

Mechanic defines illness behaviour as the manner in which persons monitor their bodies, define and interpret their symptoms, take remedial action, and utilize various sources of help as well as the more formal health-care system (Mechanic, 1962, 1978, 1984). The concept of illness behaviour was initially proposed as a framework to account for somatization tendencies. In more recent years, illness behaviour has been proposed as a dynamic process to explain help-seeking behaviour (Mechanic, 1983). Other than Fabrega (1973), who specifically referred to illness behaviour as a staged model accounting for the decision-making processes of persons considering themselves unwell, illness behaviour per se has not been accorded the status of a theoretical model. In this chapter it will be argued that the concept of illness behaviour deserves consideration by medical practitioners, social and behavioural scientists and the lay public as a general model of health disease relationships. As a theoretical model, the concept of illness behaviour can integrate the biological, psychological and social dimensions of individuals' experiences in such a way as to constitute a practical elaboration of Engel's (1977) biopsychosocial model. Not only would an illness behaviour model permit the compatible integration of current social and behavioural science concepts of man/woman as social organisms but it also allows for the future incorporation of new information of the interaction between biological state, psychological processes and social functioning. In this model the biological, psychological and social context are considered as equally important dimensions, with none having a priori superiority in understanding the nature of human behaviour in health and disease. As such, an illness behaviour model may have greater utility for present and future interdisciplinary research, education and clinical practice than exists presently.

## The Biomedical Perspective

Much of medical practice continues to be guided by what has come to be known as the biomedical model. According to this model, an individual's complaints and ailments are understood as the result of disordered biology, and the interventions are guided by biological principles and mechanistic thinking based on "either/or" and single-cause explanations (Engel, 1977). Although referred to as a model, it is more a post hoc heuristic which has become reified through the single-minded scientific pursuit of greater understanding and harnessing of the human biological processes. Engel (1977), after decades of thought regarding the relationships between health and disease, has argued that the biomedical model has assumed the status of "cultural imperative", with fusion (and confusion) of scientific and folk models. Further, he argues that the biomedical model no longer fulfills the basic requirements of a scientific model because of intransigence to consider, recognize and incorporate new ideas and concepts of the socio-cultural determinents of illness. Biomedical thinking has "acquired the status of dogma ... [which] requires that discrepant data be forced to fit the model or be excluded" (Engel, 1977, p.130).

Engel has not been alone in reaching such conclusions. Many other behavioural (defined and used in a broad sense) and medical science writers have critiqued the biomedical model (the reader is referred to the works of Mechanic, 1978, 1980; Fabrega, 1973, 1975 and 1976; Fabrega and Van Egeran, 1976; Kleinman, 1980; Kleinman, Eisenberg and Good, 1978; Eisenberg, 1977; Eisenberg and Kleinman, 1981; Barondess, 1979; Lipkin, 1981; Chrisman and Kleinman, 1983; Marsella and White, 1984; Leigh and Reiser, 1985; Levine, Feldman and Elinson, 1983). Common themes with reference to Biomedicine include: (a) that health in the social sense (and according to World Health Organization definition) is determined by public health measures, social conditions and personal health behaviours (e.g., smoking); (b) that much medical help-seeking results from distress associated with "problems in living", occurs in the absence of disease processes, and is shaped by cultural background and past learning experiences; (c) that Biomedicine deals poorly with the illness experience of patients generally (and particularly in the absence of disease), and through its biomedical focus can worsen the distress experience; (d) that the Western health care system is hospital-based and oriented around acute-care medicine; and (e) that other social science disciplines and health care professions should be integrally involved in the provision of health care services, and that barriers exist to this involvement through the organization and practice of medical care.

These criticisms of Biomedicine should not be construed as undervaluing the tremendous success achieved by medical technology in understanding the pathophysiological basis of diseases and new treatments aimed more precisely at causal "lesions" (Fabrega, 1975; Engel, 1977; Eisenberg, this volume). There is considerable advantage when the biomedical machinery can be quickly mobilized to deal with a society-threatening disorder such as AIDS (acquired immuno-deficiency syndrome, see Eisenberg, this volume, for discussion of the rapid advances in the understanding of AIDS). However, from the perspective that much of human suffering and illness arises outside the defined interest of Biomedicine, the emphasis on biomedical advances is less impressive.

The conceptual limitations of a biologically-based model has lead to increased difficulty for the medical practice in distinguishing between "diseased" and "non-diseased" states. Biomedicine accounts for illness occurring in the absence of, or disproportionate to, the severity of disease in a variety of ways. Physician opinion has ranged from the view that there is a biological explanation for all conditions, including mental disorders to the labelling of many complaints as functional: "Common slang is that the patient has 'no pathology', and it carries the double implication that he is not sick and often also that he is not worthy of help or that he is 'fooling' the physician" (Engel, 1960, p. 471). As non-disease based complaints are widely recognized as comprising more than 50% of primary care visits it is hardly surprising that medicine's faulty conceptions are associated with unsatisfactory treatment outcomes and the persistence of patients' complaints. Marsella and White (1984) have criticized medicine in general, and psychiatry in particular, for ignoring what they consider the overwhelming evidence that sociocultural factors are a major determinant of the expression of mental disorder and for failing to incorporate new information regarding these relationships:

"The major reason for this is psychiatry's continued commitment to a DISEASE conception of mental disorder, which assumes that mental disorders are largely biologically-caused illnesses which are universally represented in etiology and manifestation." (p. ix)

In this light, it is interesting to note that the evidence for a clear biological basis in mental disorders exists only for schizophrenia, affective disorders and organic brain syndromes. While the biological basis of other disorders (e.g., panic) currently receives much attention, the importance of non-biological factors (e.g., social learning theory) should not be underemphasized. Equally important, one must not implicitly endorse a mind-body dualism as all human behaviour whether generated by biological or psychological factors, is manifested at an organic level. Increased focus on biological research may also reflect the fact that in some ways it is easier to isolate and study biological processes (in the experimental sense) than psychological processes. However, the exploration of the various dimensions of the biological framework (e.g., dexamethasone suppression tests) may have less utility and importance than exploring the role of social learning theory.

The identification of disease processes is often approached in a relatively straightforward manner as though competing explanations could be definitively excluded. However, this is not the case. Feinstein (1979) cites the ability of medicine to identify with "unprecedented specificity and consistency, the principle <u>lesion</u>" (p.4) of a given disease, but that diseases are now recognized by a spectrum of clinical manifestations which may be quite diverse, resulting in individuals with the same diagnosis but quite different clinical manifestations. As a result, the identification of diseases from nonspecific or vaguely presented symptom reports often presents difficulties for physicians. As well, Helman (1985) cites a number of physician-related variables which affect the diagnosis of disease processes:

"... a closer examination of the biomedical model - its theory and its practice - suggests that far from being homogeneous, it is rather a cluster of Explanatory Models which vary greatly according to specialty, context, audience, and type of condition, as well as the personal characteristics of the physician, and his or her position in the medical hierarchy" (p. 294).

Helman (1985) illustrates these points in his description of a middle-aged man, recently under some "stress", who experiences episodic chest pain and sees five physicians, each of whom has a different explanation regarding the cause and seriousness of his symptoms. (1) Not surprisingly, the man had difficulties formulating a satisfactory explanation for himself as to the

---

1. See Lock and Lella's (this volume) discussion of physicians' conceptualizations of postmenopausal symptoms for insights into the degree of variability in these conceptualizations and the resultant treatments.

cause of his symptoms and distress. Helman described the variation in these conceptualizations, and the resultant treatments, on the basis of the physicians' training, their previous clinical experience, the highly variable clinical presentations of many diseases, and even the physicians' personalities (Balint, 1957).

The process by which nonspecific symptoms are erroneously labelled as disease has been called "pseudo-disease" (Helman, 1985), "diseasization" (Kleinman, see Helman, 1985) or "medicalization" (Cott; Zola; this volume). Specifically, these terms refer to the process whereby disease attributes are applied to problems which do not have an organic basis and to which medicine is looked to for a "cure". As Cott (this volume) discusses, the reason why some of these problems are presented to physicians is obvious, since on some occasions the symptoms are indicative of disease processes (e.g., fatigue). However, when these symptoms are treated as if there was a disease basis (e.g., with medications), when in fact they represent some form of psychological distress or dysfunctional behaviour, then Cott would argue that physicians are practicing inappropriate "medicalization".

Inappropriate "medicalization" is not benign as it is often associated with unnecessary medical investigations, expensive and even harmful treatments, and confusion between what is disease and illness (Cott, this volume). Another example of "medicalization" occurs when a constellation of common complaints is classified as a "syndrome", with the untested and often unsubstantiated implication that there is an underlying biological disturbance causing the symptoms. Non-organic pelvic pain, non-cardiac/non-gastrointestinal chest pain, irritable bowel syndrome or historically archaic conditions such as chronic brucellosis (Eisenberg, this volume) illustrate this phenomenon. What is most striking in these syndromes is the associated chronic illness behaviour (Blackwell and Gutmann, this volume) which challenges the biomedical approach that leads to such reification. Within the behavioural medicine literature, there is increasing evidence to suggest that alternative approaches, incorporating educative strategies, might be preferable and more efficacious than biomedical treatment of hypothetical "diseases" (Bradley and Kay, 1985).

Barondess (1979), has recommended distinguishing between disease and illness states more rigidly. He defines <u>disease</u> as "a biologic event, characterized by anatomic, physiologic or biochemical changes, or by some mixture of these. It is a disruption in the structure and/or function of a body part or system "... due to a variety of causes, may persist, advance or regress ... and may or may not be clinically apparent." <u>Illness</u> is defined as the subjective experience consisting "... of an array of discomforts and psychosocial dislocations resulting from interaction of a person with the environment. The environmental stimulus may be a disease, but frequently it is not" (p.375). The <u>disease-illness distinction</u> cannot be over-emphasized, particularly with respect to avoiding the treatment of either dimension as if it were the other. Promoting this distinction, Cott (this volume) suggests that physicians should limit their interests and activities to the treatment of disease and that other health professionals should treat the patient's illness. While the disease-illness distinction model might form the basis for interdisciplinary teams in specialized units dealing with chronic pain and disability it is not practical for physicians in the majority of general medical practice settings to adopt such limited interests. Further, there are historical, social, and even public policy reasons (Mechanic, 1980) why it may not be desirable for physicians to adopt a role limited to a biomedical approach. While physicians are taught largely to deal with disease and not illness experience they would do well to consider the disease-illness distinction as part of a biopsychosocial approach to patients' problems. To do more good than harm, they need to learn when to not treat biomedically, but instead, to consider psychosocial issues and treatment alternatives.

## The Evolution of an Alternative Model

The problems with the biomedical model have been known for a long time. Attempts to develop alternative models has lead to the development of the fields of psychosomatic medicine, and more recently, behavioural medicine.

Lipowski (1977), in reviewing the state of psychosomatic medicine refers to it as "...a reformist movement in medicine and a distinct approach to the prevention, diagnosis, and management of disease. It is an approach antithetical to reductionism, one that affirms the uniqueness, complexity, and systems view of man" (p. 234). Engel (1977) restated the psychosomatic approach in proposing a systems theory based biopsychosocial model. While few would discount the psychosomaticists' objectives or Engel's formulation of the biopsychosocial model, psychosomatic medicine on the whole has not lived up to its "reformist" character. There are many reasons why this has been the case, not the least important of which is the fact that medicine has been heavily committed to the biomedical model. The authors contend that the biopsychosocial model has been envisioned as the domain of medicine with no active recruitment or role for the other social and behavioural sciences. Further, the biopsychosocial model has often been portrayed (as in Ross, Schultz and Edelstein, 1982) as three overlapping domains (biological, psychological and social). While such a portrayal (see Fig. 1) identifies that relationships do exist between the variables (see Feinstein, 1967), it does not define the nature of the relationships between these variables. This failure to define the nature of these interactions may be one of the reasons why the biopsychosocial model has not been more widely received or implemented (Molino, 1983; Cott, this volume).

In the past decade, the objectives of the psychosomatic school have been subsumed by proponents of what has come to be known as behavioural medicine. This field has been defined as:

> "the interdisciplinary field concerned with the development and integration of behavioural and biomedical science knowledge and techniques relevant to health and illness and the application of this knowledge and these techniques to prevention, diagnosis, treatment and rehabilitation" (Schwartz and Weiss, 1978, p. 250).

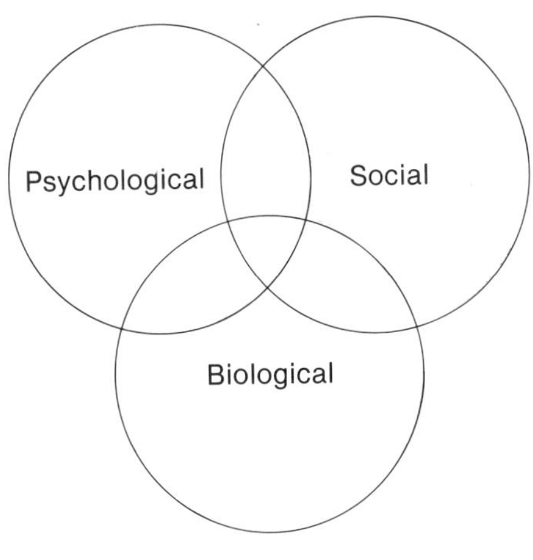


**FIGURE 1.** Schematic representation of Engel's biopsychosocial model.

While different people mean different things by the term behavioural medicine, the essential feature is that this field represents the interdisciplinary collaboration of the behavioural sciences (defined in the broad sense) and medicine with the purpose of developing and implementing a comprehensive approach to illness behaviour. Schwartz (1982b) contrasts the Biomedicine approach which is "either-or" and single-cause, with the behavioural medicine approach, which involves "more dynamic, relatively continuous, multi-category, multi-cause approaches to viewing health and disease" (p.1041). One might question how this differs from the views put forward by the psychosomaticists. The differences seem to lie in the fact that psychosomatic medicine seems to be the domain of consultation psychiatry whereas behavioural medicine has arisen as a more truly collaborative venture with the behavioural sciences being accorded an equal partnership with medicine.

The biopsychosocial approach of the psychosomaticists has been criticized by Molino (1983) and Cott (this volume) because it does not include the means for applying the model in everyday practice. Whether behavioural medicine is more successful than psychosomatic medicine will only be proven in the future. However, given the diversity and richness of approaches of the behavioural sciences for application to the study and treatment of illness (as witnessed by the various chapters in this volume), there is reason for some optimism.

## Current Trends in Medicine to Incorporate the Biopsychosocial Model

The Diagnostic and Statistical Manual of Mental Disorders (DSM-III) classification system. Psychiatrists, charged with the responsibility for dealing with patients' psychological and social problems, are often criticized by their non-psychiatric colleagues for failing to develop new conceptual approaches to assist in the management of "difficult" patients. The generally perceived failure of the psychosomaticists has done little to counteract such criticisms. However, there have been substantial shifts in mainstream psychiatry over the past several decades as evidenced by the departure from previous psychiatric classification systems and the evolution of the of DSM-III classification system (American Psychiatric Association, 1981).

Linn and Spitzer (1982) have identified the DSM's multi-axial system as containing the seeds of the biopsychosocial model advocated by Engel. The DSM-III is cited as an attempt to construct a composite of the individual experiencing mental distress so as to better reflect the relevant biopsychosocial dimensions (Linn and Spitzer, 1982; Williams, 1985). To appreciate the advantages and limitations of DSM-III it is necessary to describe the five axes of which it is comprised. Axes I and II deal with an atheoretical psychiatric label or diagnosis of the mental disorder. Axis III identifies any physical disease relevant to the presenting problem. If there are psychological factors affecting this disease, then this is recorded on Axis I (i.e., psychological factors affecting physical condition). Axis IV and V in the DSM-III code are optional for research or special clinical purposes. Axis IV is to note the presence and severity of psychosocial stressors on a single seven point global stress scale. However, the description of these stressors is limited and lacking a standardized format. Axis V is used to categorize the highest level of functioning in the past year, but again is limited by the vagueness and paucity of meaningful descriptors.

On the whole, and despite its intent, the DSM-III classification does not capture all the relevant factors of either mental disorder or physical distress. Kaplan (1985) has criticized the vagueness of Axis III and IV and its inability to describe mind-body relationships, specifically through deletion of previous (DSM-II) diagnostic categories (i.e., psychophysiological autonomic and visceral disorders). While recognizing that a behavioural or psychological problem, not attributable to mental disorder, may be the focus of attention, the possibilities cited with the DSM-III classification system are very limited. (2) Its validity unproven one can argue that the DSM-III in its present form contributes little to describing illness behaviour through its failure to provide a framework for consideration of non-disease factors. Further, DSM-III fails to provide a common language for communication between the medical, helping and social sciences. In the latter part of the chapter some suggestions for revision to this classification system are discussed.

The patient evaluation grid: A systems-contextual approach. Leigh and Reiser (1985) have provided one of the few operationalizations of the biopsychosocial model. They have suggested that specific biological and psychosocial data needs to be gathered in order to define and understand the context of patients' complaints. They organize this data in a format that they refer to as the Patient Evaluation Grid (PEG; see p.62, this volume, for an outline of the PEG). A medical history, as routinely derived, comprises but a small part of the necessary data base. The PEG dimensions include the: (a) biological - data regarding the current physical symptoms, past and family medical history; (b) personal - data regarding the patient's psychological state and particularly his/her level of distress, his/her personality and coping styles, expectations and attributions, and the way his/her symptoms have interfered in daily life; (c) environmental - data about the actual physical environment including occupational status, family relationships and social supports, and cultural background. Each of these dimensions is elaborated according to three time frameworks, namely current events, recent events and the background context. According to Leigh and Reiser, synthesis of the PEG data base permits the definition of the patient's current suffering, the contribution of disease states to the symptoms, and the patient's attitudes and attributions to his/her illness state. Additionally one can appreciate the context of the patient's complaints, the limitations posed by their own resources (both physical and psychological) and the health care options available to him/her. This patient contextual approach highlights the individual's perceived distress as the final determinant of both help-seeking and the assumption of the patient role.

Few people interested in illness behaviour would have trouble accepting the validity and nature of this systematic enquiry. The specification of these precise data are useful from an educative point of view, particularly as a reminder of the multiple determinants of illness experiences. However, the PEG is lacking as a theoretical model, because while the various dimensions are assumed to be interactive, the nature of these interactions is not specified. As well, the allocation of certain attributes and historical factors to the various dimensions has unproven validity and utility (e.g., the model involves the partitioning of important factors with little accounting for dynamic interactions). Finally, the PEG framework seems overly detailed and cumbersome to be applied on a daily basis for every patient and perhaps is best reserved for the more chronic or complex situations. The previous comments notwithstanding, the PEG represents an admirable attempt to operationalize the biopsychosocial model and deserves further investigation and evaluation.

---

2. Examples include: malingering, borderline intellectual functioning, adult, or childhood or adolescent antisocial behaviour, uncomplicated bereavement, academic, occupational, marital, phase of life, or parent-child problems.

## Illness Behaviour: Manner of Enquiry

In the following section, several of the ways in which illness behaviour have been treated are discussed. This includes the consideration of health and illness as separate states. Then models proposed to account for illness states are reviewed.

Health-illness continuum. Kasl and Cobb (1966, a & b) have elaborated upon three types of health-related behaviour. They distinguish illness behaviour (the behaviours aimed at identifying the cause and treatment for perceived symptoms) from health behaviour (those behaviours aimed at preventing disease or designed to detect it at an early stage) and from sick-role behaviour (behaviours associated with treatment of defined diseases to restore health). While these distinctions might be useful on occasion, it is clear that these behaviours are not independent of each other and that many of the factors that affect one type of behaviour also influence the other. Kasl and Cobb suggested that health and disease reflected a continuum with illness state and behaviour beginning when an individual identified themselves as unwell. It follows that if sense of well-being and unwellness do reflect a continuum (as logic and clinical experience would support) that the distinction between health and illness behaviours is arbitrary and often impossible.

Instead of artificially categorizing peoples' behavioural responses into categories of health, illness and sick role behaviour it may be more meaningful to consider illness behaviour itself as a continuum in response to perceptions of wellness or unwellness (see Figure 2). This proposal would view illness behaviour broadly but still according to the definition proposed by Mechanic (1978, 1983, 1984) as the manner in which persons monitor their bodies, define and interpret their symptoms, take remedial action, and utilize various sources of help as well as the more formal health care system. To define illness behaviour broadly does not destroy its meaning but enhances its utility since all types of illness behaviour responses are then viewed as normative.

While on occasion it may be useful to examine the social implications of being ill and how people behave in these circumstances, the sick role construct sometimes is extended beyond a practical and meaningful sense. For example, Pilowsky (this volume) defines illness behaviour in an non-normative sense, as abnormal, when patients behave in a fashion that physicians would consider as inappropriate and socially unacceptable. While decisions of normative behaviour are required on occasion for legal and social purposes, to define individuals' behaviours according to a hypothetical construct such as a sick role seems inappropriate, particularly considering the potential for individual bias (Mayou, 1984). This is not to mean that value judgements are to be avoided, but they might better be limited to the degree to which the behaviours appear proportionate or disproportionate to defineable

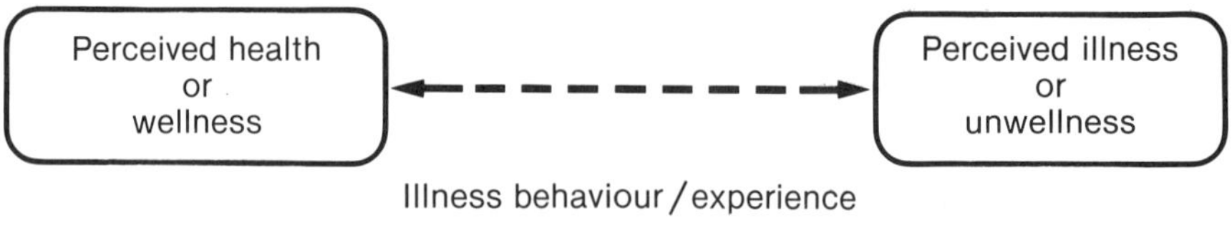


**FIGURE 2.** Perceived states of well-being.

diseases. The authors suggest that there is more utility in being descriptive, rather than applying a value-laden label which by itself has no explanatory value.

Past Illness models. Becker and Maiman (1983) have reviewed existing models of health-related behaviour. These models covered the four approaches to illness behaviour outlined by Mechanic (this volume). Specifically, Mechanic considers illness behaviour as: (a) a disposition of the person; (b) the result of an interaction between personal and environmental factors; (c) a decision-making process; and (d) as determined by the health-care services system. Becker and Maiman had the authors of the existing models judge the similarity of 109 variables extracted from their models to identify the major determinants of help-seeking. The common features included:

"(1) items pertaining to accessibility of health services, such as the individual's ability to pay for health care and awareness of health services; (2) items dealing with the individual's attitudes toward health care, such as beliefs in the benefits of treatment and beliefs about the quality of medical care provided; (3) items concerning the threat of illness, such as the individual's perception of symptoms and beliefs about susceptibility to, and consequences of, disease; (4) items pertaining to knowledge about disease; (5) items dealing with the individual's social interactions, social norms, and social structure; and (6) items on demographic characteristics (social status, income, and education)." (Becker and Maiman, 1983, p. 561, underlining added).

Considering the breadth of the common features noted above, it is not surprising that models limited to only some of these features will lack explanatory value and predictiveness. Cleary (this volume) in his discussion of the health belief model further illustrates this problem. Several shortcomings associated with these models warrant attention. First, the majority are culture-specific. Their lack of predictability may be associated with the fact that even within a single country there is a rich mosaic of ethnic backgrounds that produces a composite of sub-cultures whose health interests and behaviours vary substantially. Second, the majority of the models assume consistent rational decision-making based upon a variety of alternatives. Third, the models presume a staged progression through multiple steps.

The limitations of these health-related models for application in cross-cultural settings, has been noted by Fabrega (1975), Garro (this volume) and others. Within anthropology, appraisals of illness behaviour have been more varied and have incorporated ideas proposed by social psychologists (e.g., decison-making theory). Alternative modes of help-seeking (see Garro, this volume) and particularly the phenomenology of the illness experience have been emphasized and studied within specific cultures (Kleinman, 1980). These anthropological approaches stand out in sharp contrast to the more general approaches outlined above. They address cognition and belief systems in a manner overlooked by other approaches. Further, they also consider self-care and the use of non-medical alternatives.

## AN ILLNESS BEHAVIOUR MODEL

As with many contemporary areas of research there exists a variety of theoretical models to account for a given phenomenon. If the illness behaviour model proposed in this chapter is to be considered an improvement on the biopsychosocial model, it must represent the medical, psychosocial and cultural perspectives in such a way as to be both accurate and interactive. It must serve the purpose of providing a framework that different disciplines can relate to by providing a language that allows for translation of a given phenomenon into the terms or constructs of another perspective. From the practitioners' point of view, the model should be useful as an explanatory model for their clients or patients. When the practitioner suggests that there appears to be psychosocial factors underlying the patients' complaints, the patient need not interpret this as indicating a "mental" disease (the biomedical model) and a disvalued state.

There are four areas of the illness behaviour model that in their own right have attracted the interest of the various social science disciplines. These include: (a) the monitoring of somatic or visceral signals (symptoms); (b) the cognitive processes whereby bodily symptoms are interpreted; (c) the processes whereby individuals attach meaning to their experience (in the context of their emotional state and concurrent environmental events) in such a way as to result in perceived distress or sense of being unwell; and, (d) the ethnocultural influences that pervade all facets of human behaviour, including the nature of cognitive processes, the types of coping responses and the form of help-seeking behaviour. While this literature has provided much of the evidence on the limitations of the biomedical model, it has not been incorporated into a single model. Instead, the areas tend to stand relatively independently from each other. In order to offer a viable alternative to the biomedical model, the above areas need to be integrated into a single model, with enough specificity to be theoretically relevant, practical, and to guide future research.

The illness behaviour model detailed in this chapter (see Figure 3), attempts to incorporate the previously cited factors in a comprehensive and meaningful fashion. Each factor or dimension is considered to be equally important. The model is interactive and it is the interaction between the factors which deserves emphasizing. While the model is portrayed as a linear interactive process, this should not be taken to imply that there is a lock-step progression into and out of stages. In fact, this is not a staged model at all. All factors are presumed relevant in any given situation, although different factors would have differential relevance in particular situations. The relevance of each factor can be considered on a continuum, where it is the health practitioners task to determine which factors are more important in a given situation.

Any process must have a starting point. Flexibility is necessary as to where the process begins given the complexity of illness behaviour and the various factors contributing to it. As outlined in Figure 3, the process usually has a beginning somewhere in the interaction between changes in physiological activity, autonomic arousal, affective integration, and the cognitive interpretive processes. The interaction of these factors results in the attachment of meaning to the experience, which may lead to some form of subjective distress, which in turn leads to some form of adaptational behaviour - coping (including non-action and dysfunctional action; see Breznitz, this volume). It should be apparent that psychological processes are central and inextricably involved with the biological milieu and social-cultural environment and therefore cannot be considered in isolation from these contexts.

At this point the model will be articulated in more detail with each of the key factors described in turn.

## Physiological Function

Earlier criticisms of the biological emphasis within the biomedical model do not mean that such biological factors are not important in

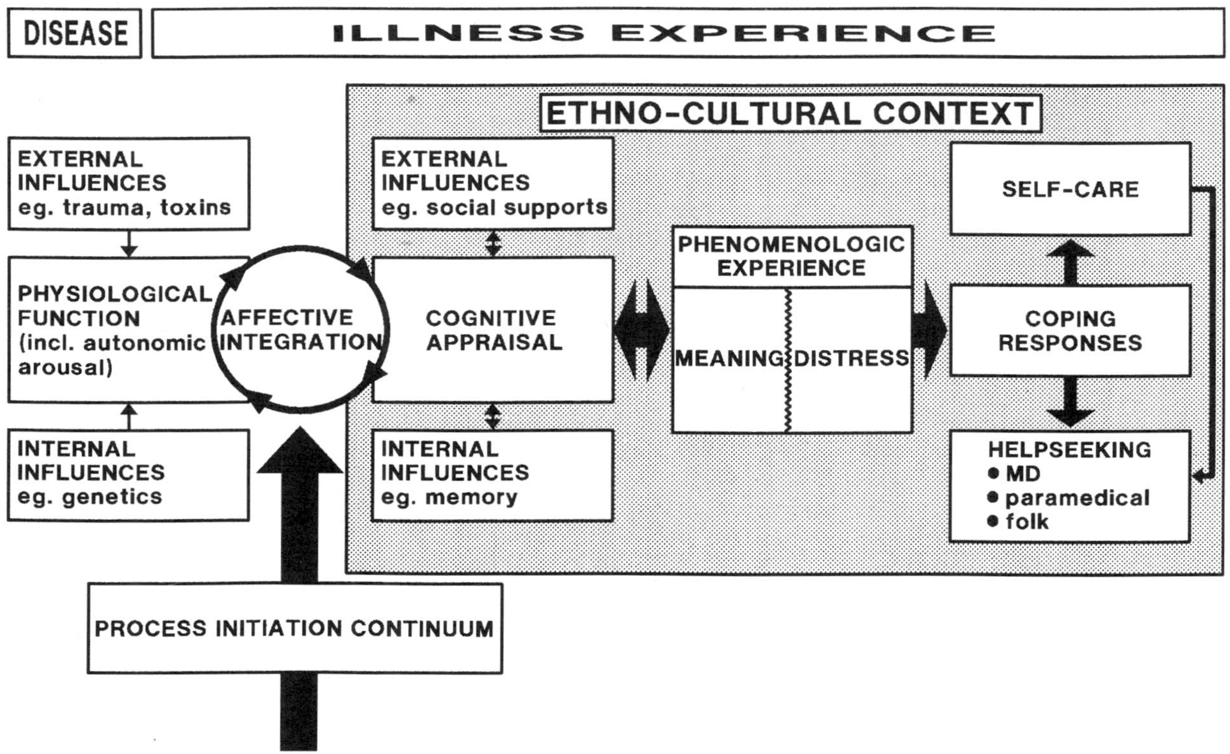
DISEASE
ILLNESS EXPERIENCE
ETHNO-CULTURAL CONTEXT
EXTERNAL INFLUENCES eg. trauma, toxins
PHYSIOLOGICAL FUNCTION (incl. autonomic arousal)
INTERNAL INFLUENCES eg. genetics
AFFECTIVE INTEGRATION
EXTERNAL INFLUENCES eg. social supports
COGNITIVE APPRAISAL
INTERNAL INFLUENCES eg. memory
PHENOMENOLOGIC EXPERIENCE
MEANING
DISTRESS
SELF-CARE
COPING RESPONSES
HELPSEEKING
• MD
• paramedical
• folk
PROCESS INITIATION CONTINUUM

FIGURE 3

evaluating illness presentations. No one would argue against the value of medical investigation in determining whether symptoms reflect an underlying disease process. However, relevant biological processes should not be restricted to disease processes. It is equally important to determine the contribution of variation in homeostatic function or states of heightened autonomic arousal in any illness presentation, as determined historically or through direct observations. How such variables interact with other factors at any given moment, and as mediated by cognitive processes, has become an important area of enquiry. (3)

According to an illness behaviour model, disturbance in body function can result from a variety of processes: a disease process (external agent or intrinsic organ dsyfunction); an over-attentiveness to variation in normal function; or a state of altered autonomic arousal (or a combination of the three factors). Attributional theory (Schachter and Singer, 1962) or cognitive processing theory (Leventhal, this volume) suggest ways in which individuals can respond to external cues (their environment) or internal cues (illness schemata) in such a way as to be concerned about the meaning or implication of their symptoms and then to seek help.

Thus it is maintained that non-disease physiological processes (such as autonomic arousal, response system variability and genetic endowment) are sufficient to elicit troublesome symptoms and deserve greater attention (Pennebaker, 1982). The autonomic concommitants of emotional states are commonly attended to and processed so as to lead to the perception of symptoms. Attentional and affective factors thus become important aspects in the perception of these non-disease symptoms. Consider the following example. An account executive, seriously overweight and living a stressful lifestyle, is distraught about a personal relationship. He has been losing sleep, having trouble concentrating and eating poorly. On the way to an important meeting, the individual rushes up some stairs to avoid being late. The interaction between his emotional state (and accompanying autonomic arousal) and the physiological effects of the physical activity, leave the individual feeling weak, winded and dizzy. An individual may attend to this experience in a variety of ways. His or her perception of these physiological changes may be associated with help-seeking reflecting the overall life distress situation (for example, the individual may attribute his/her symptoms to an impending heart attack). Leventhal (this volume) presents a model of symptom reporting that organizes the interaction between perceptual, cognitive and affective factors. He discusses illness and emotion schematas that can play a major role in symptom experience irrespective of the presence or absence of specific disease processes.

A major problem for clinical practice, when guided by the biomedical model, involves the assumption that somatic complaints do not have a physiological basis in the absence of disease. Distress, associated with an emotional event, has physiological consequences which are often attributed by patients and physicians to some (undefined) disease process. This tendency is misleading at best and harmful at worst (see the previous discussion on disease-illness distinction). It is misleading in part because the distinction ignores the fact that treatment should be directed at the

---

3. Recent conceptualizations of the etiology of panic disorder highlights such processes. Specifically, the hyperventilation model of panic disorder maintains that hyperventilation (clearly not a disease) is associated with either normal homeostatic variation or general arousal in the context of fear cues and fear-relevant cognitive processes and is sufficient to elicit panic attacks and the resultant panic disorder (Ley, 1984; Clark, Salkovskis and Chalkley, 1985).

source(s) of distress. Blackwell and Gutmann (this volume) warn against first visit medication prescribing in the assessment and treatment of chronic illness behaviour. The same caution can be applied more generally to include most symptom assessments, until the role and contribution of potential stressors has be clarified.

## Cognitive Appraisal

Within the biomedical framework, specific cognitive processes are not usually treated as important avenues of enquiry for understanding help-seeking behaviour. While the biopsychosocial model has included such processes as general psychological factors, they have not been articulated in a theoretically meaningful or practically applicable manner. The illness behaviour model outlined here considers cognitive processing as a central process in illness behaviour. This is supported by a cognitive revolution in the past decade, at least in psychology, where much research has been devoted to the identification and articulation of the role of cognitive factors in perception, affect, and behaviour. Much of this work has direct implications for illness behaviour and its treatment. For instance, Mechanic's concept of introspection (Hansell and Mechanic, this volume) has been demonstrated to be related to symptom reports, perception of distress and help-seeking.

The cognitive model highlights the fact that individuals are not passive recipients of information from their environments but instead actively process information. Knowledge is not received, as in a radio receiver, but is actively constructed (Merluzzi, Rudy and Glass, 1981). Thus, illness behaviour is not only the result of concerns of a disease state but is based on many factors, and may be quite independent of any disease process since the amount of information available to the senses quickly outstrips even the most astute individual's attentional abilities. Since not all available information can be processed, some form of selective processing is required. There are numerous factors which influence this selective filtering and the identification of these factors has greatly advanced our understanding of human behaviour.

Lazarus and Folkman (1984) have articulated the concept of cognitive appraisal as the manner in which an individual appraises his/her situation and determines his/her adaptive responses. They identify several stages to this appraisal process. The first stage involves the assessment of the significance of specific events in terms of threat, loss, or challenge. The second stage involves assessment of coping strategies for dealing with an environmental event and one's ability to implement such coping strategies. A third phase, termed reappraisal, identifies the fact that the processes operating in the first two phases continue in a dynamic fashion, in which events are constantly appraised and reappraised.

Focus on cognitive appraisal affords a non-pejorative examination of an individual's phenomenology regarding an illness episode. It becomes highly appropriate to inquire about the way an individual interprets his/her situation and their usual patterns of coping. For example, a young individual with a previous myocardial infarction may complain to his/her physician of a variety of somatic complaints and profess an inability to work, or to engage in any demanding physical or emotionally arousing activity (e.g., sexual activity). Focus on the cognitive appraisal factors might reveal that the individual interprets certain symptoms as life-threatening. He/she may believe that the only option is restriction of activity as any exertion might bring on further heart damage and death. Thus, identification of specific appraisal processes can help account for a given individual's presentation and faulty attributions can become the target for therapeutic intervention.

Bandura (1977) has identified an important cognitive process, self-efficacy, which has been demonstrated to be highly predictive in a variety of situations. Self-efficacy refers to personal judgements as to how well an individual can organize and implement patterns of behaviour in situations that may be novel, unpredictable and contain stressful elements. Bandura finds that self-efficacy is best considered as a state variable, rather than a trait variable. High and low self-efficacy states are currently the subject of much research as it appears that high self-efficacy judgements are good predictors of behaviour. For instance, self-efficacy judgements have been shown to be good predictors of behaviour in specific situations such as coping with acute pain (Vallis and Bucher, 1986) as well as more general situations such as maintenance of smoking cessation over time (Condiotte and Lichtenstein, 1981). Turk and Rudy (this volume) describe a study of the role of cognitive appraisal in the relationship between pain and depression in a mixed group of chronic pain patients. They found that the relationship between pain and depression was mediated largely by judgements of self-control. This type of data provides validation as to the importance of cognitive appraisal factors in illness experience.

In addition to appraisal and self-efficacy processes, considerable data has been gathered concerning the importance of specific cognitions in coping with physical problems. This work is illustrated by Meichenbaum and his colleagues (Meichenbaum, 1977; Turk, Meichenbaum and Genest, 1983). Assessment of specific cognitive activity (thoughts and images) has resulted in the identification of a variety of self-statements that are related to increased distress and decreased ability to cope (Segal, this volume). Such self-talk, or statements, is frequently referred to as catastrophizing. For example, a chronic pain sufferer might experience a variety of self-statements when faced with the task of preparing for work in the morning under time pressures. Examples of his/her self-statements might include: "I can't cope" or "I'll end up in bed for a week" or "If I don't slow down I may never recover." Such cognitions can have a direct impact on behaviour and subjective distress (Turk et al, 1983).

Recent research on cognitive factors in illness and emotional disorders has moved beyond the identification of conscious cognitive content (self-statements, self-efficacy judgements, catastrophizing cognitions), to the identification of the ways in which individuals organize information, referred to as cognitive schemata. It is hypothesized that such schemata guide attentional processes such that information consistent with the schemata are more easily and efficiently processed than information inconsistent with the schemata. For instance, an individual who has a schema of him/herself as an invalid will pay more attention and process more quickly information consistent with this schema (e.g., pain upon exertion, behavioural limits). Behaviours or cognitions contrary to the schema construct would be attended to less or ignored (e.g., nonimpaired activities, behavioural accomplishments). These unconscious processes serve to exacerbate or maintain chronic illness behaviour (e.g., Kuiper, Olinger and MacDonald, in press). (4)

These cognitive schemata constitute only a proportion of unconscious processes. While much has been written about unconscious dynamic processes, particularly from a psychodynamic perspective, cognitive psychology further challenges this perspective (see Lang, et al: Leventhal; this volume). It is beyond the scope of this chapter to explore these challenges more directly (see Bowers and Meichenbaum, 1984).

---

4. Much of the work in cognitive therapy is aimed at changing negative schemata (e.g., Beck, Rush, Shaw & Emory, 1979; Turk et al, 1983).

The identification of cognitive mediational (processing) factors has more value than simply advancing our understanding of illness behaviour. A wide variety of therapeutic interventions have been developed to alter dysfunctional cognitions. Many of these interventions rival alternative and more traditional interventions in terms of effectiveness. For example, cognitive behaviour therapy has been shown to be effective for pain syndromes (both acute and chronic), chronic diseases, coping with surgical preparation, and generally altering maladaptive behaviour. Interested readers are referred to Bradley and Kay (1985), or Turk, et al (1983).

Clearly, cognitive processing characteristics play an important role in the illness behaviour models represented by these major research thrusts within psychology. It is important to understand that such processing does not occur in a vacuum and is not necessarily guided by logic. Instead, cognitive processing is influenced by many factors including: ongoing environmental events (such as stressors or social supports), background dispositional factors (such as past learning or sociocultural influences), as well as physiological status and affective state. These moderator variables have a major impact on cognitive processing and thus warrant brief discussion.

Environmental stressors. Although a precise definition of the term stress, one that would be agreed to by all, is not possible, one definition states that stressors are "external events or conditions that affect the organism" (Goldberger and Breznitz, 1982, p.3). This definition highlights stress as a stimulus variable (Zegans, 1982). The work of Holmes and Rahe (1967), who developed the Social Readjustment Rating Scale to assess the severity of stressful life events, best illustrates this perspective. With this scale, specific life events are assigned a numerical value (life change units). Accumulation of life change units over a one year period is studied to evaluate relationships between degree of stress (as measured in life change units) and risk for illness.

While there is support for this research hypothesis, the paradigm is not without its critics (Zegans, 1982). A major problem is defining stress in terms of stimulus variables. Zegans (1982) reviews the literature which conceptualizes stress as a response variable (in which cognitive appraisal is an important component). He goes on to outline a model linking stress to illness. The stress response is defined in multiple stages including alarm, appraisal, search for coping strategies, the stress response itself, and finally, a stage in which the stress response relates to alteration in body functioning. The outcome of the stress response is mastery (successful coping with stress), exhaustion (coping response appropriate but not sufficient in degree), and disorganization (inappropriate coping or interference with implementation of coping). While all stages of the stress response are associated with physiological responses, failure to cope is most likely to lead to illness. Zegans goes on to develop seven hypotheses of how the stress response can be transformed into organ pathology. These hypotheses are reproduced below:

"... (1) The acute body response itself may cause damage, particularly if an already compromised organ is involved. (2) The acute body response may cause transient insult to a tissue, but repeated occurence of the stress may cause permanent tissue damage. (3) The acute physiological reaction can become chronic if it becomes conditioned to a benign stimulus resembling the stressor. Such a stimulus may be a more regular part of the individual's environment and provoke an unneccesary coping response. (4) A coping strategy may be used successfully but the physiological component is not terminated when the challenge is mastered. A reverberating circuit [italics replaced] is established, which puts unusual strain on the body. (5) A minor stress provocation releases an inappropriately severe physiological response. Modulation is lacking that grades the body's reaction according to the nature of the threat. When all stresses are responded to as major assaults, abnormal physiological reactions are possible. (6) A physiological response appropriate and adequate to cope with a given threat may result in damage to some other aspect of the body through inhibiting benign but vital body process or stimulating an imitating one. (7) Coping strategies can misfire when the behavioural component is inhibited but the physiological aspect is expressed (fight behaviour inhibited but not its physiological component). The physiological aspects of a blocked action can be continuously repeated since no appropriate cut-off signal is perceived." (p.145)

Social supports. There is a large literature that demonstrates relationships between social support variables and illness (mental illness, physical illness, recovery, etc.). A recent volume by Cohen and Syme (1985) provides an up-to-date evaluation of this area highlighting many of the current conceptual and methodological issues. Social support variables have been investigated as etiological factors in mental and physical disease (e.g., Kessler and McLeod, 1985; Kasl and Wells, 1985), as well as in adaptation to coping with illness (Wortman and Conway, 1985). (5)

Much attention has been devoted to the investigation of the mechanisms through which social supports have their effects. Cohen and Syme distinguish the direct effects hypothesis from the buffering hypothesis. According to the direct effects hypothesis, social support reduces illness by directly influencing variables such as perception of control, perception of available coping responses, etc. These variables in turn lead to positive feelings, the physiological concommitants of which reduce vulnerability to illness. According to the buffering hypothesis, social supports exert their influence at times of stress by functioning to reduce the stress level. Availability of social supports more often leads to appraisals of lower stress than occur in the absence of social supports. Similarly, the presence of social supports can increase one's sense of efficacy for coping with stress and in this way reduce the impact of stress. Cohen and Syme note that both the direct effects and buffering hypotheses have received empirical support and each may be the primary operating mechanism in different situations.

While many questions remain unanswered with respect to the role of social supports in illness behaviour, no model would be complete without including the mediating influence of social support, particularly as support interacts with the cognitive appraisal processes. Cohen and Syme pose a series of questions that need to be addressed by future research. For example, they enquire as to what effects are attributable to who is providing support, of what kind, to whom, when, and for what problem. As these questions are answered, social support variables will likely become more prominent in illness behaviour discussions.

Past learning experience. The subjective experience of illness does not occur in isolation of the history of an individual's past learning experiences. Knowledge of previous illness-related experiences (both for the

---

5. The term social support should not be taken to refer to a single construct. Social support can take the form of multiple behaviours and processes. Methodologically, Cohen and Syme distinguish the structural from the functional perspective on social support. Structural measures can include: marital status, number of relationships, and frequency of contact. Functional measures assess variables such as the affective quality of a relationship, subjective feelings in a relationship, financial aid, etc. The social supports are not differentiated in this chapter, due to space limits.

individual and for their significant others) is useful in understanding a current illness presentation. The usefulness of this information is not limited to the usual "past medical history". Instead, inquiry of past experiences with illness through direct and vicarious learning, provide the context in which current experience is interpreted. Exposure to certain illness states has an influence on the meaning that is attached to a given symptom (Kleinman, 1980). Leventhal (this volume), discusses how an individual's learning history is stored in memory as illness schemata. Symptom experience that matches (sometimes loosely) a given schemata will elicit the active processing of the schemata. For example, an individual with a schemata for skin cancer (which could be developed by past history of skin cancer or exposure to a signficant other with skin cancer) may react more strongly to an atypical mole than an individual without such a schema. In this manner, past learning has a direct impact (at the level of appraisal and meaning) on present and future illness presentations.

Past learning experiences are also important from the perspective of coping and competency with various coping strategies. There are a wide variety of means of coping with distress (e.g., denial, reliance on physician, lifestyle change, diet, emotional support) and individuals vary greatly on the repetoire of coping skills that they bring into a given illness episode (Goldberger and Breznitz, 1983). Knowledge of an individual's repetoire is useful in terms of developing intervention strategies. Turk et al, (1983) illustrate how a thorough assessment involving identification of current coping strategies (and factors that block the effective implementation of these strategies), can be used in treating illness episodes non-medically.

## Affective Integration

While physiology and cognition capture essential aspects of an illness experience, they are not all inclusive. The important contribution of emotion in the phenomenological experience of any given individual is undeniable, even though the autonomous and causal role of affect may be controversial and less clear from a theoretical perspective (Lazarus, 1984; Zajonc, 1984). In the illness behaviour model proposed in this chapter, the integrative nature of emotion in the ongoing process of an illness experience is emphasized. Indeed, the experience of emotion is, by definition, an integrative experience. This is clearly illustrated by the three-systems model of emotion (Hughdahl, 1981). Instead of being a unitary experience, emotion is indexed by multiple co-parallel (partly independent) systems; the physiological, behavioural and subjective (Rachman and Hodgson, 1981). Despite criticism on theoretical (Hughdahl, 1981) and practical grounds (Matthews and Johnston, 1981), the multiple systems model has generally been well received. The majority of clinical and theoretical investigation has been focused on the emotion of fear. The works of Lang (this volume), Leventhal (this volume), Rachman and Hodgson (1974), as well as others, illustrate how the different aspects of emotion inter-relate, albeit in a relatively loose manner. Recent work on fear reduction (Himaldi, Boice and Barlow, 1985) has attempted to identify the clinical potential of identifying synchronous and desynchronous changes across these multiple systems.

The fact that physiological and cognitive factors are essential aspects of an emotional reaction has direct and important implications for an illness experience. As states of high emotional arousal can be associated with increased physiological activity, affect becomes a direct pathway to increased autonomic arousal or to homeostatic variations in physiological function. Increased physiological activity may be perceived in ways that lead to illness perception, as has already been identified. Further, emotional factors have been directly implicated as relevant causal variables in disorders such as headache, cardiovascular problems, etc. (Bradley & Kay, 1985; Krantz, this volume). Another avenue to symptom perception results from physiological reactivity, itself eliciting an emotional reaction which in turn may escalate the degree of physiological reactivity.

As outlined in the present model, emotion is not considered separate from the non-affective factors (cognition, physiology and behaviour). There has been recent debate on whether emotion can occur without causal cognitive processing. Lazarus (1984) is an advocate of cognitive primacy, claiming that "... an emotional experience cannot be understood solely in terms of what happens inside the brain, but grows out of ongoing transactions with the environment that are evaluated ..." (p.124). Zajonc (1984) represents an opposing position, claiming that emotion can occur independent of cognition. Among his arguments he cites data suggesting separate neuroanatomical structures for emotion and cognition, how affect and cognition can be uncorrelated in some situations, and how non-cognitive processes can be used to elicit emotion.

While this debate has rekindled an interest in the role of emotion in the human experience, resolution of this cognition-affect primacy debate may not have a major impact on the role of emotion in illness behaviour. The two processes cannot be separated for any given individual. Further, physiological, cognitive and affective experience represent an ongoing interactive process, each factor affecting the other in a dynamic manner. Regardless of how the process starts, once set in motion each factor impacts on the other and a dynamic feedback loop is established.

Safran and Greenberg (in press) propose a model that circumvents the theoretical impass of the affect-cognition primacy debate. They discuss an alternative to the information processing model of emotion, the ecological model. In this model, emotion is considered an integral part of perception itself (and in this sense is independent of cognitive appraisal). Further, emotion, behaviour and cognitive processes are fused and require no prior cognitive appraisal (even though cognitive appraisal occurs concurrently). Safran and Greenberg go on to discuss the relevance of their ecological model for dealing with emotional factors in psychotherapy. Their model offers a fresh and insightful look at the role of emotion in human functioning, and it supports the contention that emotion must be considered as an interactive factor in the illness behaviour model. (6)

## The Ethnocultural Context

The limitations of a strict biomedical approach to an illness experience as well as the complexity of the same process should be obvious. To this point, the focus has been on individual factors and processes only. Equally important is the individual's social context. Rosen and Kleinman (1983) describe how social structure, defined as "... a society's institutional arrangement of social relationships" (p.86), influences the illness experience. For instance they cite data that demonstrates relationships between illness experience and socioeconomic status. Such arrangements place

---

6. The information processing model is based on a computer analogy, in which an individual passively receives information and then processes it in a step-wise fashion. Conversely, the ecological model is functional and deals with interactions between the individual and the environment, including such concepts as selection and adaptation (Safran and Greenberg, in press).

individuals in certain positions whereby they are more or less likely to experience a particular form of illness.

Sociocultural influences on illness experience are by no means limited to structural variables. The specific beliefs and norms that define a particular cultural group are equally, if not more, important influences. While these beliefs are experienced at an individual level, the culture or subculture which forms the context in which the individual exists, is responsible for the development of such beliefs. The role of culture in an illness experience is totally outside the usual biomedical model enquiry, under which a symptom takes on a different meaning only in the context of a different disease process. To limit meaning to disease process is to exclude much of what is important in terms of causality and what is important to ensure effective intervention. Rosen and Kleinman (1983) present a case history which illustrates this point.

"Mr. N. is a 28-year-old Chinese American male with 'impotence' referred by his primary care physician for psychiatric evaluation. The patient reports to the psychiatrist nocturnal emissions and several episodes of masturbation with ejaculation. Hence by biomedical definition he is not 'impotent', but he is culturally 'impotent' in the eyes of his family, since he has never had sexual relations with his wife of 6 months. Assessment by an anthropologist reveals that the patient was forced into the marriage by his family against his strong objections and that the patient strongly dislikes his wife whom he resents for going along with the family pressure and whom he believes is educationally and socially inferior to him. Furthermore, he holds the widespread belief among traditionally oriented Chinese that intercourse leads to loss of 'vital essence', which weakens the body's constitution and leads to progressive illness. Hence, besides refraining from intercourse so as not to comply with the forced marriage, he also fears becoming ill if he does so. Such illness, he reasons, will make him 'weak' and less able to stand up 'strongly' to his authoritarian parents. Finally, by avoiding intercourse he can avoid making his wife pregnant, which would make divorce more difficult, and try to have the marriage annulled. From knowledge of Chinese culture, the anthropologist is able to inform the primary care physician not only about these facts, but also about the tremendously stressful situation the patient's wife and parents are in. Without this knowledge a social problem is converted into a narrow biomedical complaint and the possibilities for intervention are greatly limited." (p.87)

This example clearly illustrates the importance of cultural factors in an illness experience and the direct implications for health care practitioners. It is important to be mindful that all individuals exist in a social environment, with specific sets of norms, beliefs and behaviour. Such norms need to be incorporated into the interventions proposed for a given individual where cultural factors may predominate. Further, cultural factors should not be considered only for an individual of a different race, or from a different country as a cultural mosaic exists within most countries (especially North America) and most health practitioners are involved with individuals of diverse cultural backgrounds. Mechanic (1972, 1978) has reviewed the significance of cultural background on illness presentations and he has also noted that age, class, location (urban or rural) influence certain beliefs which in turn can impact on the illness experience.

The concept of explanatory models, introduced by Kleinman (1980), is a useful framework to identify the meaning that a particular illness experience holds for an individual. Kleinman suggests that health practitoners systematically elicit from the individual his or her personal view of the illness: "This explanatory model (EM) usually includes a lay view of the etiology (why?), onset, pathophysiology (how it works), expected course (what to anticipate), and desired or expected treatment" (Rosen and Kleinman, 1983, p.91). Kleinman notes how the explanatory models of a patient and his/her physician may not be the same and recommends that explanatory models be made as explicit as possible for both parties. As well, the identification of patients' explanatory models allows a glimpse at personal and cultural beliefs that when combined with other biomedical information, is important to optimize patient care. By identifying the explanatory models of both patients and practitioners, discrepancies can be identified and explicit negotiation of explanatory models can then occur. In this way issues of compliance and maximal impact of treatment (be it biomedical or psychosocial) can be facilitated.

Despite the influence of ethnocultural variables upon illness experience, these areas typically receive little attention in traditional biomedical education. As a result, health practitioners must educate themselves as to the types of cultural beliefs common to their patient population (Rosen and Kleinman, 1983). Knowledge of general cultural and subcultural beliefs, along with specific explanatory models, may then be combined with all other information to understand an individual's illness experience. This may not be a small task and it highlights the importance of the multidisciplinary team approach to health care where physicians don't have to assume the impossible task of becoming an expert in all fields. Instead, by working with practitioners of the other health and social sciences, a higher level of understanding and care may be possible.

The role of cultural factors in illness behaviour is not limited only to the individual. Gaines and Hahn (1985) describe Biomedicine itself as a sociocultural system rather than a "reality". In making this claim, they cite three related criteria that identify a sociocultural phenomenon. These criteria refer to: a specific body of knowledge and associated practices that can be differentiated from other bodies of knowledge; a system characterized by clear definition of roles with division of labour and specific rules of practice for individuals with different roles in the system; and, a specific means by which the system is evaluated and altered. Clearly Biomedicine meets all the criteria. Conceptualizing Biomedicine as a sociocultural system allows for its revision without discarding the insights and successes engendered by the model. As stated by Gaines and Hahn:

"That the system of Biomedicine is a sociocultural system implies that Biomedicine is a collective representation of reality. To claim that Biomedicine is a representation is not to deny a reality which is represented which affects and is affected by what it represents. It is rather to emphasize a cultural distance, a transformation of reality; an ultimate reality cannot be known except by means of cultural symbol systems. ... Our representations of reality are taken to be reality though they are but transformations, refracted images of it." (p.6)

## The Phenomenology of Action: Translating Component Processes Into Action

Beyond the various factors of the proposed illness behaviour model two additional constructs are required in order to understand the connection between these hypothetical constructs and the individual's behaviour during an illness episode. The first concept has to do with illness meaning and is discussed in detail by Kleinman (this volume). Meaning refers to the significance that a particular body state (whether caused by a disease or non-disease process) has for the individual. While illness meaning for a given individual incorporates cognitive appraisal processes, it is more than simply the outcome of these processes.

Kleinman illustrates how meanings vary for the individual and for the clinician trying to make sense out of illness and how these meanings further shape the experience. The meaning behind a particular illness may have a symbolic meaning, shaped by special cultural salience; personality and perceived life trajectories. These types of illness meanings are more subjective and more difficult to assess, however "... to leave the meanings out of the paradigm greatly impoverishes the subject and the findings." (Kleinman, this volume). Further, Kleinman argues that identification of which specific illness meanings that are important for an individual in a given illness experience are necessary to determine the most appropriate type of intervention, whether clinical, social, or educational.

In addition to the concept of meaning, the concept of distress is a further, final common pathway to understand illness behaviour and particularly to the type of action taken by an individual. Mechanic (this volume) has identified specific symptoms (perception of unusual body process), social stress, and introspectiveness as factors which determine the level of distress. If an individual identifies somatic dysfunction, and attaches certain meanings (either directly or by virtue of cultural factors, social pressures, past experience, etc.) that results in perceived distress he/she will likely take some form of remedial action or coping. These actions become an important part of the illness experience and may include some form of help-seeking, self-care or even inaction. It is important to recognize that help-seeking is not limited to consultation with Western medical practitioners. Rather, the use of alternative help-seeking is ubiquitous, both in industrial and non-industrial countries, and is significantly influenced by sociocultural factors (see Garro, this volume). As an alternative to medical professionals, both paramedical and folk-healers are commonly visited. Paramedical resources would include such individuals as chiropractors, and folk-healers which include shamans, herbalists and individuals who engage in combinations of folk and western medicine.

More often than formal help-seeking, most individuals rely on themselves, family members, or friends in attempts to cope with somatic dysfunction or perceived distress. Self-care or self-help has received relatively little attention in illness behaviour research to date which is unfortunate, as self-care factors may be important in preventative health care. These informal self-help efforts may precede and determine the nature of help sought, or occur concurrently with more formal help-seeking. Finally, in response to perceived distress individuals may take no specific steps toward amelioration of their condition, instead preferring denial. It is common for individuals experiencing symptoms of a heart attack to perceive a serious problem but deny anything is wrong until the symptoms become too severe to tolerate, or others intervene.

Coping has become a major focus with respect to treatment of illness behaviour, as witnessed by the contributors of this volume, as well as many other current volumes dealing with illness behaviour (e.g., Bradley and Kay, 1985; Turk et al, 1983). No attempt is made here to systematically outline this research. The reader is referred to chapters in this volume by Lazarus, Folkman, Turk and Rudy, and Breznitz, for more details. In considering the construct of coping, Breznitz cautions that there may be reason to suspect that conditions necessary for positive coping (e.g., choice, ability to plan) may not be met.

## Translation of distress into action

The translation of distress into action has been examined by a variety of illness behaviour researchers (e.g., Fabrega and Van Egeran, 1976; Suchman, 1965; Chrisman, 1977). Suchman (1965) identifies five sequential stages which comprise the action taken subsequent to the perception of distress. Stage I refers to the symptom experience, the perception that something is wrong. The behaviours associated with this stage include use of folk medicine, self-medication, denial of symptom or delay in seeking assistance. Stage II refers to assumption of the sick role, in which normal role behaviours are suspended and lay interventions are continued. Stage III in the model refers to medical care contact, in which professional advice is sought. Stage IV is termed dependent-patient role and signifies acceptance of professional treatment. Finally, stage V refers to recovery and rehabilitation, the stage in which sick role is relinquished and normal roles resumed. At each stage in the model the individual could respond with acceptance or denial/refusal. The implication of Suchman's model is that acceptance leads to progression through stages, whereas refusal/denial leads to illness behaviour problems (e.g., multi-physician involvement, non-compliance and malingering; see Blackwell and Gutmann, this volume).

Fabrega and Van Egeran (1976) present an even more complex model of the decision-making processes. The model identifies 8 stages which deal only with cognitive aspects of decision-making. As a result the model is highly complex and therefore difficult to apply in a clinical context and narrow in focus. The specific stages outlined by Fabrega and Van Egeran include: illness recognition and labelling, illness disvalues, treatment plans, assessment of treatment benefits, treatment costs, net benefits or utility, selection of treatment, and set-up for recycling.

Locking oneself into a complex staged model limited to only certain types of factors (e.g., cognitive) is a reductionistic approach which may lose the essence of the illness experience and resultant behaviour. Further, a locked-step progression through stages may have less explanatory value for a given individual than a process where factors have differential relevance and may not even be acting to influence outcome. The staged models proposed by Suchman and Fabrega illustrate that the explanations attempting to connect distress and action are not straightforward. The utility of a staged model is unproven. There may be greater explanatory value in a linear interactive illness behaviour model where factors have differential relevance rather than in the staged models. The multiple factors mediating distress and action outlined in this chapter suggest that a reductionist approach focussing solely on cognitive factors may account for lack of predictability.

## Application of an Illness Behaviour Model

It is untenable that the promulgation of the biomedical perspective and its associated manner of practice should continue given the existing body of knowledge. Few physicians have difficulty accepting the concept that psychosocial distress is a major reason why many people seek medical attention. At the same time, relatively few physicians are sufficiently knowledgeable, have the therapeutic skills or feel that they have the time to handle problems outside the biological focus of medicine. While increased awareness of the biopsychosocial framework may be having some impact on individual physician's practices, the advance of medical technology and innovation progresses far more rapidly than is possible within the social sciences. Therefore, it is difficult for new concepts and ideas from the social sciences to be incorporated into medical education and practice. It follows that considerable change is required to alter the biological focus and bias of medical education. Further, physicians must see the social sciences as an equally important area as the biological sciences for their continuing medical education. Those individuals who are optimistic would look towards changes presently being made within medical school curricula as positive signs; those individuals who are pessimistic would counter that these changes are insufficient to deal with the magnitude of the problem, counter the biomedical focus, or are inadequate to develop the skills required for physicians of the future.

The focus of attention on physicians is in accord with their historical role as the dominant and most influential health-care provider. It is beyond the scope of this chapter to discuss changes required in the health-care system in order to accommodate new approaches to health and disease care. However, several points deserve mentioning. First, the transition from a biomedical perspective to a broader biopsychosocial perspective may be opposed by some medical practitioners, who may perceive their self-interests and autonomy as being threatened by new and more active roles being accorded other health-care professionals. Second, the structure of the health-care delivery system has considerable bearing upon the manner of medical practice. This structure is determined by health and social planners and politicians who establish both the financial base and method of remuneration for institutions and health-care providers. Examples of how recent changes in health and social policy affect the structure of the delivery system include: the trend to de-institutionalized care of chronic schizophrenics; medical insurance reimbursement of some, but not all, health professionals; administrative decisions as to the priority areas for allocation of AIDS research funds.

## Revising Medical Assessment

Common terms of reference. There is little experience to fall back upon to consider the impact of restructuring the biomedical approach to problems of ill health. It is clear that the implications are far reaching and should be considered systematically. A useful place to start in the institution of an illness behaviour model would be a reconsideration of the manner in which illness behaviour problems are described.

Pilowsky (this volume) has suggested that revisions to DSM-III might include a 6th axis, an illness behaviour axis, which would be assessed according to the severity of the behaviour and the "degree of cooperation with treatment". On the other hand, Mayou (this volume) has examined the ways in which psychiatrists have used the illness behaviour terminology ("illusion of meaning") and criticized applications such as Pilowsky's as value-laden, idiosyncratic and failing to provide insights into the etiology of the psychosocial interactions.

An alternative approach for revision to the DSM-III comes from Leigh, Price, Ciarcia and Mirassou (1982) who model their approach on the Patient Evaluation Grid (Leigh and Reiser 1982, 1985). These revisions would include four axes as follows: Axis I - Biological dimension: disorders of anatomy, biochemistry and constitutional factors; Axis II - Personal dimension: affective, cognitive, and behavioural syndromes which would include personality traits (current Axes I and II); Axis III - Environmental dimension: enumeration of environmental stressors or life circumstance factors affecting other dimensions; Axis IV - Interactive dimension: elaboration of how biological, psychological and environmental factors interact to affect each other. Leigh et al's suggestions for revision to the DSM-III would have a significant impact on modifying the biomedical model. They acknowledge that the etiological factors for some psychiatric disorders (e.g., affective disorders) would be defined on more than one axis as the interactions between biological and cognitive factors are more precisely defined. Their suggestion for a new Axis IV would require some creativity to allow for a flexible, yet standardized approach for elaboration of factor interactions, an area where little work has been done. Despite the evolution of the DSM-III along more atheoretic and descriptive lines than its psychoanalytically oriented predecessor, DSM-II, Leigh et al's proposal might represent too radical a shift for the present popular biological orientation of psychiatry. Whatever assessment schema is finally adopted, it should be broad enough to accommodate all the factors known to influence illness behaviour.

## Reframing the Emphasis of Inquiry

In presenting an illness behaviour model, it is has been the authors' intention to organize existing models and constructs into a single model by reframing the emphasis of inquiry. A major advantage of this model is that it is broadly applicable to health-care practitioners, researchers and patients alike. As noted throughout this volume, there is a plethora of evidence highlighting the limitations of a pejorative and hierarchical biomedical model.

In contrast, the illness behaviour model presented here is non-hierarchical (all health-care professionals can work collaboratively within the model; see Shaw this volume) and less value-laden. Examination of Figure 3 allows for an appreciation of the implications of the model. Perhaps the most obvious of which is that many more areas of inquiry are appropriate and relevant as compared to the biomedical model of inquiry. Various degrees of sophistication can be employed in the application of the illness behaviour model. Physicians, experts in the disease process and in biomedical interventions, can continue to focus in greater detail on the physiological and related aspects of the illness presentations. However, they should not stop here. They can explore factors such as meaning (explanatory models), cognitive appraisal (distressing and dysfunctional cognitions, attributions and other beliefs), social supports, sociocultural background, level of distress, and coping strategies without considering these areas as the exclusive domain of psychiatry. In settings where physicians practice independently, he/she can establish a network of referral sources who can be consulted for a more intensive assessment of a particular factor. In multidisciplinary settings where the physician is but one member of a team, the responsibilities for assessment of illness behaviour factors may be shared according to interest, training and skills, with treatment plans developed in a collaborative fashion.

The proposed illness behaviour model opens up a broad area of inquiry that usually goes unexamined by medical practitioners. Physicians need not become expert psychologists, sociologists or anthropologists in order to use the model. In fact, a series of questions or probes could easily be added to routine medical history taking. Obviously, the nature and depth of enquiry into these areas will depend on the presenting complaints and whether there is repetitive help-seeking, disproportionate complaints or excessive distress apparent. In these latter circumstances a more extensive enquiry of life circumstances is warranted. Examples of such probes include:

<u>Interference in daily life</u>: What are you not doing now that you would otherwise be doing if it weren't for your current problems?; How have these problems interfered in your relationships with other people? <u>Tendency to psychologize or introspect</u>: Are you a person who thinks much about or who analyzes the things that go on in everyday life? <u>Attributions/explanatory models</u>: What do you think is the cause of your symptoms?; Are you worried that these symptoms represent cancer?, heart disease?, AIDS?, or some other serious illness?; What does your family or those close to you think is going on?; How have each of your other doctors or healers explained your symptoms? <u>Self-care</u>: How have you treated yourself for this problem up until now?; Have you taken any pills, medications, vitamins or supplements, or other treatments?; Who suggested these? <u>Non-medical help-seeking</u>: Have you asked someone else other than doctors for assistance with your problem? i.e., family members, neighbours, clergy, counsellors, herbalists, chiropractors, or other healers? <u>Social supports</u>: Who is there in your daily life that you can count on to help should you encounter problems that you need some assistance with?; Do you have someone that you are close to or intimate with? <u>Coping responses</u>: Give an example of a recent situation or problem where you have coped well?; Where you didn't cope so well?; How do

you think you "cope" generally? Stress responses/relationships: Most people respond to "stress" or tension with changes in bodily function (e.g., stomach upset, diarrhea, headache, feeling anxious, fatigued or sleeping poorly). How do you typically respond?; Is there any relationship between your current symptoms and "stress"? What are the current, or most recent, stressful situations in your life?

In this volume a number of the authors make specific suggestions regarding patient management emphasizing aspects of illness behaviour management. Kleinman outlines important clinical issues with respect to understanding which, of many, illness meanings are important at a given time. Cott emphasizes the importance of separating out disease and illness issues and directing attention and treatment accordingly. Blackwell and Gutmann outline important considerations in the overall management of patients who display chronic illness behaviour.

Refocussing educational emphases. Few would dispute that the current emphasis in medical education and training is on the identification and treatment of disease processes. Even in medical schools where greater attention is directed to the psychosocial dimensions of how and why patients seek medical attention, there is insufficient teaching time accorded to social scientists to train future physicians to manage non-biological issues. Lock and Lella (this volume) describe the frustrations associated with a comprehensive program of behavioural sciences taught to medical students in competition with the "basic" medical sciences. Any footholds gained in undergraduate training are lost during hospital-based internship and residency training where relatively less effort is spent to develop the skills needed to deal with the non-biological aspects of patients' problems than in learning the skills of disease management. Undergraduate and post-graduate training is associated with a paucity of effective clinical role models with major interests in the psychosocial dimensions of patients. As well, Schwartz (1982) describes the realities of the "real world" where medical care is fragmented and poorly coordinated:

"Unfortunately, strict adherence to a specialty perspective (rather than a systems perspective) by the people and/or the professionals leads each person to be dissected as if he or she consisted of totally independent parts, each diagnosable and treatable as if they were completely separate entities." (p.132)

The nature of medical education in the future will depend upon the models held and the context of social and health care systems in which physicians will work. Unless a biopsychosocial model is more clearly articulated then medical education will change only to reflect biotechnological advances and to meet the constraints of the political and economic system.

## New Directions Require Evolving Roles

Mechanic (1978) has suggested that "... one might reasonably argue that the technical-scientific aspects of medicine ought to be separated from sustaining and caring aspects of patient care" (p.413) given the nature of Biomedicine. However, given the historical role of physicians as "healers" and the inability to divorce the psychosocial and behavioural dimensions of patients from their biology, he argues that this separation would be difficult and undesirable from a public policy perspective (Mechanic, 1978).

One alternative is to involve other health and helping professionals to assist or manage the non-biological aspects of patient illness presentations. However, the structural organization of physician practice (solo or group) is a significant factor as to whether it is feasible for non-physicians to take on these roles. In addition, the manner in which the various health and helping professionals are remunerated for their services (whether financial incentives or disincentives or competition for fees exists) will strongly influence the nature of interprofessional collaboration. As a rule, multi-disciplinary patient management most often is restricted to specialized treatment facilities dealing with chronic pain or disability. The trend towards community health centers and HMO's (Health Maintenance Organization) may present a viable multi-disciplinary setting where non-physicians (e.g., nurses, social workers, psychologists) can be involved more directly in patient care.

Johnson (1985) argues that consultation-liaison psychiatry serves the role of bridging the "dominant biomedical and marginal psychosocial 'traditions' within our plural medical 'culture' "(p.269). Within the hospital setting where consultation-liaison psychiatry is practiced, he calls for:

"further exploration [of] ... its relationship with natural 'allies' such as hospital social work, clinical psychology, psychiatric nursing, and perhaps even medical anthropology, in promoting the perspectives of the psychosocial tradition. While there is a history of some competition among these fields, collaboration might be mutually beneficial." (p.289)

Cott (this volume) has proposed using a disease-illness distinction model as one means by which the roles of medical and non-medical health workers can be defined and by which they can work together. This model exists co-parallel with the biomedical model and restricts "medical" care to the biological domains. The distinction between disease and illness may be useful in everyday practice to avoid "medicalization" although many would contest that physician roles should not be so restricted. However, this model may have much usefulness as a conceptual framework for multidisciplin-teams dealing with chronic pain and disability.

The relationships between traditional medicine and non-physician healers deserves greater attention (see Garro, this volume). The use of accupuncture is a recent example where folk-medicine has interfaced and even gained credibility within traditional medical practice. Depending on the nature of the problem, the individual's cultural background and explanatory models, "non-medical" treatments may be equally effective and appropriate. Much more research is required in order to examine and compare the effectiveness of self-care and folk-healers with traditional medicine.

To summarize, multi-disciplinary team efforts are sporadic, exist around specialized problems such as chronic pain, are extremely heterogeneous in terms of structure and relationships within the team and are largely dependent upon the personalities of the individuals involved. This exists in part because of the lack of good theoretical models which articulate the relationships by which health professionals work together and the processes by which "psychosocial problems" are approached (see Shaw; Cott; this volume).

## CONCLUSIONS

So much of what Medicine deals with is beyond disease process, medical model of inquiry and a biological approach to treatment. As noted throughout this chapter a significant proportion of the problems taken to physicians might be more accurately considered as <u>problems in living</u>, what Mechanic (1980) refers to as the abundant frustrations, problems and disillusionments that people experience as part of everyday life.

What then is the role of physicians in patients complaints arising from problems is living? Some would argue that according to a disease-illness distinction model, physicians should confine their interests and treatment to the biological or disease aspects of patients' complaints. Mechanic (1980), on the other hand, argues that physicians are in a strategic position to assess people's psychosocial needs and then refer them to the appropriate community support network or service. Physicians who consider psychosocial and cultural factors as important will be motivated to explore these dimensions in their patients, to be aware to their community resources, and lastly, to refer these patients to non-medical helping professionals who are better trained to deal with these problems. Unemployment, job dissatisfaction, child rearing difficulties, role dissatisfaction, interpersonal conflicts, and loneliness are but a few examples of such problems in living for which Biomedicine has few solutions. Although anxiety and depressive symptoms are common accompaniment of problems in living, these symptoms most often do not justify a medical (DSM-III) diagnosis or pharmacological treatment. Obviously then, the conceptual framework of physicians will be of critical importance determining whether this strategic position is fully used to reduce patient distress and its associated help-seeking.

Many would support the idea that "Much of medical care has encouraged the patient to assume a dependent stance relative to the professional and has failed to support the patient's ability to struggle for mastery over his/her problems" (Mechanic, 1983; p.604). Following this thesis, much of what is referred to as chronic illness behaviour has a significant iatrogenic component. To reduce this chronic help-seeking physicians might consider changing some of their own behaviours. As well, they might want to consider educational strategies with objectives aimed at fostering independence, self-initiative, self-mastery and self-care. While these objectives at first perusal appear outside the usual interests of Biomedicine they have the potential for increased social functioning through better coping and thereby lessening subjective distress. Such strategies are as applicable whether dealing with situations of chronic disease (e.g., chronic renal failure, chronic respiratory disease, chronic neurological diseases, etc.) as with situations where there is no disease present but the patient is behaving in a disabled fashion and displaying much help-seeking behaviour. Thus rests the challenge for Medicine if a biopsychosocial model is to be truly adopted and the "whole" person treated.

It is obvious that the implications of an illness behaviour model, extend well beyond the boundaries of a hospital-based medical service industry. The issues of what constitutes illness and mental health from a medical and non-medical perspective need to be dealt with more explicitly at health and social policy levels with much debate involving health and helping professions and the general public. Failure to undertake such a debate and review may result in greater problems in the future, with fewer options available for patients and physicians as cost-control efforts predominate to influence health care.

<u>In summary</u>, this chapter represents an attempt to integrate and synthesize current knowledge of illness behaviour and disease into a broad conceptual model that might be used to guide education, research and clinical practice. Where many of the facets of the model have been demonstrated to have theoretical and practical merit, its usefulness will depend on its ability to guide the thinking (explanatory models) and behaviour of the various health and social sciences practitioners. In order for this to occur, practitioners must conceptualize and approach the illness experience in a broader and more flexible fashion, recognizing the equal contributions of biology, psychology and culture.

ACKNOWLEDGEMENTS

The authors would like to thank Drs. N. E. Diamant, J. Howes, G. Rodin and M. Olioff for their helpful suggestions in revising this chapter.

REFERENCES

American Psychiatric Association. (1981). Diagnostic and Statistical Manual of Mental Disorders. Washington: American Psychiatric Association.

Balint, M. (1957). The doctor, his patient, and the illness. London: Pitman Medical.

Bandura, A. (1977). Self-efficacy: Toward a unifying theory of behavioral change. Psychological Review, 84, 191-215.

Barondess, J. (1979). Disease and illness - A crucial distinction. American Journal of Medicine, 66, 375-6.

Beck, A. T., Rush, A. J., Shaw, B. F. & Emery, G. (1979). Cognitive therapy of depression. New York: Guilford Press.

Becker, M. H. & Maiman, L. A. (1983). Models of health-related behaviour. in D. Mechanic (Ed.) Handbook of health, health care and the health professions. London: Free Press.

Bowers, K. S., and Meichenbaum, D. (1984). The unconscious reconsidered. Toronto: J. Wiley & Sons.

Bradley, L. & Kay, R. (1985). The role of cognition in behavioral medicine. In P. Kendall (Ed.) Advances in cognitive-behavioral research and therapy. Vol. 4. New York: Academic Press.

Breznitz, S. & Goldberger, L. (1982). Stress research at a crossroads. In L. Goldberger and S. Breznitz (Eds.) Handbook of stress. New York: Free Press.

Chrisman, N. J. (1977). The health seeking process. An approach to the natural history of illness. Culture, Medicine, and Psychiatry, 1, 301-377.

Chrisman, N. J. & Kleinman, A. (1983). Popular health care, social networks and cultural meanings: The orientation of medical anthropology. In D. Mechanic (Ed.) Handbook of health, health care, and the health professions. New York: Free Press.

Clark, D., Salkouskis, P. & Chalkley, A. (1985). Respiratory control as a treatment for panic attacks. Journal of Behavior Therapy and Experimental Psychiatry, 16, 23-30.

Cohen, S. & Syme, S. L. (1985). Issues in the study and application of social support. In S. Cohen and S.L. Syme (Eds.) Social support and health. New York: Academic Press.

Condiotte, M. & Lichtenstein, E. (1981). Self-efficacy and relapse in smoking cessation programs. Journal of Consulting and Clinical Psychology, 49, 648-658.

Eisenberg, L. (1977). Disease and illness. Distinctions between professional and popular ideas of sickness. Culture, Medicine and Psychiatry, 1, 9-23.

Eisenberg, L. & Kleinman, A. (1981). Clinical social science. In L. Eisenberg and A. Kleinman (Eds.) The relevance of social science for medicine. Boston: Reidel.

Engel, G. (1960). A unified concept of health and disease. Perspectives in Biology and Medicine, 3, 459-85.

Engel, G. (1977). The need for a new medical model: A challenge for biomedicine. Science, 196, 129-36.

Fabrega, H. (1973). Toward a model of illness behaviour. Medical Care, 11, 470-484.

Fabrega, H. (1975). The position of psychiatry in the understanding of human disease. Archives of General Psychiatry, 32, 1500-1512.

Fabrega, H. & Van Egeren, L. (1976). A behavioral framework for the study of disease. Annals of Internal Medicine, 84, 200-8.

Feinstein, A. (1967). Spectrums of disease and other "mathemedical" constructions. (pp. 173-228) In Clinical judgment. New York: Kreiger.
Feinstein, A. (1979). Science, clinical medicine and the spectrum of disease. In P. B. Beeson, W. McDermott, and J. B. Wyngaard (Eds.) Cecil textbook of medicine. Toronto: Saunders.
Gaines, A. D. & Hahn, R. A. (1985). Among the physicians: Encounter, exchange and transformation. In R.A. Hahn and A.D. Gaines (Eds.) Physicians of western medicine. Boston: Reidel
Gentry, W. D. (1984). Behavioral medicine: A new research paradigm. In W. D. Gentry (Ed.) Handbook of behavioral medicine. New York: Guilford Press.
Helman, C. G. (1985). Disease and pseudo-disease: A case history of pseudo-angina. In R.A. Hahn & A.D. Gaines (Eds.) Physicians of western medicine. Boston: Reidel.
Himaldi, W., Boice, R. & Barlow, D. (1985). Assessment of agoraphobia: Triple response measurement. Behavior Research and Therapy, 23, 311-23.
Holmes, T. & Rahe, R. (1967). The social readjustment rating scale. Journal of Psychosomatic Research, 11, 213-218.
Hughdahl, K. (1981). The three systems model of fear and emotion - A critical examination. Behavior Research and Therapy, 19, 75-85.
Johnson, T. M. (1985). Consultation-liaison psychiatry: Medicine as patient, marginality as practice. In R. A. Hahn & A. D. Gaines (Eds.) Physicians of western medicine. Boston: Reidel.
Kaplan, H. I. (1985). History of psychosomatic medicine. In H. I. Kaplan & B. J. Sadock (Eds.) Comprehensive textbook of psychiatry. (4th ed.) Baltimore: Williams and Wilkins.
Kasl, S. V. & Cobb, S. (1966). Health behaviour, illness behaviour and sick-role behaviour. Archives of Environmental Health, 12, 246-66.
Kasl, S. V. and Cobb, S. (1966b). Health behaviour, illness behaviour and sick-role behaviour. Archives of Environmental Medicine, 12, 531-41.
Kasl, S. V. & Wells, J. A. (1985). Social support and health in the middle years: Work and family. In S. Cohen & S. L. Syme (Eds.) Social support and health. New York: Academic Press.
Kessler, R. C. & McLeod, J. D. (1985). Social support and mental health in community samples. In S. Cohen & S. L. Syme (Eds.) Social support and health. New York: Academic Press.
Kleinman, A. (1980). Patients and healers in the context of culture. Berkeley: University of California Press.
Kleinman, A., Eisenberg, L. & Good, B. (1978). Culture, illness and care: Clinical lessons from anthropologic and cross-cultural research. Annals of Internal Medicine, 88, 251-58.
Kuiper, N., Olinger, L, and MacDonald, M. (in press). Depressive schemata and the processing of personal and social information. In L. B. Alloy (Ed.) Cognitive processes in depression. New York: Guilford Press.
Lazarus, R. S. (1984). On the primacy of cognition. American Psychologist, 39, 124-9.
Lazarus, R. S. & Folkman, S. (1984). Stress, appraisal, and coping. New York: Springer.
Leigh, H., Price, L., Ciarcia, J. & Mirassou, M. M. (1982). DSM-III and consultation-liaison psychiatry: Toward a comprehensive medical model of the patient. General Hospital Psychiatry, 4: 283-89.
Leigh, H. & Reiser, M. F. (1985). The Patient: Biological, psychological and social dimensions of medical practice. New York: Plenum Press.
Levine, S., Feldman, J. J. & Elinson, J. (1983). Does medical care do any good? In D. Mechanic (Ed.) Handbook of health, health care and the health professions. New York: Free Press.
Ley, R. (1984). Agoraphobia, the panic attack, and the hyperventilation syndrome. Unpublished manuscript, State University of New York at Albany.
Linn, L. & Spitzer, R. L. (1982). DSM-III : Implications for liaison psychiatry and psychosomatic medicine. Journal of the American Medical Association, 247, 3207-9.

Lipkin, J. O. (1981). Understanding illness behaviour and its importance in the practice of medicine. Behavioral Medicine Update, 2, 15-18.

Lipowski, Z. (1977). Psychosomatic medicine in the seventies: An overview. American Jounal of Psychiatry, 134, 233-44.

Mayou, R. (1984). Sick role, illness behaviour and coping. British Journal of Psychiatry, 144, 320-22.

Maretzki, T. W. (1985). Including the physician in healer-centered research: retrospect and prospect. In R. A. Hahn & A. D. Gaines (Eds.) Physicians of western medicine. Boston: Reidel.

Marsella, A. J. and White, G. M. (1984). Introduction: Cultural conceptions in mental health research and practice. In A. J. Marsella and G. M. White (Eds.) Cultural conceptions of mental health and therapy Boston: Reidel.

Mathews, A. and Johnston, P. (1981). Agoraphobia. New York: Guildford Press,

Mechanic, D. (1962). The concept of illness behavior. Journal of Chronic Diseases, 15: 189-94.

Mechanic, D. (1978). Medical sociology. (2nd ed.) New York: Free Press.

Mechanic, D. (1980). Mental health and social policy. (2nd ed.) Englewood Cliffs, NJ: Prentice-Hall.

Mechanic, D. (1983) The experience and expression of distress: The study of illness behavior and medical utilization. In D. Mechanic (Ed.) Handbook of health, health care, and the health professions. New York: Free Press.

Mechanic, D. (1984). Illness Behaviour. Paper presented at the First International Conference on Illness Behaviour. Adelaide, Australia.

Mechanic, D., Cleary, P. D. & Greenley, J. R. (1982). Distress syndromes, illness behavior, access to care and medical utilization in a defined population. Medical Care, 20, 361-72,

Meichenbaum, D. (1977). Cognitive-behavior modification: An integrative approach. New York: Plenum Press.

Merluzzi, T., Rudy, T. & Glass, C. (1981). The information-processing paradigm: Implications for clinical science. In T. Merluzzi, C. Glass and M. Genest (Eds.), Cognitive assessment. New York: Guilford Press.

Molino, J. (1983). Understanding the biopsychosocial model. International Journal of Psychiatry in Medicine, 13, 29-36.

Pennebaker, J. (1982). The psychology of physical symptoms. New York: Springer-Verlag.

Rachman, S. & Hodgson, R. (1974). Synchrony and desynchrony in fear and avoidance. Behavior Research and Therapy, 12, 311-318.

Rittenberg, W. (1985). Mary; patient as emergent symbol on a pediatrics ward: The objectification of meaning in social process. In R. A. Hahn and A. D. Gaines (Eds.) Physicians of western medicine. Boston: Reidel

Rosen, G. & Kleinman, A. (1983). Social science in the clinic: Applied contributions from anthropology to medical teaching and patient care. In J. E. Carr & H. A. Dengerink (Eds.) Behavioral science in the practice of medicine. New York: Elsevier.

Ross, W. D., Schultz, J. R. & Edelstein, P. (1982). The biopsychosocial approach: Clinical examples from a consultation-liaison service. Psychosomatics, 23, 141-51.

Safran, J . & Greenberg, L. (in press). Hot cognition and psychotherapy process: An information processing ecological approach. In P. Kendal (Ed.) Advances in cognitive-behavioural research therapy. Vol. 5. New York: Academic Press.

Schachter, S. & Singer, J. (1962). Cognitive, social and physiological determinants of emotional state. Psychological Review, 69, 379-99.

Schwartz, G. E. (1982a). Integrating psychobiology and behavior therapy: A systems perspective. In G. T. Wilson & C. M. Franks (Eds.) Contemporary behavior therapy: Conceptual and empiral foundations. New York: Guilford.

Schwartz, G. E. (1982b). Testing the biopsychosocial model: The ultimate challenge facing behavioral medicine. Journal of Consulting and Clinical Psychology, 50, 1040-53.
Schwartz, G. E. & Weiss, S. (1978). Behavioral medicine revisited. An amended definition. Journal of Behavioral Medicine, 1, 249-52.
Strauss, J. S. (1975). A comprehensive approach to psychiatric diagnosis. American Journal of Psychiatry, 132: 1193-7.
Suchman, C.A. (1965). Stages of illness and medical care. Journal of Health and Social Behaviour, 6, 114-128.
Turk, D., Meichenbaum, D. & Genest, M. (1973). Pain and behavioral medicine: A cognitive-behavioral perspective. New York: Guilford Press.
Vallis, T. M. & Bucher, B. (1986). Individual difference factors in the efficacy of covert modelling and self-instructional training for fear reduction. Canadian Journal of Behavioural Science, 18, 146-58.
White, G. M. & Marsella, A. J. (1984). Introduction: Cultural conceptions in mental health research and practice. In A. J. Marsella & G. M. White (Eds.) Cultural conceptions of mental health and therapy. Boston: Reidel.
Williams, J. B. (1985). The multiaxial system of DSM-III: Where did it come from and where should it go? I. Its origins and critiques. Archives of General Psychiatry, 42, 75-180.
Wortman, C. B. & Conway, T. L. (1985). The role of social support in adaptation and recovery from physical illness. In S. Cohen & S. L. Syme (Eds.) Social support and health. New York: Academic Press.
Zajonc, R. B. (1984). On the primacy of affect. American Psychologist, 39, 117-23.
Zegans, L. Stress and the development of somatic disorders. In L. Goldberger & S. Breznitz (Eds.) Handbook of stress: Theoretical and clinical aspects. New York: Free Press.

# IS THERE TOO MUCH SCIENCE IN MEDICINE OR NOT ENOUGH?

## A POSITION PAPER

Leon Eisenberg

Department of Social Medicine and Health Policy
Harvard Medical School

The purpose of this chapter is to discuss the interface between science and the practice of medicine. A frequent complaint made about contemporary physicians is that they are not sufficiently kind and understanding. The implication, sometimes a bald statement and other times implicit, is that physicians are overly scientific and insufficiently empathic. This chapter critically addresses this position. A series of propositions will be made and each of these discussed.

Specifically, the following are advanced:

(a) It is the application of science to the clinic which has advanced medicine to its current state.

(b) Only a continued commitment to the scientific method will permit medicine to improve its present capabilities.

(c) Much of the criticism of science in medicine mistakes the technology made possible by science, and the way that technology is employed, for science itself. What has hampered progress is too narrow a view of the sciences relevant to medicine, rather than "too much" science.

(d) The concepts and methods of the social sciences are essential if physicians are to be enabled to understand and respond effectively to illness as a human experience, an experience whose dimensions are not specified by biology and chemistry.

### The Application of Science to the Clinic

Physicians trained around World War II have lived through a time in which the therapeutic powers of the physician have grown in an extraordinary fashion as the basic sciences have been applied to medicine. To encounter a public increasingly dubious about those benefits and nostalgic about a halcyon past is disconcerting. To hear critics maintain that there is too much emphasis on science in medical education and practice strains one's credulity. Why does the very public which clamors for liver and heart transplants in the same breath lament the disappearance of the "kindly old-fashioned family doctor"? Prior to the application of scientific discoveries the physician was able to do little for his/her patients. Any implication that in medical transactions personal style is more important than competence has no basis in fact.

To list the therapeutic gains that have occurred during the last few decades requires a volume in itself. One example will suffice. At one time the diagnosis of acute leukemia in children was tantamount to a death warrant. Doctors could do no more than support families in their bereavement (Richmond and Waisman, 1955), an honourable role, but one far less needed in today's pediatrics. Even a generation ago, less than 20 percent of children with acute lymphocytic leukemia survived two years after the diagnosis and far fewer at five years. With today's treatments, there is a 90 percent survival at two years and 70 percent at five years (Smithson, Gilchrist, and Burgert, 1980). The extent of progress in medical therapeutics is evident in Paul Beeson's comparison of the effectiveness of the treatments recommended in the first (1927) edition of Cecil's Textbook of Medicine with those in the fourteenth (1975) edition. Beeson rated the value of 60 percent of the remedies in the first edition as nil, harmful, useless, questionable or at best symptomatic; only three percent provided fully effective treatment of prevention. In the half century between the two editions, effective regimens had increased sevenfold and dubious ones had decreased by two-thirds (Beeson, 1980).

These accomplishments were due to the systematic application of the basic biomedical sciences to the investigation of disease. Furthermore, the speed of advance of these accomplishments can be expected to accelerate. Consider only such imminent possibilities as safer vaccines prepared from cloned fragments of the antigenic surface of infectious agents; better prenatal diagnosis by restriction-endonuclease analysis of fetal DNA obtained by chorionic biopsy; enzymatic correction of genetic disorders, already accomplished in tissue culture and in transgenic animals; monoclonal antibodies and gene mapping for the diagnosis of malignancy; and new measures for the prevention and treatment of cancer based on an understanding of the role of oncogenes in malignant transformation.

I do not suggest that all has been progress. Premature introduction of therapeutic agents has led to unacceptable morbidity and mortality. Because physicians can do more, doing all too easily becomes mindless; decisions to discontinue life support systems when recovery is no longer possible are surrounded by moral disputes and threats of litigation. But surely this is not the fault of the methods available, but of the way those methods are used. This point will be dealt with more fully below. Suffice it to say that balanced appraisal of what has been accomplished must conclude that the gains have been quite extraordinary even after all the costs have been taken into account.

## The Continuing Need for Research

Despite the progress made possible by the application of science to medicine, the current level of knowledge is only a beginning on what we will need to know to control persisting sources of morbidity and mortality. Consider the following examples: the epidemic of AIDS; smoking and cancer; and the marked variation in the use of "standard" treatments. These issues illustrate the range of scientific competencies needed to analyze health problems.

The epidemic of AIDS. The first reports of unusual opportunistic infections and rare sarcomas arising in young men were published in 1981 (Centers for Disease Control, 1981). Because cellular immunodeficiency was common to these disorders, they were named acquired immunodeficiency syndrome (AIDS). As cases accumulated, it was noted that some three-quarters occurred in homosexual or bisexual males and one-fifth in IV drug users. Other groups observed to be at risk were hemophiliac patients treated with factor VIII concentrate derived from pooled blood, recipients of blood transfusions, and infants born to infected mothers. The number of cases reported to the Centers for Disease Control had reached 10,000 by April 30, 1985, 5,000 having been reported within the previous year. Half of all patients are now dead (Centers for Disease Control, 1985) and the total cases reported continue to escalate. Costs for care have been estimated at some $50,000 to $100,000 per case, the total approximating one billion dollars to date.

Well before the extent of the threat to public health became apparent, AIDS attracted the attention of researchers, who recognized the syndrome as an "experiment of nature" able to shed light on the basic mechanisms of the immune response. Vigorous research began in laboratories all over the world. The pattern of transmission - from one sexual partner to another (Auerbach, Darrow, Jaffe, and Curran, 1984), through shared IV drug paraphernalia, and by the infusion of blood products - clearly implicated an infectious agent. Laboratory studies identified an inverted ratio of helper to suppressor T lymphocytes in patients and in populations at risk (Terhost, van Agthoven, Reinherz, and Scholossman, 1980). By 1984, two independent laboratory groups (Gallo, Salahuddin, Popovic, et al, 1984; Barre-Sinoussi, Chermann, Rey, et al, 1983) had isolated a retrovirus as the presumptive cause of the disease and antibodies reactive to the virus had been identified in the serum of AIDS patients (Sarngadharan, Popovic, Bruch, Schüpbach, and Gallo, 1984). The tropism of the virus for helper (T4) lymphocytes has been shown to be due to a cell surface receptor unique to those cells (Dagleish, Beverly, Clapham, et al, 1984). The origin of the virus has been traced to central Africa, with green monkeys as a presumptive animal reservoir (Newmark, 1985). This is an extraordinary set of accomplishments in three short years. It was possible only because of the scientific capabilities in place <u>before</u> the crisis arose.

Nonetheless, there is still no effective treatment. Scientific puzzles abound. Among high risk populations, some individuals who are asymptomatic are antibody positive (Landesman, Ginzburg, and Weiss, 1985); others have no antibodies but carry the virus (Salahuddin, Groopman, Markham, et al, 1984). AIDS in Africa is equally distributed in men and women and appears to be transmitted heterosexually, with risk increasing with the number of sexual partners (Clumeck, Van de Perre, Carael, et al, 1985). Is the difference in sexual distribution accounted for by geographic variation in viral characteristics or does it reflect no more than the chance that the initial entry of the virus came through the homosexual community in the West?

The institution of a national program to screen blood for antibodies (Budiansky, 1985) will reduce the risk of transfusion-acquired AIDS (though it will not eliminate it because of the false negative test results). The decision to inform donors who are test positive has been challenged. Concern has been expressed that present policy may lead to a decrease in the pool of voluntary blood donors because of the fear of being stigmatized (Osterhold, Bowman, Chopek, et al., 1985). Those who are false positives will suffer altogether unnecessary anxiety about their future; those who are true positives cannot be given an accurate estimate of the risk of future illness because not all will become ill. In the absence of treatment, there is no way to use the "information" for personal benefit. Can donors be fully assured of confidentiality, given current difficulties in protecting computerized data banks?

As many as one million Americans may have been infected by the AIDS virus thus far; cases of clinical disease may total 100,000 within two years. Without a treatment to reverse the disease or a vaccine to prevent it, the public health scenario looks ominous. Hope of halting the epidemic rests on further scientific progress.

<u>Smoking and cancer</u>. Cigarette smoking has been implicated in as many as 40 percent of all cancer deaths in the United States (Ravenholt, 1984). Despite the high risk, not all smokers succumb; in addition to intensity and duration of smoking, individual variation in biological susceptibility must be an important determinant. One current hypothesis is that individuals at high risk carry a gene for an inducible form of an enzyme which is a key to carcinogenesis. Aryl hydrocarbon hydroxylase (AHH) is one of a large family

of heme-containing enzymes known as cytochrome P 450's. The P 450 system plays a major role in detoxifying foreign chemicals; unfortunately, it also can transform a certain number of them into active carcinogens. Some years ago, Kellerman, Shaw, and Luyten-Kellerman (1973) reported that lung cancer patients exhibited more rapid induction of AHH. This observation proved difficult to replicate because of the unreliability of the biological assay then in use. Subsequent research has demonstrated heritable variation in AHH inducibility in man (Nebert, 1980). Recent reports, based on an antibody to AHH, show higher rates of inducibility among patients with lung cancer than in comparison groups (Marx, 1985). Because of the major role of P 450 enzymes in detoxification, the design of AHH inhibitors does not appear to be a feasible strategy. However, if AHH inducibility characterizes persons at risk for smoking-induced cancer, then population screening could make it possible to target anti-smoking campaigns at vulnerable individuals, thereby increasing efficiency and perhaps efficacy.

There is a major element common to these two public health problems, that is, the social mediation of the disease process. If effective social interventions could be implemented the incidence of both would be markedly reduced. Yet this goal is far from being reached (McKusick, Horstman, and Coates, 1985; Surgeon General, 1982). The search for a technological "fix" continues because of the relative poverty of the social measures at our command. Yet, the stakes are so high that all avenues must be pursued. Recall that although high rates of smallpox were associated with poverty and underdevelopment, the disease was entirely eliminated, despite the persistence of social disadvantage, by a modest improvement in technology (a freeze-dried vaccine), a new set of social strategies (case identification and vaccination of potential contacts), and an international commitment of the necessary resources (Breman and Arita, 1980).

Variation in the use of "standard" treatment. This third example is quite mundane in comparison to the other two. It occurs in daily medical practice where physicians make decisions to recommend "standard" surgical procedures which have been in use for many years. The problem became apparent when clinical epidemiologists studied the rates at which these procedures were being used and found marked variability from one area to another. The variability made it evident that, in the absence of a solid data base, physicians were following local "fashions". The worst of it was that doctors had been unaware that a problem existed until the epidemiologic studies were undertaken.

Wennberg and his colleagues (1982) have documented the extent of variation in rates for surgical procedures among small geographic areas with comparable populations. In a survey of the New England states, rates for tonsillectomy were found to vary sevenfold and those for hysterectomy and prostatectomy fourfold from one area to another. The investigators concluded: "the amount and cost of hospital treatment in a community have more to do with the number of physicians there, their medical specialties and the procedures they prefer than with the health of the residents." Consider also the remarkable parallel between the number of surgeons per population and the rates for operative procedures across countries: both figures are about twice as high for the U.S. as for the U.K., with Canada about halfway between the two (Vayda, Mindell, and Rutkow, 1982). That, however, does not tell us whether the U.S. is oversupplied, the U.K. undersupplied, or Canada about right.

The problem is not simply the pecuniary interest of physicians working in a fee-for-service system. In a comparison among Norway, the U.K., and the New England States, surgical rates showed similar variability within each country despite the differences in total rates and in the methods of organizing and financing medical care among them (McPherson, Wennberg, Hovind, and Glifford, 1982). These findings contrast with relatively small variations in rates for appendicectomy, regarded as the only acceptable treatment for a presumptive diagnosis of appendicitis. Further evidence against a financial motive as the sole determinant of overuse is the behaviour of physicians when they or their wives are the patients. Bunder and Brown (1974) found that rates of elective surgery on doctors' families were higher than on other professional families. Physicians clearly believe in what they recommend to their patients; they apply the same judgements to themselves.

Vayda and Mindell (1982) have reported similar findings for Canada. Variations in age- and sex-standardized surgical rates per 100,000 population in Ontario counties in 1977 ranged from more than twofold for cholecystectomy to almost tenfold for colectomy. The investigators found no evidence that differing operative rates reflected differences in disease prevalence. That there are differences between surgeons is evident, not only from area variation, but also from second opinion studies which have found that about one-quarter of patients for whom surgery is recommended by one surgeon have that opinion reversed by a second (McCarthy and Finkel, 1978). If U.K. rates for the seven common operations examined by Wennberg and his colleagues had applied to the U.S., deaths associated with surgery would have decreased by one-third to one-half (Wennberg, Bunker, and Barnes, 1980).

What options are there to change this unsatisfactory state of affairs? In 1972, the College of Physicians and Surgeons of Saskatchewan appointed a study committee when it was reported that the annual number of hysterectomies in the province had increased at a rate ten times greater than the increase in the number of adult women in the population. By stipulating the approved indications for hysterectomy, the College succeeded in reducing the number performed by one-third over a four-year period (Dyck, Murphy, Murphy, et al, 1977). In similar fashion, Wennberg, Blowers, Parker and Gittelsohn (1977) found that the feedback of information on disproportions in the number of tonsillectomies to the Vermont State Medical Society was associated with a significant reduction in rates.

Yet these steps, laudable as they are, do no more than reify expert opinion. That opinion can be no better than the quality of the evidence on which it is based; for many medical and surgical procedures the available data are at best equivocal. As Vayda and Mindell (1982) point out, "the issue of necessary versus unnecessary surgery will not be resolved until the question of efficacy or effectiveness of competing treatments (or treatment versus nontreatment) is answered." Thus, the following steps are needed: systematic collation of existing information from properly controlled studies; randomized clinical trials to evaluate treatments of uncertain efficacy; a mechanism to change physician behaviour to accord with the evidence.

Unnecessary and unduly prolonged hospitalization in itself results in serious health risks. More than three million infections are acquired each year in U.S. hospitals, afflicting almost one patient in every 18 admitted to an acute care facility (Haley, Culver, White, et al, 1985). In one study of 815 consecutive patients on a general medical service of a university hospital (Steel, Gertman, Crescenzi, and Anderson, 1981) 36 percent experienced iatrogenic illness, most instances arising from drugs or invasive procedures. In nine percent of all patients admitted, a major untoward incident occurred; in two percent, it was thought to have been a contributing factor in the patient's death!

Excessive reliance on test findings is apparent in outpatient practice as well. Its inappropriateness is indicated by a British study (Almy, 1981) of the relative contributions of the history, the physical examination, and laboratory investigations to the diagnosis and management of medical outpatients. On 80 newly referred clinic patients, participating physicians recorded a tentative diagnosis after taking the history, reassessed it after the physical examination and, again, after laboratory findings were in. A diagnosis in accord with the final diagnosis was established in 82 percent of the cases by the history alone and in a further nine percent after the physical examination had been performed. In only seven of the 80 patients did the laboratory findings change the diagnosis based on history and physical. Although 24 percent of the tests ordered yielded abnormal results, in most cases they served only to confirm the clinical diagnosis.

Technology or Science?

Some critics conclude from the same data sets - on the over-use of surgery and the over-reliance on laboratory tests - that medical practice suffers from "too much science". That criticism confuses science with the technologies scientific findings make possible and with the ways those technologies are employed. Lewis Thomas (1984) stresses that:

> " ... These technologies are, in their very existence, the best of arguments for more basic biological research ... Unless we learn the ... causes of coronary occlusion, and ... how to prevent it, the artificial heart will be in production ... costing the moon and impossible to prohibit."

The misuse of technology stems from such factors as: a medical payment system which pays doctors more, the more they use technical procedures; the legal and moral controversies which make it difficult for doctors to withdraw so-called life-saving measures when all they prolong is the process of dying; and the failure of medical education to prepare doctors to weigh competing claims.

The current payment scales of the fee-for-service system of reimbursement reward procedures with fees far higher than those for time spent in clinical assessment. A gastroenterologist realizes a net hourly income from endoscopy which is more than six times greater than from the general management of the patient's illness (Spiro, 1974). The disproportion between the fees paid for procedures and those for a thorough history and physical examination is transforming gastroenterologists into endoscopists (Phibbs, 1979) and cardiologists into "catheterologists" (Hampton, Harrison, Mitchell, et al, 1975). The fact that the net income of technically oriented specialists is much higher than that of primary care practitioners influences the career choices of young physicians and contributes to the disproportion in the ratio between generalists and specialists. A change in the relative fee schedule is necessary to provide an economic incentive to expand primary care, including a greater emphasis on disease prevention and health promotion.

Therapeutic advances accentuate moral dilemmas. Whereas once doctors could do nothing for a patient with pneumococcal pneumonia but await the outcome of the disease process, we now possess powerful antibiotics that make a decisive difference. This is an extraordinary accomplishment when the life saved is a life of quality. But is it for the good when medicine intercepts the terminal illness that might have brought a merciful end to pain and misery?

Demographic changes in the age structure of the population in Western countries, resulting from much more than medical progress, but including that as well, foretell ever-increasing numbers of elderly people. In the United States, by the year 2000 there will be 30 million persons over 65 and by 2030 there will be 50 million, even without further increases in longevity. Such projections imply many more individuals with chronic brain disease, a thus far unavoidable consequence of the aging process. The ability of cardiorespiratory support to maintain vegetative existence in such patients has confronted society with unprecendented ethical dilemmas. Now that death can be postponed almost indefinitely, it has been transformed from an event of nature to a human decision. Families shun the responsibility, even when the doctor is willing to share it with the family and the law intervenes. Yet, does it make sense to indict the technology which can restore meaningful life because it can also be employed to make death an agonizing process? The issues at stake are not technical, but moral and legal; the resolution of the dilemma requires input from doctors, but ultimately rests with society at large.

## The Role of the Social Sciences

Most patients treated by most doctors get well most of the time. That good fortune for patients - and for doctors' reputations - creates a problem for the practitioner. It is difficult for the doctor to avoid concluding that the patient improved because of what he or she has done. The difficulty is compounded because existing patterns of medical practice do not provide information on the denominator; that is, the relevant population in the community from whom the sample seen in the office is drawn. The ultimate measure of the effectiveness of medical care is its impact on the health status of the population it serves.

Unfortunately, the education doctors receive is so narrowly focused on organs and tissues as the locus of disease that they have lost sight of the purpose of the medical enterprise: to maintain the health of the population. Even in Britain, where all citizens are assured coverage by a national health service, general practitioners limit their concern to the patients who consult them and overlook those in their patient panel who are silent (Hart, 1983). The remedy must lie in a broadening of medical education to include the concepts and methods of the social sciences.

Recognition that the way men and women live matters to their health is hardly new. Indeed, the Hippocratic Treatise: Airs, Waters, Places (Hippocrates, translated by Jones, 1973) enjoins "whoever wishes to pursue properly the science of medicine" to consider, among other features of the place of practice, "the mode of life ... of the inhabitants." Yet academic medicine remains indifferent to this injunction. This is a legacy of the emphasis on single causes and single effects in 19th century bacteriology; its spectacular accomplishments made it the paradigm for medical theorizing. Yet, even in its own domain, this mode of analysis does not account fully for disease pathogenesis. Though infection by the tubercle bacillus is a necessary condition for tuberculosis, it is not a sufficient condition. Of individuals with a primary infection, as evident from the positive tuberculin skin test, only a minority exhibit the symptoms and signs of clinical disease. Susceptibility to tuberculosis varies not only with age, sex, and race but also with housing and social class (Glassroth, Robins, and Snider, 1980). Indeed, during the 40 years before Koch discovered the bacillus, the mortality rate from tuberculosis had fallen by half because of improvements in nutrition and housing; it was to fall by more than half again during the next 60 years, before effective chemotherapy was discovered (McKeown, 1976).

The pattern of disease characteristic of a particular society is a function of its level of development. Consider the changes in disease epidemiology in the United States. In 1900, the three leading causes of death were infectious: pneumonia, tuberculosis and diarrheal disease. By 1940, they declined sharply and had been displaced by increasing rates of heart disease, cancer and cerebrovascular disease (Levy and Moskowitz, 1985). The decline in mortality from infectious disease resulted from improvements in sanitary engineering and nutrition during an era when there had been few advances in medical therapeutics; the new pattern of mortality arose from changes in diet, activity, and exposure to environmental toxins, as well as a rising age distribution in the population.

But if heart disease, cancer and stroke remain the three leading causes of death in the 1980's, mortality rates in themselves do not provide a full picture of the greatest threat to public health. When we compare potential years of life lost by specific causes (a figure computed by multiplying the number of deaths from each cause by the number of years between the age of death and age 65), the focus changes. Such a calculation reveals that deaths from violence (accidents, homicides and suicides), because of the relative youth of the victims, accounts for 39 percent of the potential years of life lost in the United States (Centers for Disease Control, 1984), an amount equal to that produced by heart disease, cancer and cerebrovascular disease.

Confronted by lives lost in such epidemic proportions, we would do well to recall the words of Rudolf Virchow, written almost one and one-half centuries ago (cited by Rosen, 1947):

> "If disease is an expression of individual life under unfavorable conditions, then epidemics must be indicative of mass disturbances of mass life."

The resolution of such "mass disturbances of mass life" demands measures well beyond those of medicine as such. Yet, medicine, which Virchow recognized as a social science, has a role to play in identifying their consequences, studying their sources, and advocating the social remedies (Eisenberg, 1984).

Just as sociology can help physicians to recognize the role of class, caste and social organization as disease determinants at the macro level, social anthropology enables the physician to understand that illness, patienthood, and health-related behaviours are social constructions which are not explicable at the biological level. The usefulness of distinguishing between "disease" and "illness", terms used synonymously in ordinary usage has already been articulated (Eisenberg, 1977). Physicians have been taught to conceptualize diseases as abnormalities in the structure and function of body organs and tissues. But patients suffer illnesses; that is, experiences of disvalued changes in states of being and in social function. Disease and illness do not stand in a one-to-one relationship. Similar degrees of organ pathology can generate quite different reports of pain and distress; illness may occur in the absence of detectable disease; the course of the disease is distinct from the trajectory of the accompanying illness. A visit to the doctor may be more likely, on average, when disease is present; although being diseased, feeling ill and being a patient may overlap, they are not coterminous (Eisenberg, 1980).

The way a given culture conceptualizes illness and the behaviours it prescribes for curing or preventing it must be taken into account if even the best of what medicine has to offer is to be effective. Chen and his colleagues (Rahman, Chen, Chakraborty, et al, 1982) have reported the disappointing results when they applied an effective and appropriate technology, tetanus vaccine, for the prevention of infant deaths in Bangladesh. Two years after its introduction, the vaccine, a simple measure which can be delivered to pregnant women in their homes with a biologic efficacy of 100 percent, had reduced net infant mortality by less than three percent; yet, epidemiologic studies had demonstrated that neonatal tetanus accounts for 26 percent of all infant deaths. Village surveys revealed that less than a quarter of the pregnant women had accepted the vaccine. Some were reluctant to take it for fear of damage to the fetus. Moreover, local experience did not persuade the villagers of the effectiveness of the vaccine. Bangladeshi folk terms for diseases which afflict infants do not distinguish neonatal tetanus from other fatal conditions. Because deaths from these other causes continued despite vaccine administration, its "perceived efficacy" was far less than its actual efficacy against tetanus.

Postneonatal mortality is higher among female than among male children in Bangladesh, a reversal of the sex ratio found in the West. Field studies of parental behaviour indicate that the explanation lies in the preference extended to sons in the allocation of the limited resources available to the family. In apportioning family meals, mothers give smaller rations to their daughters than to their sons, who contribute more to family earnings and who will be the economic support for their parents in old age. In an area where undernutrition is endemic, this additional restriction on food intake leads to greater malnutrition in girls and to lower resistance to infection. Further, parents are more likely to take a sick son than a sick daughter to the clinic, even when it is free, because of the hours of work lost during travel (Chen, Huq, and D'Souza, 1981).

A third finding from the field research station in rural Matlab Thana illustrates a phenomenon also seen elsewhere in the world; namely, the dysjunction between behaviour and belief. Better education, particularly of the mother has consistently been associated in the Third World with improved child survival (with income held constant). However, this is not, as one might have surmised, because education leads to a "modern" understanding of disease causation. Education is associated with upward social mobility. Educated women marry and have their first child at later ages. They are more assertive on behalf of their children, shift household resources toward child needs, and utilize health services more effectively. These mothers retain their traditional beliefs, despite adopting the hygienic practices associated with higher social class (Lindenbaum, 1983).

These examples make clear the vital importance of understanding the complex interactions between technology and culture, if the methods of biomedicine, so successful in a Western context, are to meet the health needs of the Third World. As Chen (1984) summarizes the issue:

> "Future research should attempt to combine the relative strengths of the natural and social sciences. Absent is a broad theoretical framework incorporating the essence of both sciences for policy application. The biomedical sciences focus on medical causes of disease and death often in a vacuum regarding the sociopolitical, environmental, and behavioural forces which powerfully shape disease risk and therapeutic response. The social sciences, in contrast, usually correlate mortality with socioeconomic indicators in the absence of understanding of how such forces operate to generate disease risk and the biological processes leading to disease outcome. One consequence of this disciplinary isolationism are policy prescriptions following either a (biomedical) technology approach or a broad (and often vague) social change approach. Tapping into the combined strengths of the biomedical and social sciences could lead to more powerful policy approaches."

In addition to the above, other concerns could be noted, including: economic analysis for an understanding of resource allocation; history for an essential perspective on the development of medical theory and practice; social psychology for the illumination of the doctor-patient relationship, and so on. Collectively, these issues illustrate the relevance of the social sciences for medical research and practice (Eisenberg and Kleinman, 1981).

In conclusion, recall a question raised at the beginning of this chapter: is it true that the "old-fashioned family doctor" was more responsive to patient needs than his successors have proved to be? It is important to keep in mind that doctors today - or yesterday, for that matter are not as aware of the personal and social issues in patient care as they should be. But were things better once upon a time? If not, whence stems the belief that they were?

The fact is that complaints about practitioners being "too scientific" date from well before applied science had any appreciable impact on medical practice. Professor Francis W. Peabody, to whom we owe the moving sentence: "the secret of the care of the patient is in caring for the patient" (1927) wrote in 1923 (1930):

> " ... Older practitioners complain that young graduates have been taught

'a great deal about the mechanism of disease, but very little about the practice of medicine' - or to put it more bluntly, they are too scientific and do not know how to take care of patients." (p. 27)

> "The layman of the older generation ... who feels that something has been lacking in the way of warmth, sympathy and understanding ... is very apt to hark back to earlier days. 'What we need,' he says, 'is a general practitioner!'" (1) (p. 7)

If the criticism levelled by the "older practitioners" can be dismissed as reflecting the threat to their status by physicians competent in methods they had not mastered, this does not account for lay complaints. What was changing? Peabody provides the clue:

> "The more a doctor knows of his patient's general background, the greater advantage he has in handling the case ... [The general practitioner] knows the patient from childhood up - his physical health, the nervous and mental strain to which he has been subjected, the conditions of his social, business and domestic life, and more even than this, he may have the same detailed knowledge of the patient's parents and of the circumstances of their lives ..." (p. 30).

The virtues of the family doctor Peabody spoke of stemmed from an intimate acquaintance with patient, family and community over years of practice, and not from formal instruction received in medical school. Those virtues were inherent in the doctor's role in an America of small towns, family farms and multigenerational families, an America which was disappearing as he wrote. Generalist or specialist, today's physician no longer has the chance to know the extended family over several generations, with one in five American families moving every year. Familiarity with "the conditions of the patient's social, business and domestic life" is no longer automatically accessible to "neighbourhood" doctors now that our population has shifted to a predominantly urban locus, with its anonymity and fragmentation. Indeed, doctors themselves no longer spend their professional lifetimes in a single place.

The task for contemporary medical education is to teach physicians to obtain, through systematic and sensitive inquiry, that knowledge of the patient's "social, business and domestic life" which astute practitioners once acquired through long acquaintance with family and community. The problem is not with what doctors are taught but what they are not taught and never were: to understand the intimate interconnections between health and illness, on the one hand, and the way men and women live in society and what they believe, on the other. That goes well beyond what Peabody's idealized general practitioner mastered. His/her values were paternalistic and his/her sensibilities extended only to patients who shared a common background with him/her. Preparation for medical practice in an increasingly pluralistic society requires knowledge of and respect for group differences. More than that, it demands the acquisition of skills in assessing needs and negotiating common understandings with individuals and families. It is not enough to mean well. The doctor must know enough to <u>do</u> well for the patient.

---

1 Indeed, a century before Peabody, we find in Balzac's novel <u>Pere Goriot</u>, written in 1834, a passage which might have been written today: Bianchon, reassuring his friend Rastignac that he cares for the dying Goriot, comments:

> "Doctors already in practice see only the illness; I can still see the sick man, my boy."

It is not too much science, but a narrow and impoverished view of science, which handicaps contemporary medicine.

REFERENCES


Almy, T. P. (1981). The role of the primary physician and the health care "industry." New England Journal of Medicine, 304, 225-228.

Auerbach, D. M., Darrow, W. W., Jaffe, H. W., & Curran, J. W. (1984). Cluster of cases of the acquired immune deficiency syndrome: patients linked by sexual contact. American Journal of Medicine, 76, 487-492.

Barre-Sinoussi, F., Chermann, J. C., Rey, F., et al. (1983). Isolation of a T-lymphotropic retrovirus from a patient at risk for acquired immune deficiency syndrome (AIDS). Science, 220, 868-871.

Beeson, P. B. (1980). Changes in medical therapy during the past half century. Medicine, 59, 79-99.

Breman, J. G., & Arita, I. (1980). Confirmation and maintenance of smallpox eradication. New England Journal of Medicine, 303, 1263-1273.

Budiansky, S. (1985). Blood test trials inconclusive. Nature, 316, 96.

Bunker, J. P., & Brown, B. W. (1974). The physician-patient as an informed consumer of surgical services. New England Journal of Medicine, 290, 1051-1055.

Centers for Disease Control. (1981). Kaposi's sarcoma and Pneumocystis pneumonia among homosexual men - New York City and California. The Morbidity and Mortality Weekly Report, 30, 305-308.

Centers for Disease Control. (1984). Years of potential life lost. The Morbidity and Mortality Weekly Report, 32, 109.

Centers for Disease Control. (1985). Update: acquired immunodeficiency syndrome - United States. The Morbidity and Mortality Weekly Report, 34, 245-248.

Chen, L. C. (1984, March 18). Primary health care in the developing world: technological and social interactions. Delivered in the Takemi Lecture Series at the Harvard School of Public Health, Boston.

Chen, L. C., Huq, E., & D'Souza, S. (1981). Sex bias in the family allocation of food and health care in rural Bangladesh. Population and Development Review, 7, 54-70.

Clumeck, N., Van de Perre, P., Carael, M., et al. (1985). Heterosexual promiscuity among African patients with AIDS. New England Journal of Medicine, 313, 182.

Dagleish, A. C., Beverly, P. C. L., Clapham, P. R., et al. (1984). The CD4 (T4) antigen is an essential component of the receptor for the AIDS retrovirus. Nature, 312, 763-767.

Dyck, F. J., Murphy, F. A., Murphy, J. K., et al. (1977). Effect of surveillance on the number of hysterectomies in the Province of Saskatchewan. New England Journal of Medicine, 296, 1326-1328.

Eisenberg, L. (1977). Disease and illness: distinctions between professional and popular ideas of sickness. Culture, Medicine and Psychiatry, 1, 9-23.

Eisenberg, L. (1980). What makes persons "patients" and patients "well"?. American Journal of Medicine, 69, 277-286.

Eisenberg, L. (1984). Rudolf Ludwig Karl Virchow, where are you now that we need you? American Journal of Medicine, 77, 524-532.

Eisenberg, L., & Kleinman, A. (1981). The Relevance of Social Science for Medicine. Boston: Reidel.

Gallo, R. C., Salahuddin, S. Z., Popovic, M., et al. (1984). Frequent detection and isolation of cytopathic retroviruses (HTLV-III) from patients with AIDS and at risk for AIDS. Science, 224, 500-503.

Glassroth, J., Robins, A. G., & Snider, D. E. (1980). Tuberculosis in the 1980's. New England Journal of Medicine, 302, 1441-1450.

Haley, R. W., Culver, D. H., White, J. W., et al. (1985). The nationwide nosocomial infection rate: a new need for vital statistics. American Journal of Epidemiology, 121, 159-167.

Hampton, J. R., Harrison, M. J. G., Mitchell, J. R. A., et al. (1975, May 31). Relative contributions of history-taking, physical examination, and laboratory investigation to diagnosis and management of medical outpatients. British Medical Journal, i, 486-489.

Hart, J. T. (1983). A new type of general practitioner. Lancet, ii, 27-29.

Hippocrates. Airs, Waters, Places. (1973). (pp. 71-72). Translated by W.H.S. Jones. Cambridge: Harvard University Press.
Kellerman, G., Shaw, C. R., & Luyten-Kellerman, M. (1973). Aryl hydrocarbon hydroxylase inducibility and bronchogenic carcinoma. New England Journal of Medicine, 289, 934-937.
Landesman, S. H., Ginzburg, H. M. & Weiss, S. H. (1985). The AIDS epidemic. New England Journal of Medicine, 312, 521-525.
Levy, R. I., & Moskowitz, J. (1985). Cardiovascular research: decades of progress, a decade of promise. Science, 217, 121-129.
Lindenbaum, S. (1983). The influence of maternal education on infant and child mortality in Bangladesh. Bangladesh: International Center of Diarrheal Disease Research.
Marx, J. L. (1985). The cytochrome P 450's and their genes. Science, 228, 975-976.
McCarthy, E. G., & Finkel, M. L. (1978). Second opinion elective surgery programs: outcome status over time. Medical Care, 16, 984-994.
McKeown, T. (1976). The Role of Medicine: Dream, Mirage or Nemesis?. London: Nuffield Hospitals Trust.
McKusick, L., Horstman, W., & Coates, T. J. (1985). AIDS and homosexual behaviour reported by gay men in San Francisco. American Journal of Public Health, 75, 493-496.
McPherson, K., Wennberg, J., Hovind, O., & Glifford, P. (1982). Small area variations in the use of common surgical procedures: An international comparison of New England, England and Norway. New England Journal of Medicine, 307, 1310-1314.
Nebert, E. W. (1980). The Ah locus, a gene with possible importance in cancer predictability. Archives of Toxicology. (Suppl. 3), 195-207.
Newmark, P. (1985). Trailing AIDS in Central Africa. Nature, 315, 273.
Osterhold, M. T., Bowman, R. J., Chopek, M. W., et al. (1985). Screening donated blood and plasma for HLTV-III antibody. New England Journal of Medicine, 312, 1185-1189.
Peabody, F. W. (1927). The care of the patient. Journal of the American Medical Association, 88, 877-882.
Peabody, F. W. (1930). Doctor and Patient. New York: Macmillan Company.
Phibbs, B. (1979). The abuse of coronary arteriography. New England Journal of Medicine, 301, 1394-1396.
Rahman, M., Chen, L. C., Chakraborty, J., et al. (1982). Tetanus toxoid I: Reduction of neonatal mortality by immunization of non-pregnant women and women during pregnancy in rural Bangladesh. Bulletin of the World Health Organization, 60, 261-267.
Rahman, M., Chen, L. C., Chakraborty, J., et al. (1982). Tetanus toxoid II: Factors related to immunization acceptance among pregnant women in a maternal-child health program in rural Bangladesh. Bulletin of the World Health Organization, 60, 269-277.
Ravenholt, R. T. (1984). Addition mortality in the United States, 1980: Tobacco, alcohol and other substances. Population and Development Review, 10, 697-724.
Richmond, J. B., & Waisman, H. A. (1955). Psychologic aspects of management of children with malignant diseases. American Journal of Diseases of Children, 89, 42-47.
Salahuddin, S. Z., Groopman, J. E., Markham, P. D., et al. (1984). HTLV-III in symptom-free seronegative persons. Lancet, 2, 1418-1420.
Sarngadharan, M. G., Popovic, M., Bruch, L. Schupbach, J., & Gallo, R. C. (1984). Antibodies reactive with human T-lymphotropic retrovirus (HTLV-III) in the serum of patients with AIDS. Science, 224, 506-508.
Smithson, W. A., Gilchrist, G. S. & Burgert, E. O. (1980). Childhood acute lymphocytic leukemia. Cancer, 30, 158-181.
Spiro, H. M. (1974). My kingdom for a camera - some comments on medical technology. New England Journal of Medicine, 291, 1070-1072.
Steel, K., Gertman, P. M., Crescenzi, C., & Anderson, J. (1981). Iatrogenic illness on a general medical service at a university hospital. New England Journal of Medicine, 304, 638-642.
Surgeon General. (1982). The Health Consequences of Smoking: Cancer.

Rockville: Office on Smoking and Health, Public Health Service.
Terhost, C., van Agthoven, A., Reinherz, E., & Scholossman, S. (1980). Biochemical analysis of human T lymphocyte differentiation antigens T4 and T5. Science, 209, 520-521.
Thomas, L. (1984, December 5). Whitehead Institute Inaugural Address.
Vayda, E., & Mindell, W. R. (1982). Variations in operative rates. Surgical Clinics of North America, 62, 627-639.
Vayda, E., Mindell, W. R. & Rutkow, I. M. (1982). A decade of surgery in Canada, England and Wales and the United States. Archives of Surgery, 117, 846-853.
Virchow, R. (1947). Cited in Rosen, G. What is social medicine? Bulletin of the History of Medicine, 21, 674-733.
Wennberg, J. E., Blowers, L., Parker, R., & Gittelsohn, A. M. (1977). Changes in tonsillectomy rates associated with feedback and review. Pediatrics, 59, 821-826.
Wennberg, J. E., Bunker, J. P. & Barnes, B. A. (1980). The need for assessing outcomes of common medical practices. Annual Review of Public Health, 1, 277-295.
Wennberg, J. E., & Gittelson, A. (1982). Variations in medical care among small areas. Scientific American, 126, 120-134.

# REFORMING MEDICAL EDUCATION: TOWARDS A BROADENING OF ATTITUDES

Margaret Lock and Joseph Lella

Department of Humanities and Social Studies in Medicine
McGill University

## SOCIAL SCIENCE AND VALUES

About ten years ago, in an attempt to alleviate the financial insolvency associated with writing a Ph.D. thesis, one of us became part of a team of four people employed as raters of mother/infant behaviour. The study, done in California, made use of home movies taken during the first six months in an infant's life. It was known that some of the babies had become diagnosed as schizophrenic in later childhood, and our job was to rank episodes of mother/infant interaction, eye contact, holding and feeding techniques, and so on, on a five point scale. Mother and infant were evaluated separately. It was hypothesized that the behaviour of some mothers and some infants (not necessarily in the same family), would allow one to predict by the age of six months which children were at serious risk for becoming schizophrenics in the future. We could then check our experimental findings against what had actually become reality.

One of the major assumptions in this study was that mother/infant interaction has certain features which are universally true and not subject to historical and cross-cultural variation. The study soon ran into trouble because one mother (a European) was filmed in the bath together with her baby (a male) enjoying close body contact with the infant while she bathed it. The other three raters gave this woman very low marks for this episode since they perceived incipient dependency problems. Lock had just returned from two years in Japan where it is essential for an adult to bathe with an infant to prevent it from drowning in the deep, hot water. It is also customary there, as in most parts of the world, for adults to sleep with babies. Feelings of dependency in Japan are in general encouraged, valued, and not abhorred. Lock ranked the mother high, but was castigated by the other raters and the principal investigator when "anomalies" in the rating procedures were being investigated.

To some extent, poor scientific design was the problem with this study, but tightening criteria for evaluation would not have provided a lasting solution since values and beliefs of both investigators and subjects were involved. The isolation and assessment of little pieces of behaviour served to reduce an ongoing, intimate, and complex process to a game of charades in which the raters tried to create a whole picture from small contrived scenarios using value-laden criteria.

## The Biopsychosocial Model in Medical Education

Over the past ten years, some rather important changes have taken place in the teaching of medical students, among them the introduction of board examinations in behavioural sciences in medicine, and the systematic expansion of teaching in medical schools to include courses in behavioural sciences (Kennedy, Pattishall, and Baldwin, 1983). The biopsychosocial model elaborated by Engel (1977, 1980) and others, has been widely promoted as a theoretical framework to facilitate a new approach in medicine, and is frequently used as the organizing principal for these courses (Simons, 1985; Lella, Gill, and McGlynn, 1985). While this approach has facilitated the process of change and stimulated a much broader approach in medical training we believe that it has not encouraged any radical shift in medical thinking, but has instead tended to fall into difficulties similar to those which arose in the mother/infant study cited above.

Engel's original 1977 paper in Science, subtitled "A Challenge for Biomedicine" is an innovative and highly influential document. He suggests that by applying to medicine ideas derived from systems theory developed by biologists such as Von Bertalanffy and others, one can broaden the reductionistic and biologically oriented biomedical model, the characteristic "dogma" of modern medicine, as Engel describes it. He calls for a scientifically rational approach to behavioural and psychosocial variables in which data carefully collected from the patient's verbal accounts are given due weight (1977). He stresses that biological changes are necessary but not sufficient variables in the onset of disease; that illness is the result of complex interactions of environmental, social, psychological and biological variables which together account for variation in the onset, severity and the course of a disease. He also emphasizes that it is important to establish why simple "problems of living" for some become "illness" for others. He hopes that these and other insights will ensure a more scientific approach to patient care, the scope of which is "determined by the historic function of the physician to establish whether the person soliciting help is 'sick' or 'well'; and if sick, why sick and in which ways sick; and then to develop a rational program to treat the illness and restore and maintain health" (1977, p. 132).

Changes in the epidemiology of disease, spiralling costs in health care, and the recognition that access to modern medicine has not been the prime contributor to greater longevity or improved quality of life (McKeown, 1979), have promoted some receptivity to the biopsychosocial model in most medical faculties, and with it has come a change in the way that diseases are conceptualized.

## The Model in Historical Context

A brief review of the evolution of clinical medicine can place this development in historical context and help us understand its significance for broadening medical attitudes through education. It is our thesis that the biopsychosocial model alone is not as significant as it may seem.

Up until the early 19th century, the outward manifestations of disease on the body surface, combined with what symptoms the patient described, provided the raw data with which the physican worked (Foucault, 1963). The patient was indispensible to the task of diagnosis and little distinction was made between the subjective experience of the illness and its evaluation by the physician. Gradually, however, with the adoption of Cartesian philosophy and the development of medical technology, the human body came to be seen as a discrete entity, objective, passive, and analysable through a combination of induction and deduction. At the same time it became generally accepted that the goal of medical science was to describe the body in ever finer and more precise terms. "The core task ... became not the elucidation of what the patient said but what the doctor saw in the depths of the body" (Armstrong, 1984, p. 738). Textbooks from the early part of this century stress the importance of "looking behind" the patient's words. Bourne, for example, stated that "The human being is a recording instrument of uncertain and variable power" (1931), and it was believed that the physician should only use this instrument to get at the "character" and "life-history" of the symptom" (Stern, 1933).

Armstrong documents how, from the late thirties onwards, there was another gradual change in the content of clinical texts in light of the emergence of psychiatry as a discipline. The concept of "mental hygiene" became prevalent; the psychiatric examination was acknowledged as important, and the illness was now perceived, by some at least, to be located not solely inside the tangible body but also partially in the patient's less tangible psychology and social relations. As Armstrong notes, it became necessary once again to pay close attention to the patient's account of the problem (1984).

With the rise of medical sociology and survey techniques through which to elicit patients' views, and with the development of sophisticated statistical models, the concept of "multi-causality" was firmly established. Thus the earlier and rather clear distinction between a state of health and illness was radically modified to include the idea of a person "at risk". In addition the community, rather than the individual patient, became the focus of analysis for many sociologists, epidemiologists, anthropologists, and allied physicians (Ruffini, 1983; Berkman, 1981).

What has characterized much of this type of research is quantification and concern for prediction and hence control over potential illness behaviour. Studies based on the Health Belief Model (Becker, 1974), and those oriented toward patient compliance (Haynes, Taylor, and Sackett, 1979) perhaps most clearly embody these characteristics. Both approaches attempt to use an understanding of patient attitudes, beliefs and behaviour to predict and channel patient behaviour toward clearly and professionally conceptualized, health-related goals. Knowledge of the "normal" aging process is also recognized as important if populations "at risk" are to be defined. Dimensions of time and space are therefore made more central in the concept of illness which is now rather difficult to view as a static entity. These attempts to overcome the "mind-body" duality of biomedicine have made the notions of variability, "borderline cases", and "illness as process" more respectable. Engel's work is of great significance because he garnered this rather diffuse interdisciplinary work and applied the results rigorously to clinical practice and medical education while promoting his insights through scientific and clinical journals.

## The Biopsychosocial Model as Cultural Construct: Problems and Implications for Medical Education

Recently, and with increasing vigor, a more critical assessment of medical practice has emerged. Aided by insights gained from the history, sociology, and anthropology of knowledge (Freidson, 1970; Foucault, 1963, 1965) it has become clear that not only the experience of illness, but also medical knowledge and practice, are historically, socially, and culturally constructed (Kleinman, 1980: Hahn and Gaines, 1985; Lock, 1980; Wright and Treacher, 1982). Engel himself is not unaware of this issue. He notes that the physicians' approaches to patients is modified by "their teachers, their mentors, the texts they use, the practices they are encouraged to follow, and even the medical institutions and administrative organizations in which they work [which] all reflect the prevailing conceptual models of the era" (1980, p. 535). He also stresses that the patient should be considered as a person and that the clinical encounter should be seen as involving two subjects in negotiation.

In the adoption of the biopsychosocial model into medical education, however, these crucial but perhaps painful insights for physicians seem to have been given rather short shrift. Four points illustrate the problem.

First, the teaching of medical history is far from being a universally established and well-accepted part of the medical curriculum (Bylebyl, 1982). Even in medical schools where professional medical historians are present, the subject is often regarded as relatively unimportant by all but a small minority. Students are frequently left with the unexamined idea that medical "progress" (a 19th century concept in itself) has traced a path from superstition to mastery of nature, and that they are privileged to be close to the end of the journey (Osler, 1932). Such a notion is, of course, no longer generally accepted by serious students of the biological and social sciences. Thus, medical students remain relatively unaware and unreceptive to the idea that, historically and comparatively speaking, there have been and are many ways of conceptualizing and dealing with health and illness. In <u>all</u> medical systems some ideas are rubbish, some are iatrogenic, and others are highly effective for a variety of reasons, which may not be amenable to scientific evaluation. Modern "technomedicine" is clearly superior in many ways to all that has gone before it. But numerous critics have shown that environmental and social factors have a more profound effect on the health of populations than do medical techniques (McKeown, 1979; Starr, 1982). A knowledge of the social history of medicine including its political struggles for power and control, if sensitively taught, can serve to encourage a more sceptical, open-minded, and realistic understanding of modern medicine and its practices, many of which are surely not the result of scientific progress.

Further, it is not at all clear, when looked at in this perspective, that a psychosocially altered or "fixed" biomedical model is all "progress". Some analysts (Illich, 1975; Arney, 1982; Foucault, 1963; Zola, 1972) have seen it as a mere extension of the medicalization of life, subjecting even the patient's internal states, family relations, and community life to the expert "gaze" and interventions of an all-powerful professional outsider. Viewed in such a way, the biopsychosocial model can be seen as a lever to reduce the patient's autonomy rather than one which might lift him toward wholeness and health.

Secondly, the basic structure of medical education itself has not been changed in any fundamental fashion, despite the introduction of behavioural science teaching and the adoption of the biopsychosocial model. This is in part because students are now expected to imbibe knowledge from psychology, sociology, and anthropology in addition to the biomedical sciences. They are, moreover, taught this information as though it were a basic science. A body of supposedly testable knowledge is imparted and multiple choice questionnaires are used in the Board examinations and also in medical faculties. This means that information which is often contextually relative is treated as absolute fact, and as suitable subject matter for study through testable hypotheses. Further, the student is not required to reflect upon or debate this information. On the contrary, the use of multiple choice questions tends to encourage the idea that one is dealing with <u>the truth</u>.

With the addition of behavioural sciences, time pressure and stress upon the student has not been relieved but increased. For example, the authors' group was recently castigated a few years ago by a visiting faculty accreditor when he discovered that standard examinations were not administered in the McGill behavioural science course. His opinion was that medical students should be under great stress since, as future physicians, they must learn how to deal with it - a not uncommon viewpoint.

It is paradoxical that students are encouraged to think of the patient as a whole person while at the same time, faculty take away the few hours in the week left to these students, just out of adolescence, to develop into well-rounded adults. Furthermore, by turning the biopsychosocial approach into a "scientific" endeavour students are not encouraged, any more than they were in the past, to explore their subjective responses to the patient as a person, to the process of becoming a physician, or to the organization and structure of the hospital or other dimensions of professional life. Emotion, ambiguity, uncertainty, reflection - these are states which are to be avoided and circumscribed in patient care, and student and professional life. They have no place in the "quest for scientific excellence" which brings us to the third point.

The biopsychsocial model draws upon ideas developed principally in ecology, and although it promotes an integration of biological and social variables, it nevertheless does so with the ultimate objective of developing a more scientific, rational, and controlled medical knowledge and practice. Using this approach careful studies in social epidemiology such as those of Brown and Harris (1978) on depression, Marmot and Syme (1976) on coronary heart disease, and Kaufert (1984) and McKinlay and McKinlay (1986) on menopause, can be incorporated into medical education and contribute to a broadening of the physician's frame of reference. Research such as this demonstrates, for example, normal variation in non-clinical populations and serves to reduce the bias of education based almost exclusively on clinical samples. However, the major problem with the biopsychosocial approach remains since survey research usually stays within a deterministic paradigm and does not incorporate the creative, symbolic powers of human beings into its analysis.

People everywhere construct conceptual maps of their natural and social worlds and try to explain change, expecially misfortune (Durkheim and Mauss, 1963; Evans-Pritchard, 1937; Geertz, 1973). Viewed within a deterministic paradigm, such insights can lead physicians to look for "the" conceptual model held, for example, by Greek immigrants or native Canadians for a particular biological condition. Such an approach ignores the rather commonplace social science insight that such models are in constant flux and that individuals and groups are always creatively revising and adapting their conceptual model to newly evolving social contexts and events.

Finally, remaining within a deterministic paradigm suppresses the awareness that much professional medical knowledge and practice is also socially constructed and handed down. It too is a cultural product. Thomas (1970, p. 172) calls medicine the "youngest science", and partly because explanations for a broad range of clinical phenomena are minimal, there is room for different schools of thought. In clinical practice, however, one must act. Freidson has commented that since the focus of medicine "is on the practical solution of concrete problems, it is obliged to carry on even when it lacks a scientific foundation for its activities; it is oriented towards intervention irrespective of the existence of reliable knowledge". We would add, even when there is reliable knowledge or scientific "facts", that in clinical practice all medical knowledge is subject to value judgements and interpretations. However, medical students, interns, and residents are usually led to justify their clinical judgements as scientifically based decisions. The example given below based on the management of menopause will illustrate this point.

The following statement comes from "Understanding Human Behavior" in

Health and Illness (Simons, 1985, p. 480), a text widely used in medical schools: "the menopause is relatively simple to discuss because the picture is fairly clear". In fact, all that is clear about menopause is that endocrine changes do eventually precipitate the end of menstruation and female reproductive life. Beyond this there is no end to speculation about almost every aspect of research and clinical care. For example, next to nothing is known about the cause, duration, incidence, or frequency of "hot flashes." Furthermore, no connection has ever been scientifically established between psychological variables and declining estrogen levels although this association is widely accepted by physicians, patients, and the general public and is often used to justify therapeutic choices. Similarly, no statistical relationship has been clearly established between changing social roles, departure of children, loss of parents, husband's infidelity, greying hair, wrinkled skin, or anything else and the experience of physical symptoms at menopause. The use of estrogen replacement therapy has, of course, been heatedly debated. Its effectiveness in preventing hot flashes is reasonably well established, but associated difficulties are widely discussed including possible dependency and withdrawal problems (Coope, 1975). This plethora of speculation and uncertainty should be acknowledged in medical texts and lectures. It should also be made clear that practising gynecologists, family and general practitioners have each evolved working models of menopause which are constructed in light of their own clinical experiences, their particular patient populations, personal and professional perspectives, and whatever stereotype they may hold about middle-aged women and aging (including their own). These culturally constructed working models are subject to modification and change by factors as far-reaching and unscientific as what the physician's wife or husband thinks about menopause, to television programmes on the subject.

In a study of Montreal physicians, Lock (1985) found great variation in knowledge of, attitudes toward, and treatment approaches to the menopause. There were at least five clear perspectives which will be presented in simplified form for the sake of brevity. One group felt that menopause should be viewed as a deficiency disease; that physicians should strive for greater scientific understanding of the topic at the somatic level, and that psychosocial variables are unscientific and should not be considered by physicians, who are scientists. Estrogen replacement therapy (ERT) is prescribed for about 60 percent of the patient population by this group of physicians, often with the addition of androgens.

The second group felt that the majority of women who seek medical care at menopause are suffering from depression, and that they are principally concerned about aging, loss of sexuality and libido. These physicians frequently prescribe ERT which they believe relieves not only debilitating hot flashes, but also depression; these clinicians also frequently recommend psychological counselling.

The third group stated that trouble at menopause usually arises out of role conflict, the "empty nest", a spouse's retirement, and so on. Family counselling was seen to be in order, at which time somatic symptoms, if present, should decline and diminish in importance to the patient. ERT was used rarely by members of this group - on about two percent of the menopausal patient population. Some physicians avoid use of medications altogether.

The fourth, "stiff upper lip school", asserted, along with some feminists, that altogether too much fuss is made about menopause. Healthy menopausal patients are usually referred to "my colleague down the corridor who likes to do a bit of counselling".

Finally political/feminist physicians (either male or female) considered the debate over menopause as a distraction, perpetrated by the media, by bored middle-class women, and by physicians seeking an easy income. Many of their patients were said to have more serious health problems to deal with and hence did not report menopausal symptoms.

To experienced clinicians these findings should come as no surprise. Similar variations in perspective could be described for physicians treating other medical problems. Taylor, for example, found two basic approaches to patients with breast cancer among oncologists which could be linked to their underlying acceptance or not of randomized clinical trials (Taylor, 1985). Such differences in opinion have profound consequences for power and dependency relationships between physician and patient, and for the medicalization of many areas of life and, therefore, should be explicitly discussed throughout medical education. Should molecules and organs, the whole body, person, family, or society, be the focus for therapeutic change? What are the implications of these choices for symptom relief, for attribution of responsibility, for coping, and life-style, and for future generations?

If the physician is to be educator and psychotherapist as Engel recommends (1977, p. 132), then value judgements are involved. If today he or she chooses to adhere closely to the biomedical model, that too is a value judgement. The inevitability of value judgements <u>and their consequences</u> need to be carefully considered.

## <u>Encouraging Self-Reflection</u>

Students can be encouraged to move from a "value-laden" through a "value-free", to a "value-committed" position during the course of their education. At present most medical education can be seen as perpetrating what can be called "value-laden" attitudes. The biopsychosocial approach, in its present form, can inadvertently reinforce these attitudes since there is a tendency in all of us to move easily from percentages, to absolutes, to stereotypes, when presented with statistical data without considerable pause for reflection. The student can, however, be taught to appreciate the idea of cultural relativism both before and during medical school, through exposure to the medical systems and ideas about health and illness of other cultures, and will then perhaps arrive at a "value free" position which is similar to the experience of many anthropologists in their early days of doing fieldwork in an exotic setting.

A "value-free" position could logically imply, to give an extreme example, that as a physician one would be willing to do clitorodectomies on North and East African immigrant female children, or check the virginity of the adolescent daughters of Greek immigrants, should their parents request it.

The goal of all education, however, in medicine and other disciplines, should be for the student to arrive at an informed "value-commitment" - a flexible and reflective stance which, in the case of a future medical practitioner, can facilitate an assessment of his or her own values and knowledge in light of each new case. It is within this approach that patient-negotiation and therapeutic alliance models can be used successfully. The clinical encounter then becomes one where, as far as possible, pre-formed suppositions on the part of <u>both</u> practitioner and patient are mutually examined. More scientific research is needed as suggested by Eisenberg (this volume), but its appropriate application cannot be determined through purely scientific or logical principles.

Many physicians survive medical school and reach an intelligent value-committed position on their own, but for large numbers, medical education needs _radical_ reform if patient care and therapeutic choices are to be improved.

## _Reforming Medical Education: Toward a Broadening of Attitudes_

How can such reform be effected? How can attitudes be truly broadened? It is surely not by adding more facts to the same old deterministic paradigm of patient and physician functioning. The content cannot simply be changed while leaving underlying assumptions intact. Such change, of course, will not come easily since assumptions are deeply embedded in social and cultural contexts over which there is little control. Physician educators tend to manipulate students, patients, and each other toward fixed and supposedly enlightened goals often irrespective of the context and the "will" of the manipulated. Despite this, there are certain directions toward which one can work using leads supplied by imaginative, humanistically oriented precedents (Novak, 1972; Gregory, 1984).

Historical, cross-cultural, and sociological study of health care and medical institutions can inform students about the variety of medical practices and the factors which have conditioned their emergence. Such study can also promote respect for this variation. Academic tomes such as those of Freidson, Starr and Foucault have their place, but historical novels, diaries, and drama concerning medical culture can teach the student to appreciate how and on what grounds that culture is continually being invented by people like themselves. Novels such as Solzhenitsyn's _Cancer Ward_, Sinclair Lewis' _Arrowsmith_, Eliot's _Middlemarch_, Moliere's and Shaw's, "doctor plays", Osler's and Lewis Thomas' "lay sermons", and many other works are suitable material. If taught with a sensitivity to the student's own reactions and insights, such materials can promote self-respect, a capacity to reflect on the issues involved, and to adapt creatively to the ambiguities and uncertainties ever present in medicine.

While students are being taught about the various pathways to health and illness which behavioural science has discerned through the application of a biopsychosocial model, he or she should also be helped to _appreciate_ and respect what it feels like to be a patient. This is not easy to do today. As Thomas (1983, p. 221) has said:

> "The high technologies which are turned on to cope with serious disease - the electronic monitors in intensive care units, the chemotherapy drugs for cancer, the _tour de force_ accomplishments of contemporary surgery, and the mobilization of increasingly complex procedures for diagnosis in medicine - are matters to be mastered only from lecture notes and books, and then by actual practice on patients, but very few doctors have more than an inkling of what it is actually like to go through such experiences. Even the childhood contagions are mostly gone, thanks to vaccines for measles, whooping cough, chicken pox, and the like, thanks especially to the easy control of streptococcal infections. Today's young doctors do not know what it is to have an earache, much less what it means to have an eardrum punctured."

However, students can be given the time and encouragement to get to know patients in their social and cultural contexts in some depth before, and while they are being given clinical responsibilities. They can be taught to explore and appreciate patients "explanatory models" (Kleinman, Eisenberg, and Good, 1978; Helman, 1985; Good and Good, 1980), and strategies for coping with illness. For example, students can be given long-term responsibility for home and hospital visits with particular patients; they can participate in tutorials concerning such visits in which the student is required to examine what biopsychosocial information means when applied to a particular case or cases. Such tutorials can also allow the tutor and student to explore the student's own feelings about and reactions to the patient (Bates, 1973).

During the clinical and residency years, students can be encouraged to participate in Balint groups in which the dilemmas of their own professional development and relations with patients are considered and in which they are made aware of the choices in patient care which are open to them. They can be given support in making their choices and in working through the difficulties which result. Finally, service rounds and seminars, tutorials and consultations can be developed in which clinical cases involving psychosocial dimensions and value judgements are prominent. The student's creative imagination often needs help to be liberated when he or she is surrounded by the organizational constraints of hospital life.

The cultivation of self-reflection and tolerance of ambiguity and uncertainty has a number of analogues in other disciplines. Training in anthropological and sociological fieldwork is oriented toward helping students become aware of their own biases and value judgements. Immersion in a situation where the dominant values are alien to one's own produces a severe shock, but reflection on this experience can be highly conducive to the development of empathy and reflection. If some medical training took place outside of clinical and academic settings, the development of a more flexible stance might be facilitated.

Training in psychoanalysis, or in counselling presents models more closely related to medicine. In these fields, student-trainees are helped by supervisors to be receptive to the needs and hopes of patients or clients. In supervisory sessions, matters concerning both the patient-client <u>and</u> the trainee's reactions to the situation are carefully considered (Rogers, 1951; Malcolm, 1981; Freud, 1910). Viewed somewhat simplistically, the goal is to move from a value-laden stance, in which one imposes one's ideas on another person, to a value-committed stance, in which one is prepared to negotiate between two differing sets of ideas and aspirations.

What is proposed is a difficult but not impossible goal. Human beings, especially members of professions, seek certainty and routines whereby they may justify their expertise and their power to themselves, to the society around them, and, in the case of health professionals, to their patients. The courage and insight necessary to cultivate expertise with empathy, and an ability to admit the limits of one's knowledge, can never be simply taught in a didactic fashion. These virtues must be constantly cultivated. Radical change will not come about through the adoption of the biopsychosocial model as such. It will come about only if those who apply it in medical education treat it not only as a kit bag of knowledge and concepts to be taught and manipulated, but also as embodying a moral and reflective approach to be continually developed throughout life (Bruyn, 1966).

When the hero of A.J. Cronin's novel, <u>The Citadel</u>, is asked in his fellowship examinations what he had learned from medical practice he replied "not to take anything for granted." Still sound advice, but not something one comes to understand easily if one is taught as Mr. Gradgrind states in Charles Dickens'(1854) <u>Hard Times</u>, "You must discard ... Fancy altogether ... You must use ... combinations and modifications ... of mathematical figures which are susceptible of proof and demonstration". Fancy, spontaneity, creativity, respect, understanding, reflection, ambiguity, are all old-fashioned, "soft" and perhaps moralistic words. However, they and the realities they represent must re-enter our vocabularies, and our lives as teachers and as scientists if we are to see medical attitudes truly broadened.

ACKNOWLEDGEMENTS

The authors would like to acknowledge their debt to Dr. Don Bates, historian of medicine and departmental colleague, for his continuing contribution to these ideas on medical education.

This paper was made possible, in part, by a grant from Formation des Chercheurs et d'Action Concertee, F.C.A.C. (Quebec).

REFERENCES

Armstrong, D. (1984). The patient's view. Social Science and Medicine, 18, 737-744.

Arney, W. R. (1982). Power and the profession of obstetrics. Chicago: University of Chicago Press.

Bates, D. (1973). Humanism in undergraduate medical education. In J. P. McGovern (Ed.), Humanism in medicine. Springfield, IL: Charles C. Thomas.

Becker, M. (1974). (Ed.). The health belief model and personal health behavior. Health Education Monograph, Vol. 2, No. 2.

Berkman, L. F. (1981). Physical health and the social environment: A social epidemiological perspective. In L. Eisenberg & A. Kleinman (Eds.), The relevance of social science for medicine. (pp. 51-75). Boston: Reidel.

Bourne, G. (1931). An introduction to medical history and case-taking. Edinburgh: Edinburgh Livingstone.

Brown, G. W. & T. Harris. (1978). Social origins of depression: A study of psychiatric disorder in women. London: Tavistock.

Bruyn, S. (1966). The human perspective in sociology. Englewood Cliffs, NJ: Prentice-Hall.

Bylebyl, J. (1982). Introduction. In J. Bylebyl (Ed.), Teaching the history of medicine at a medical center (pp. 1-12). Baltimore: Johns Hopkins University Press.

Coope, J., Thomson, J. M., & Potter, L. (1975). Effects of "natural aestrogen" replacement therapy on menopausal symptoms and blood clotting. British Medical Journal.

Engel, G. (1977). The need for a new medical model: A challenge for biomedicine. Science, 196, 129-196.

Engel, G. (1980). The clinical application of the biopsychosocial model. American Journal of Psychiatry, 137, 535-544.

Evans-Pritchard, E. E. (1937). Witchcraft, oracles and magic among the Azande. Oxford: Clarendon Press.

Foucault, M. (1963). The birth of the clinic: An archeology of medical perception. London: Tavistock.

Foucault, M. (1965). Madness and civilization. New York: Random House.

Freidson, E. (1970). Profession of medicine: A study of the sociology of applied knowledge. New York: Dodd, Mead.

Freud, S. (1910). The future prospects of psychotherapy. In P. Rieff, (Ed.), Freud: Therapy and technique, Chapter V. (pp. 77-88). New York: Collier Books, 1963.

Geertz, C. (1973). The interpretation of cultures. New York: Basic Books.

Gregory, M. S. (1984). Science and humanities: Toward a new world view. In D. S. Brock & A. Harward (Eds.), The culture of biomedicine. (Studies in Science and Culture, Vol. 1). (pp. 11-33). Newark: University of Delaware Press.

Good, B. J. & Good, M. J. (1980). The meaning of symptoms: A cultural hermeneutic model for clinical practice. In L. Eisenberg & A. Kleinman (Eds.), The relevance of social science for medicine. Boston: Reidel.

Hahn, R. A. & Gaines A. D. (Eds.). (1985). Physicians of Western

medicine: Anthropological approaches to theory and practice. Boston: Reidel.
Haynes, R. B., Taylor, D. W. & Sackett, D. L. (Eds.). (1979). Compliance in health care. Baltimore: Johns Hopkins University Press.
Helman, C. (1985). Communication and primary care: The role of patient and practitioner explanatory models. Social Science and Medicine, 20, 923-931.
Illich, I. (1975). Medical nemesis: The expropriation of health. Toronto: McLelland and Stewart.
Kaufert, P. (1984). Women and their health in the middle years: A Manitoba project. Social Science and Medicine, 18, 279-281.
Kennedy, D. A., Pattishall, E. G., & Baldwin, D. C. (1983). Medical education and the behavioral sciences. Baltimore: Association for the Behavioral Sciences and Medical Education.
Kleinman, A. (1980). Patients and healers in the context of culture: An exploration of the borderland between anthropology, medicine and psychiarty. Berkeley: University of California Press.
Kleinman, A., Eisenberg, L., & Good, B. J. (1978). Culture, illness and care: Clinical lessons from anthropological and crosscultural research. Annals of Internal Medicine, 88, 251-258.
Lella, J. W., Gill, D. G., & McGlynn, R. (1985). Basic curriculum content for the behavioral sciences in pre-clinical medical education. McLean, VA: Association for the Behavioral Sciences and Medical Education.
Lock, M. (1980). East Asian medicine in urban Japan: Varieties of medical experience. Berkeley: University of California Press.
Lock, M. (1985). Models and practice in medicine: Menopause as syndrome or life transition? In R. A. Hahn & A. D. Gaines (Eds.), Physicians of Western medicine: Anthropological approaches to theory and practice. Boston: Reidel.
Malcolm, J. (1981). Psychoanalysis: The impossible profession. New York: Knopf.
Marmot, M. G. & Syme, L. (1976). Acculturation and coronary heart disease in Japanese Americans. American Journal of Epidemiology, 104, 225-247.
McKeown, T. (1979). The role of medicine: Dream, mirage, or nemesis. Oxford: Blackwell.
McKinlay, S. & McKinlay, J. B. (1986). Health status and health care utilization by menopausal women. In L. Mastroianni & C. A. Paulsen (Eds.), Aging, reproduction and the climacteric. New York: Plenum Press.
Novak, M. (1972). The liberation of imagination. Instituting human values in medicine: Proceedings of the second session. Philadelphia: Society for Health and Human Values.
Osler, W. (1932). Medicine in the nineteenth century. Acquanimitas: With other addresses to medical students, nurses, and practitioners of medicine (3rd ed.). Philadelphia: Blakiston.
Rogers, C. (1951). The training of counsellors and therapists. In Client-centered therapy: Its current practice applications and theory. Chapter 10. (pp. 429-478). Boston: Houghton-Mifflin.
Ruffini, J. L. (Ed.) (1983). Advances in medical social science. New York: Gordon and Breach Science.
Simons, R. C. (Ed.). (1985). Understanding human behavior. Health and Illness (3rd ed.). Baltimore: Williams and Wilkins.
Starr, P. (1982). The social transformation of American medicine. New York: Basic Books.
Stern, N. S. (1933). Clinical diagnosis: Physical and differential. New York: Macmillan.
Taylor, K. (1985). Decision difficult: Physician behavior in the diagnosis and treatment of breast cancer. Unpublished doctoral dissertation. McGill University, Montreal, Department of Sociology.

Thomas, Lewis, (1983). The youngest science: Notes of a medicine-watcher. New York: Viking Press.
Wright, P., & Treacher, A. (Eds.). (1982). The problem of medical knowledge: Examining the social construction of medicine. Edinburgh: Edingurgh University Press.
Zola, I. K. (1972). Medicine as an institute of social control. Sociological Review, 20, 487-504.

# IMPROVING THE MANAGEMENT OF ILLNESS BEHAVIOUR BY CHANGING ROLES WITHIN MULTIDISCIPLINARY TREATMENT TEAMS

Brian Shaw

Clarke Institute of Psychiatry
University of Toronto

## Introduction

Clinicians interested in illness behaviour have generally accepted an interdisciplinary approach to treatment. For example, Schwartz and Weiss (1978, p.249) defined behavioural medicine as "the interdisciplinary field concerned with the development and integration of behavioural and biomedical science, knowledge and prevention, diagnosis, treatment and rehabilitation." In a later definition, Matarazzo (1982, p.8) defined behavioural medicine as "an interdisciplinary field dedicated to promoting a philosophy of health that stresses individual responsibility in the application of behavioural and biomedical science knowledge and techniques to the maintenance of health and the prevention of illness and dysfunction by a variety of self-initiated or shared activities." There are several operative concepts in these definitions besides the interdisciplinary notion. The terms "science" and "the application of knowledge" imply a deciphering of data to guide specific interventions. These data may become available through methods of bio-medicine, behavioural science, or both. This chapter addresses some of the problems and a few potential solutions in the delivery of health-care services within a multidisciplinary model of treatment. The main theme of this chapter concerns the influence of roles, expectations, and attitudes that produce significant difficulties in the integration of knowledge acquired from the observations of various disciplines. By discussing strategies to change roles, expectations and attitudes within multidisciplinary treatment teams, the hope is to improve the quality of care provided to consumers, in part by better management of illness behaviour.

Agras (1982, p.797) points out that a major strength of the field of behavioural medicine is "an emerging network of communication among an array of disciplines not previously well connected." As boundaries between disciplines become less rigid due in part to the realization that "the complex problems of health and illness were ... inherently multidimensional in nature ... researchers and clinicians from diverse disciplines have become motivated to seek better ways of building bridges between disciplines and establishing a common set of terms and principles ..." (Schwartz, 1982, p. 1041). Clearly, the hope reflected in these statements is that knowledge of the complexity of problems will lead to improved communication and, as a result, to better care. This development may occur in time but it is certainly not a given. One threat to the "building of bridges" leading to better management of illness behaviour is that with increased specialization within the disciplines the care of the patient may become fragmented. For the individual patient, communication within the various professions involved in direct health care is essential. Along with the value of "a common set of terms and prinicples", other factors that will help unite various professionals are necessary. These factors include, but are not limited to, the roles, expectations, and attitudes of the care-givers and changes in the clinical management environment.

## Interprofessional Roles, Attitudes and Expectations

As the main thrust of this chapter concerns how to change roles to facilitate changes in clinical management, it becomes important to consider the roles that develop amongst health professionals. Roles refer to socially expected behaviour patterns (Brown, 1965) and they consist of a rather substantial number of norms (Nadel, 1957) which are essentially prescriptions for behaviour. Roles are determined by norms that apply to categories of persons. As such, there is some essential characteristic that defines the membership of the category. Training in various disciplines or professions represents a major role induction procedure, specifically through controlled membership as defined by legal procedures such as licensure, certification and contracts.

Understandably, disagreements among the prescriptions create a problem for the professional. Often roles in occupational settings are designed to complement each other so that several people together may be organized to achieve certain goals (for example, a treatment team). For some roles, such as teachers or police officers, all of society is familiar with the chief requirements and expected behaviour. However, for most occupational roles, particularly the health professional roles, the definition of normative behaviours are set by members of the group. As a result, the expectations and demands of a self-interested group may overlook the concerns of the public. On the other hand, the complexity of professional responsibility often requires that the profession be given the task of monitoring or guaranteeing a satisfactory level of role performance. Sanctions rewarding proper performance (e.g., merit awards) or punishing poor performance (e.g., disciplinary hearings) are generally applied within the profession. As the allegiance to the norms set by the profession has a major influence on the maintenance of roles members are often more sensitive to their professional group than to broader concerns. The impact of this professional allegiance and organization is clear when one considers the health-care team.

The health-care team is typically part of an organization whose by-laws, policies and procedures are written in terms of role titles. Thus, many responsibilities and duties within a health-care facility are defined according to one's occupationally defined title (e.g., physician, nurse, social worker). This environmental situation has an important influence on the maintenance of traditional professional roles. The first task is to minimize hassles and/or problems for team members who want to change their roles to improve their management of illness. An openess to changing roles in multidisciplinary teams at the institutional or even governmental level will have to be developed via the usual educational and political processes. The press for cost containment in the health-care system will almost undoubtedly be the major impetus towards these role changes (Cummings, 1986).

Berg (1986, p.54) addressed the role conflict in multidisciplinary teams from the perspective of diagnostic problems but many of his points have a broad applicability. He pointed out that "Each participant brings attitudes about his or her role and the other's role; the extent to which these intertwine or clash determines whether the collaboration is successful."

Occupational roles are an important part of the way individuals define themselves. When one considers the normative behaviour of other professions, one tends to be cryptic and sterotyped in our responses. There is a further tendency to maximize differences among the occupations each with their unique contribution to the care of patients. To facilitate the functioning of a treatment team it would be best to find commonalities in roles rather than differences. Clearly, the training in the various professions provides unique skills and knowledge necessary for the management of complex cases. Equally relevant however, are the common rules that health-care providers bring to the case. Two roles that come to mind are those of observer of the patient's behaviour and educator. Each profession requires a base of information that serves both to inform the care-giver and to guide others (including the patient) in the management of the problem. The disease-illness distinction (Eisenberg and Kleinman, 1977) is particularly relevant as it provides a framework for both clinical management and communication (see Cott, this volume).

Changing roles involves introducing new normative behaviours. The introduction and acceptance of new normative behaviours will require changes in the team members' attitudes and expectations toward illness and disease. To improve health care a broad conceptual model of the patient's illness is necessary so that different professionals may develop a common base of behavioural observations and an emphasis on their roles as educators.

## Conceptualizing Care From a Biopsychosocial Perspective

One important question to be addressed is why roles developed within the treatment team need to change? After all, it may be argued each profession has unique skills and special behaviours developed within a carefully considered curriculum honed through years of experience. The point has been made that "the prevalence of the interdisciplinary model is evidence of its soundness and of its advantages for managing complex clinical tasks" (Berg, 1986, p.52). Yet, it is the push toward specialization of tasks within the teams that may in reality fragment the patient's care and impede the management of his/her illness. The argument here is not designed to promote wholesale changes in professional roles, but rather of the expansion of certain behaviours that are prescribed a part of each role. Furthermore, a generic model of interchangeable health-care providers is not intended. Instead, the approach under consideration is one which fully endorses a biopsychosocial perspective (Engel, 1977) in such a way that the different professionals provide a common set of observations along with the unique observations associated with their professional training.

The "biopsychosocial model proposes that a medical diagnosis should always consider the interaction of biological, psychological, and social factors in order to assess a person's health and to make recommendations for treatment" (Schwartz, 1982, p. 1047). As such, "it stimulates common theories and research designs, facilitates interdisciplinary thinking and research, and encourages greater synthesis among numerous variables" with the result that "it has the potential to establish a more effective, multi-cause, multi-effect approach to health and illness" (Schwartz, 1982, p. 1049).

While the value of the biopsychosocial model has not been tested against traditional models of treatment, at face value, it remains a worthy alternative to other models.

From a clinical perspective, biopsychosocially oriented clinicians may find the proposals of Leigh and Reiser (1980) to be particularly useful. They recommended a system that clinicians can use to organize their diagnoses and management (treatment) plans. The Patient Evaluation Grid (PEG) helps organize the clinician's thinking as he/she moves towards a comprehensive assessment of the patient. Three dimensions are evaluated: biological, personal (psychological) and environmental (social). Within these

TABLE 1. PATIENT EVALUATION GRID (PEG)*

| DIMENSIONS | CONTEXTS: CURRENT (Current States) | RECENT (Recent Events/Changes) | BACKGROUND (Culture, Traits, Constitution) |
|---|---|---|---|
| BIOLOGICAL | physical symptoms, signs<br>physical exam<br>medications<br>abnormal lab values | onset/change in symptoms and signs<br>change in physical conditon<br>change in medications<br>recreational drugs | past history of disease<br>family history of medical disease<br>family history of psychiatric illness |
| PERSONAL | chief complaint<br>chief psychiatric complaint<br>mental status<br>expected treatment | change in psychiatric condition<br>change in mood/behaviour<br>change in habits<br>recent help-seeking | personality traits<br>defence/coping mechanism<br>past psychiatric history |
| ENVIRONMENTAL | who lives with patient<br>occupation<br>stress<br>physical environment | change in living condition<br>change in occupation<br>LCU (Holmes & Rahe)<br>change in physical environment | parents occupation and socioeconomic class<br>schools attended<br>early relationships<br>marriage/jobs |

*Reprinted (with permisson) from Leigh, H., and Reiser, M. F. (1985). The patient: Biological, psychological and social dimensions of medical practice. New York: Plenum Press.

dimensions, three contexts (current states, recent events and changes, and background factors) are assessed. Table 1 illustrates the form used to evaluate the variables associated with these dimension and context factors. Systems like the PEG of Weed's (1968) Problem Oriented Model allow different professionals to broaden their roles by changing the tasks expected of them by the treatment team. This process is illustrated by Cott's (this volume) discussion of the practical implications of "demedicalization" - separating medical from non-medical factors. (1) Each member of the multidisciplinary team contributes to the information base thereby advancing knowledge about the patient. Regardless of the team members' specialized professional training anyone may contribute to any of the three dimensions in the information base as no one profession owns any one particular aspect of this knowledge. "The specific roles that particular persons play ... depends upon an interaction of (a) the bodies of knowledge they actually know, (b) the bodies of knowledge necessary to conceptualize and solve the problems comprehensively, and (c) legal and ethical prinicples that theoretically should reflect (a) and (b)" (Schwartz, 1982, p. 1050). Of course, any conceptual systems may be misused. Schwartz (1982) observed that with a system like the PEG it is possible to error either by thinking comprehensively and thus, missing key details but ignoring the big picture. A balance betweeen these errors in judgement is one key to quality care. The most important point is that knowledge of the patient within a broad conceptual framework as assessed from many points of view is expected of all team members. The biopsychosocial perspective is best captured when all team members have a responsibility for understanding the many factors contributing to illness behaviour. This procedure differs from the usual multidisciplinary approach in which different professionals add their piece of the clinical puzzle but look to one member to put it together. The emphasis shifts from seeking information (e.g., the social worker provides the family history) to conceptualizing how the various biological, psychological and social variables maintain the patient's illness. The clinical assessment of contributory factors may be best assigned in a context where team members are responsible to the group for this work (see Cott, this volume, for a discussion of clinical case management and accountability)

## Impact of Personality Upon Team Functioning

The desire for comprehensive health care continues to be a priority of Western societies. The development of health teams emerged as one means of facilitating comprehensive care. As Szasz (1969) has pointed out, the team concept is made possible by the acceptance of two principles. First, the basic equipment of the health professionals is not simply their specialized skills or knowledge but also their own personalities. Second, the interrelation of physical, emotional and social components of illness necessitate a planned approach to the illness resolution. Since a planned approach requires careful assessment prior to treatment this issue may become an area of potentioal conflict within the team. In this section, consideration will be given to the first principle; the importance of monitoring the personality styles of team members.

Balint in his monograph, The Doctor, His Patient, and the Illness (1957) pointed to the importance of the care-giver's own personality functioning in the understanding of patients' illnesses. One of Balint's significant observations was that the physicians' reports of difficult patients

---

(1) The term "demedicalization" may be perceived as an attack on one profession's role, when in fact an emphasis from a biopsychosocial perspective cuts across all professions.

(including those that he/she did not like) probably fell into a pattern that could be detected, in part, via an understanding of the physician's own personality. Balint identified four personality signs in physicians who may have particular difficulty treating patients. These types were the over-anxious, the superior, the obsessional and the seriously neurotic professional. Bacal, Molineux, and Shaw (1979) later extended this work and evaluated two criteria assessing a successful adaptation given these personality attributes. First, the physician engages in work commensurate with his/her felt ability, stops on the basis of appreciating his/her limits and he/she makes appropriate use of consultant help. Secondly, the interference by his own psychopathology in his work is minimal.

This particular categorization of personality is based on a simple view of a complex area. What is interesting is the emphasis on the professional's personal contribution to the treatment process. It is unwise to think of the assessment of a patient as a purely technical or mechanical exercise as many other factors influence a professional's evaluation of the clinical data. For example, the team member biased because of past experience or personal preference may ignore the cultural context of a patient's illness. If each team member has the responsibility of conceptualizing the case then he/she is dependent on unbiased information. Data from tests would have to be interpreted to group members as part of the accountability to the group. That is, rather than speaking in the jargon of the profession, team members would be expected to explain the potential impact of an abnormal finding, a process that in turn should improve the knowledge of each team member. The input from team members through their questions may aid their colleagues by challenging pre-conceived notions thereby increasing the clinical competence of the group.

Balint's proposals included a training seminar whereby family physicians could discuss their difficult patients with a group of colleagues. Recently other investigators (e.g., Steinberg and Shaw, 1986) have used this training approach with other members of the treatment team. The goal of Balint training is for group members to gain a better understanding of their personaltiy styles and thus, be able to examine potential biases in this information in their interpretation of patients' illness behaviours. For example, the obsessional health professional may undervalue the affective or social contributions to a patient's complaints. He/she may react in a logical, mechanistic fashion and be less aware of the impact of his/her inattention to the context of the patient's concerns. An overly anxious clinician may order tests and procedures without using this information to advance the understanding of the patient's illness. Through discussion the identification of these types of biases may help correct omissions or over-inclusiveness in the assessment information.

Within multidisciplinary teams, the proposal to have each team member be responsible for standard observations of illness behaviour and to be accountable for a biopsychosocial conceptualization of the patient's illness will require an open communication. A significant part of this communication will depend on feedback to each other about biases in the interpretation of clinical data. One excellent recommendation that will serve as a starting point for the identification of these biases is simultaneous assessment (Cott, 1986). Complex and difficult cases may be assessed by different professional at the same time so that the biases that emerge are not confounded by a different data base. This procedure is costly and pragmatically difficult, yet could serve as the basis for a new model of clinical management.

Attitudes and Expectations of Health Professionals

Attitudes refer to positions that people take with regard to certain facts. Traditionally, attitudes have been closely associated with one's feelings and a state of readiness to respond to a characteristic way to situations (Brown, 1965); for example: If I'm going to be legally responsible then I must have absolute authority; If they are going to make the most money, they should have the most responsibility. If I don't have control, then I may be faulted by others.

Clearly the task of changing roles within multidisciplinary treatment teams is a complex endeavour. Many factors contribute to the attitudes and expectations that health professionals have about their roles on treatment teams. One of these significant elements is the tendency of the professions to resolve identity or role conflicts by "reaffirming allegiance to the orthodox tenets of their parent disciplines and by staking claim to areas [of superiority] (Berg, 1986, p.54). Examples of the thinking of individuals taking such a stance include: "My assessments are the most (or least) important"; "Their job is to provide me with information so that I can function more effectively"; "I'm not responsible for medical decisions." While it may be unusual for professionals to disclose this type of thinking it is certainly a destructive force to the concept of multidisciplinary treatment. Consider the following attitudes: "Only physicians have the training necessary to garner a comprehensive understanding of the patient's illness" or "Only psychologists have the training to interpret research data." The point here is not simply to refute the validity of these statements but rather, to illustrate how rigid attitudes such as these alienate others and destroy the potential for communication about illness behaviour. Furthermore, these attitudes lead to resentment and withdrawal of team members, that in turn reduces the quality of patient care.

There is probably no greater stimulus for rigid professional attitudes than the patient who is not compliant with treatment recommended by the team. Clinicians, when faced with such a patient often try to control their interactions with the patient by lecturing or conversely, by withdrawing their attention. The care-givers' perception of the patient's lack of caring may be an important contributor to a sense of frustration on both sides. The multidisciplinary team when faced with this difficult situation may begin to diverge in their views of management with the result of mixed and confusing messages and advice. In this case it is critical for team members to acknowledge the potential emergence of biased attitudes and the blaming of others. Some team members may attempt to control or manipulate the patient. Taking too much control, however, may unwittingly foster a sense of helplessness and dependency in the patient.

This type of difficult case management is an excellent one for the simultaneous interview and discussion of an intervention strategy directed toward the patient's illness behaviour. The role of team members changes from one associated with the profession to the observer/educator role that was presented earlier. One strategy to decrease the patient's non-compliance is to discuss his/her <u>negative dysfunctional predictions</u> and to provide information as to what events can be anticipated, thereby giving the patient as much control of the situation as is reasonable. Information and advice may also be given on how to cope in the face of uncontrollable events (e.g., chronic pain). In this situation, each team member is put into a role that is more consistent with an educator. It demands a skilled and <u>consistent</u> communication between the health professionals and the patient, the kind of intervention that has been emphasized in many of the chapters in this volume.

When confronted with patients whose illness behaviours generate a sense of helplessness in the team, there is a strong tendency for the members to become pre-occupied with their specialized skills and knowledge. If they can discuss their feelings and co-operate to develop a shared conceptualization of the factors maintaining the illness behaviour, then they are more likely to educate the patient about his/her diffricutlies. As indicated previously, providing information to the patient about his/her condition in an emotionally sensitive way, as well as changing the contingencies leading to the patient's behaviour, may reduce both his/her sense of helplessness and/or non-compliance. In this way, the educator/counsellor role is one that is common to all team members who interact with the patient.

Shaw and Harris (1985) presented a case that illustrates some of these points. The patient was a 39-year-old man with "chronic renal failure" undergoing renal dialysis and awaiting renal transplantation. Unfortunately, because the patient did not adhere to the fluid restrictions of his diet, his dialysis treatment was problematic. His non-compliance resulted in up to a 7 kg increase in weight between three-times weekly and on two dialysis treatments his life was threatened. This behaviour resulted in extreme tension within the team with the result that the patient was openly criticized by some and cajoled by others. Individual members tended to retreat into a pattern of interaction where they would meet their "clinical responsibilites" without examining their reactions. Furthermore, a pattern of blame began to develop in an attempt to identify the team members who were responsible for the patient's condition. These difficulties lead to a sense of frustration amongst staff as well as within the patient.

When the staff were able to discuss their reactions to the patient a behavioural program emerged that returned the responsibility for treatment and change to the patient, but not in a blaming way. The extent of the patient's depression was assessed and his associated sense of helplessness was identified and gradually understood. The resolution of the staff's distress lead to a positive program of change rather than individual attempts to control his behaviour or a withdrawal from the obvious difficulties. All staff retained their responsibility to identify factors that maintained his helplessness and depression while providing information to him about his condition.

Returning now to the risk of team members becoming involved with role conflicts and the emergence of dysfunctional expectations and attitudes. These cognitive variables may impart a decidely negative set or influence into the treatment team characterized by an insistence on a return to traditional roles. Under high stress, territorial concerns and attitudinal rigidity set up barriers to effective communication. These difficulties may have been initially acquired during the person's basic professional training. Social, psychological, economic and other factors also influence the co-operative spirit necessary for comprehensive health care (Szasz, 1969).

Szasz (1969, p.451; also see Levy, 1966) discussed many of the barriers between the professions that "contribute to misunderstanding and distrust or maintain ignorance of each others' accomplishments and potentialities." These barriers include a lack of definition of areas of responsibility as a function of rapid technological developments, the public's attitudes toward various professions, and the emphasis on competition and non-cooperative behaviour within educational settings.

## Strategies to Change Behaviours

In this section strategies to change role behaviours within multi-disciplinary teams will be presented. The goal is to build reasonable expectations and functional attitudes in the mutlidisciplinary team toward an improved management of illness behaviour. The primary strategy for change requires several steps: 1) develop a common conceptual base from which to understand the patient's illness; 2) acquire necessary training to interpret clinical data; 3) identify common and separate areas of professional competence; 4) engage in research to test the effects of these ideas in the management of illness.

A limited but significant change in roles will require physicians, nurses, social workers, occupational therapists, psychologists, dietitians, and others to develop a common conceptual base. A base of mutual respect based on a developing competence within a biopsychosocial model will complement specialized skills and foster productive relationships amongst health professionals.

Eisenberg (this volume) emphasized the importance of training physicians in the evaluation of clinical data. This statement is easily applied to all health professionals including those whose clinical tradition has not emphasized assessment (i.e., interventions of care are provided generally with no specific functional goals). In order to evaluate these clinical data randomized treatment trials are required. Eisenberg discussed the construct of professional competence that cuts across stereotyped roles. The acquisition of clinically relevant data through the measurement, evaluation, and treatment of illness behaviour is an important direction in this regard. Research testing the biopsychosocial model is essential (Schwartz, 1982).

## The Process of Change

Policy analysts often examine problems from two perspectives, the "top down" and the "bottom up". Change may be precipitated from the top through the efforts of hospital administrators or leaders of professional associations. Much of the attention of these people was once dominated by their concern for the attitudes and behaviour of physicians. More recently, the concern for quality assurance procedures has opened doors to broaden roles and to emphasize the attainment of competence criteria in these roles. Specific reference to mulitdisciplinary co-operation and communication in quality assurance programs will help to facilitate change.

The "bottom up" perspective looks to foster change by providing information and pressure from the public. Through knowledge and communications a concerned public may force health professionals to alter their behaviour. The public consults these individuals with pre-existing expectations of treatment. If these expectations are limited to drugs or surgery then little change in the health care systems can be expected. Increasingly, however, the public is becoming more knowledgeable about health care. They are beginning to expect to receive information that helps them participate in their own treatment. For example, when treating depressed patients, we often refer to the therapeutic alliance of collaborative involvement of the patient in such a way that the patient and therapist are working to treat "the depression" (Beck, Rush, Shaw, and Emery, 1979).

Hopefully, the public will continue to look for ways to influence their own treatment. One important aspect of their concern involves the area of consent to treatment. In a free society the patient has the right to make the wrong decision with respect to his/her treatment. Patients also have a right to know what alternatives they face. By involving the patient in treatment decisions via a fully informed consent, health professionals take steps to minimize their patients' sense of helplessness and maximize their individual responsibility. Health professionals interested in broadening the public's involvement can become more active by letting them know about the findings of research or by other efforts in public education.

## Education

Other than two brief points the interested reader will do well to consult the chapter by Lock (this volume) for an indepth consideration of the education of health professionals. Efforts can be made in the selection of students to capitalize on those personalities and skills most closely aligned with comprehensive health approaches. Margaret Mead (1935) used the example of selecting soldiers on the basis of the trait of aggressiveness, rather than by gender. Other training programs that select students on the basis of a broader evaluation than grades or test scores may assist the development of co-operative participants in a mulitdisciplinary team.

In the area of medical education one would certainly want to consider educational programs designed to foster inter-professionalism. These programs provide a common base of academic study and frequent opportunities for social interactions amongst the students. Such an experiment was conducted in the late 1960's at the University of British Columbia (see Szasz, 1969, 1974). If such programs are to be undertaken it is essential to include an evaluative component to the work. If they prove to be effective, further educational initiatives may be worth considering within continuing education programs although the vehicle for this work is difficult to conceive.

## Government Initiative

It is difficult for governments to legislate changes in roles per se but their policies do have a significant influence on the probability that change will occur. One major stumbling block of interdisciplinary co-operation involves the economics of the health professions. A government that was interested in illness behaviour would want to provide access to practitioners who are skilled in assessing and treating illness and behaviour. Yet, access to certain health professionals may be limited by health insurance plans. For example, in the province or state where patients may be reimbursed by their health insurance plan only when they consult physicians or chiropractors, but not other health professionals such as psychologists or social workers.

On another front there is a proposal under consideration of the Canadian Federal Government to pay for "prevention initiatives" by physicians. This scheme involves a fee to physicians for taking 15 minutes to advise patients about lifestyle issues. Apparently this type of initiative is one of only a few considered by the Department of Health and Welfare to encourage physicians to promote health rather than illness. This money while intended for a worthy cause would probably be better spent on research and public education programs.

## Research

The value of clinical research in the service of improving health care is significant. It has been estimated by Mechanic (this volume) and by Cummings (1985), that somewhere between 33 percent and 75 percent of patient visits to their family doctor involve emotional rather than physical reasons. Given these estimates, efforts to understand the patient from an illness behaviour viewpoint requires little other defence. Researchers, as evidenced by the work in this volume continue to demonstrate relationships between illness and psychosocial factors. Researchers have a major responsibility to evaluate the value of a biopsychosocial model for the treatment of illness (Schwartz, 1982). The knowledge from this evaluation may in time have a powerful effect on the normative behaviour contained within the roles adopted by health professionals.

## SUMMARY

The whole of a patient's health care should amount to more than the sum of separate professionals. If the care of a difficult patient is segmented in such a way that the physician handles the biological findings, the psychologist gives a perspective on the person, the social worker speaks of the family, the occupational therpatist discusses functioning at work and the nurse presents ward behaviour, then one does not have comprehensive health care. Instead, the essence of bringing various professionals together to address the patient's distress is lost. To achieve this goal, health-care practitioners need to: establish a broad information base within a multi-disciplinary framework, provide training to improve competence evaluating these clinical data, explore knowledge from clinical trials to guide their treatment decisions, and above all, develop realistic attitudes about each other.

## REFERENCES


Bacal, H. A., Monineux, J. E., & Shaw, B. F. (1979). The assessment of training in Balint groups. In P. Hopkins (Ed.), The human face of medicine. London: Pitman Medical.

Balint, M. (1957). The doctor, his patient, and the illness. London: Pitman Medical.

Beck, A. T., Rush, A. J., Shaw, B. F., & Emery, G. (1979). Cognitive therapy of depression. New York: Guilford Press.

Berg, M. (1986). Toward a diagnostic alliance beteen psychiatrist and psychologist. American Psychologist. 41,52-59.

Brown, R. (1965). Social psychology. New York: Free Press.

Cummings, N. A. (1986). The dismantling of our health system. American Psychologist. 41, 426-431.

Eastman, C. (1976). Behavioral formulations of depression. Psychological Review, 83, 277-291.

Engel, G. L. (1977). The need for a new medical model: A challenge for biomedicine. Science, 196, 129-136.

Leigh, H., & Reis, M. F. (1980). The patient: Biological, psychological and social dimensions of medical practice. New York: Plenum Press.

Levy, L. (1966). Factors which facilitate or impede transfer of medical functions from physicians to paramedical personnel. Journal of Health and Human Behavior, 7, 50-54.

Matarazzo, J. D. (1982). Behavioral health's challenge to academic, scientific, and professional psychology. American Psychologist, 37, 1-14.

Mead, M. (1935). Sex and temperment. New York: Morrow.

Nadel, S. F. (1957). The theory of social structure. New York: Free Press.

Schwartz, G. E. (1982). Testing the biopsychosocial model: The ultimate challenge facing behavioral medicine? Journal of Consulting and Clinical Psychology, 50, 1040-1053.

Schwartz, G. E., & Weiss, S. (1978). Behavioral medicine revisited: An amended definition. Journal of Behavioral Medicine, 1, 249-251.

Shaw, B. F., & Harris, G. (1985). Affective disorders. In M. Hersen (Ed.), Inpatient behavior therapy. New York: Grune and Stratten.

Steinberg, P., & Shaw, B. F. (1986). A controlled trial of Balint training for psychiatric nurses. Manuscript submitted for publication.

Szasz, G. (1975). An experience with interprofessional education. In J.

Hamburg (Ed.), Review of allied health education. University of Kentucky Press.
Szasz, G. (1969). Interprofessional education in the health sciences. The Millbank Memorial Fund Quarterly, 68, 449-475.
Szasz, G. (1975). An experience with interprofessional education. In J. Hamburg (Ed.), Review of allied health education. University of Kentucky Press.
Weed, L. L. (1968). Medical records that guide and teach. New England Journal of Medicine, 278, 593-600.

# THE DISEASE-ILLNESS DISTINCTION: A MODEL FOR EFFECTIVE AND PRACTICAL INTEGRATION OF BEHAVIOURAL AND MEDICAL SCIENCES

Arthur Cott

Department of Medicine
McMaster University

## Introduction

In spite of significant potential, the actual impact of the behavioural sciences on medicine, the delivery of health care, and the issues of health and illness in general, has for the most part been negligible (Agras, 1982)! The purpose of this chapter is to examine some of the reasons for this failure and to present a detailed description of a model which, by providing a method for integrating behavioural and medical sciences, can help contribute to the solution.

It has been some time since Mechanic first discussed the concept of illness behaviour (Mechanic, 1962). In so doing, he illustrated the relevance of the behavioural sciences to the understanding of, and solution to, this significant area of human difficulty. Remarkably, this seems to have had little or no practical effect on the problem, despite the large volume of ensuing research on illness behaviour (Mechanic, 1978; Turk, Meichenbaum, and Genest, 1983) and the extensive body of knowledge in the various behavioural sciences of anthropology, sociology and psychology. There has been a notable lack of application of the models, principles and knowledge available from the behavioural sciences. In the related and highly applied area of Behavioural Medicine, in which the concept of illness has obvious relevance, there was not a single reference to Mechanic's work in a recent volume of 19 review articles in the area (see Garfield, 1982). The primary focus of such behavioural and integrative approaches continues to be on the factors which can control and influence disease rather than illness (Schwartz, 1982). This is consistent with the current conceptual trends in medical thinking which continue to be "anatomicopathological" in nature (Baron, 1985). In addition, there appears to be an even greater tendency to "medicalize" a broader range of human problems; that is, to formulate problems within the medical model, label them as "health" problems and look to medicine inappropriately for solutions (Barondess, 1979; Zola, this volume). Medical practitioners tend to become burdened with the non-medical as well as the medical components of problems and are often held accountable when unable to provide solutions (Lipkin, 1981).

With respect to practical application, the potential benefit of current knowledge in the behavioural sciences remains unrecognized and untapped.

Most practicing physicians, for example, barely recognize the name Pavlov and the phrase Classical Conditioning, let alone understand its significance in the development and treatment of observed involuntary physiological signs and symptoms (including such things as muscle spasm, gastrointestinal responses, and various cardiac responses), which cannot be accounted for on the basis of definable organic dysfunction or disease process).

Some of the reasons for the negligible impact of the behavioural sciences in the areas of health and illness are relatively simple and include:

(1) Many of the behavioural sciences models, particularly in areas such as anthropology and sociology, are more descriptive than truly experimental. These models tend not to translate readily into the operational terms required for practical application in health care delivery and research. It is this essential element of translating theory into practice which is critical for any substantial impact to occur. Practitioners need to be provided with a practical process for applying the knowledge and concepts and use in their day to day practices. Without such a process, there can be little progress.

(2) There is a notable absence of consistent and precise definitions of "illness", "health" and of what constitutes a "medical" problem in general. As will be discussed in this paper, this is a major cause of unnecessary health-related problems and illness behaviour. This lack of precision and ambiguity tends to mislead and cause confusion among those who look to the medical and other health-related professions for "expert" opinions, advice, and direction. The assumption is that such precision and factual knowledge exists and underlies the opinions and professed areas of expertise and jurisdictions of these professions. Health professionals often fail to understand and appreciate the effects they and their actions have not only on individuals' behaviours, but also on all aspects of their life and livelihood - access to employment, income, eligibility for assistance and benefits, and legal status (Cott and Goldberg, 1985).

(3) There appears to exist no adequate model or framework for integrating medical, behavioural, and other relevant health-related disciplines (Fabrega and Van Egeren, 1976; McWhinney, 1972). There have been some attempts to formulate relationships between services, roles of various disciplines in delivering components of the service, and team process (e.g., the notion of the "transdisciplinary" team) (Bailey, 1984; Fordyce, 1981, 1982; Melvin, 1980), but none translates readily into operational terms sufficient to be of general, practical value. The methodologies underlying the integration and co-ordination of interdisciplinary activities are often informal, poorly defined (if at all), and not well articulated. The related problems of evaluating, comparing, and replicating such efforts are obvious.

Academically, the lack of a formal model for integrating the medical and behavioural sciences has had equally negative effects, particularly with regard to research, training, and the development of new directions in health-care concepts and delivery systems. Currently, non-medical disciplines tend either to become incorporated within and subordinated under a relevant area of medicine, or to operate in total isolation and independently from medicine. For example, the perspectives imposed by various medical and non-medical disciplines such as Psychiatry or Physical Medicine, and Educational Psychology or Physical Education will have a significant effect on the manner in which something like operant learning principles would be conceptualized and applied to such topics as rehabilitation or prevention. Neither alternative is adequate or even desirable. It is obvious that any meaningful health-related efforts cannot occur in isolation from medicine.

While the importance and relevance of medicine cannot be ignored, it is equally inappropriate that the non-medical disciplines be incorporated within and subordinated under a particular area of medicine. As will be discussed, most behavioural sciences cannot easily be incorporated within the medical model because the underlying fundamental principles of the two approaches are, to a large degree, incompatible.

What is required is a model which permits: (a) the practical application of knowledge and principles from all of the behavioural sciences; (b) clear definitions of health and illness; (c) a methodology for the practical delineation of medical from non-medical issues; and, (d) an applicable formula for the effective integration of the medical and behavioural sciences.

The concepts of disease-illness distinction advanced by Eisenberg and Kleinman, 1977; Wooley, Blackwell and Winget, 1978; Barondess, 1979; Fedoravicius, 1981; Lipkin, 1981; Helman, 1985; can be imposed upon the contemporary interactive models used in experimental behavioural psychology (Estes, 1978; Hearst, 1979; Keefe and Blumenthal, 1982). The experimental focus of these models necessitates the reduction of constructs into operational terms and, consequently, is ideal for bridging the gap between theory and practice in the area of illness behaviour. Thus considered as a disease-illness distinction model, the concepts and principles of the various behavioural sciences may be translated into specific operational terms.

The disease-illness distinction model provides: (a) a conceptual framework and precise operational definition which permit the effective integration of behavioural and medical sciences, and thus the practical application of the knowledge and principles from all of the behavioural sciences; (b) a formula and formal set of procedures for interdisciplinary intervention and clinical management of complex cases; (c) a "demedicalization" process for separating the medical from the non-medical issues of a problem, and delineating the components for which clinical intervention (treatment) is indicated from those for which non-clinical (educative) intervention is more appropriate; (d) a resulting empirical methodology for defining disability; and, (e) a framework for effective communication between the professionals from various disciplines, as well as between health care professionals and patients, clients, families, insurers, employers, and other individuals and institutions for whom a person's health and illness status is relevant.

The model allows for the optimal use of medical and behavioural sciences by permitting each to be applied to the problems for which they are most effective through the workable separation of medical from non-medical components of a problem.

## EXPERIMENTAL MODELS

A significant source of difficulty in dealing with all health-related issues for which the concept of illness behaviour is relevant, is the general imprecision of terminology and absence of consistent operational definitions (e.g., such terms as "health", "illness" and "illness behaviour", "disease", and even "medicine" and, consequently, what constitutes a "medical" problem. It would appear that this area is one in which long standing dogma have dramatically influenced contemporary conceptualizations (Szasz, 1961). This seems to be particularly true with the concepts of disease, illness and the practice of medicine. In fact, there appears to be a tendency in both the medical and behavioural sciences to approach the concept of illness as though it were a phenomenon which actually exists in nature and that defining it properly is merely an exercise in discovering the most accurate description of the "true" entity - a search for the "correct" definition. Since "illness" and "illness behaviour" and, for that matter, disease are all merely hypothetical contructs the initial focus should solely be whether and to what degree these concepts are useful. The next step is to develop the measurement instruments necessary to provide adequate operational definitions of the concepts.

In general, many of the theories and models of the behavioural sciences tend not to be truly experimental. The nature of the subject matter is not readily amenable to experimental manipulations. Consequently, the general approach tends to be more descriptive and correlational in nature. The operational measures and definitions of the constructs tend to reflect this. Since intervention is not emphasized, the related body of knowledge and operational expertise are not well developed. With more experimentally oriented disciplines such as experimental psychology, there is a major emphasis on experimental manipulation; that is, attempting to produce effects through interventions. A large body of knowledge and refinement of operational issues related to intervention have been developed and it is for this reason that these models are particularly relevant and useful in the area of illness behaviour.

The so-called "medical model", as others have pointed out (Ullmann and Krasner, 1965), is currently the most dominant and accepted formulation used for dealing with any response considered to be abnormal. Before proceeding, it is important to appreciate some of these fundamental principles upon which the practice of modern medicine is based. Some of these are incompatible with the basic formulations from which most behavioural principles and related techniques are derived.

<u>Medicine versus Behaviourism - ("disorder" versus "different")</u>

In medicine, "normal" is considered to reflect a state of "order" while variability and deviance are conceptualized as states of "disorder" (as "sick" vs. "healthy" and, therefore, "right" vs. "wrong", "correct" vs. "incorrect", "functional" vs. "dysfunctional"). In the behavioural sciences, on the other hand, variability and deviance generally tend to be viewed as being on a continuum and as being merely "different". While this may be well understood and frequently stated, it is nevertheless a principle problem in preventing the integration of medical and behavioural principles and techniques. In medicine, the general formulations and focus of treatment tend to be that of "correction" and "repair". The tradition of medicine is that of a reactive, corrective practice, an attempt to restore order. Behavioural formulations and focus, on the other hand, are "alteration", "modification", and "change" rather than correction and repair.

Typically, it is only specific behavioural procedures or techniques which are incorporated into medicine in a corrective manner as a hodge podge of techniques and operations, divorced from the concepts from which they arise. Consequently, they are frequently employed inappropriately and in contexts which make no conceptual sense (Fordyce, Roberts, and Sternbach, 1985).

The following disease-illness distinction model allows for the compatible integration of these opposing conceptual frameworks by providing a clear and meaningful operational separation of "medically related" and "non-medically related" problems, defined operationally on the basis of effectiveness.

## Disease versus Illness

The key distinction of the model is that between "DISEASE PROCESS" and "ILLNESS STATE". DISEASE is a physical or organic CAUSE or DETERMINANT. ILLNESS is the EFFECT or RESPONSE. DISEASE is defined as an observable or inferred physical condition resulting from any sort of lesion, insult, infection, or other homeostatic dysfunction. ILLNESS, on the other hand, is defined as the whole array of subjective states and other overt responses and behaviours which are presented by individuals as in some way being disabling or disruptive to their normal lives and which they attribute to a disease determinant.

The general approach of experimental psychology and of experimental behavioural sciences is to treat behaviour as the dependent variable - the response (R) variable. Internal and external stimulus (S) variables, organismic (O) variables, and other behavioural response variables (R) are treated as independent variables in an effort to describe lawful relationships among these variables (i.e., R=f(S); R=f(O); R=f(R)). The organism is treated as the proverbial "black box"; that is, as the "normal" entity for which the described set of laws hold. It defines the predictable functional relationship between behaviour and stimuli, organismic characteristics, and other behaviours.

The contemporary interactive models evolved from early dualistic "isolated determinants" and "independent additive determinants" of behaviour models. In the early dualistic approaches, an individual's responses were viewed as being members of different classes of behaviour with independent isolated determinants: either psychologically determined - as functions of the mind and spirit; or physically determined - as functions of the body and physiology.

Fundamentally, medicine is dualistic in concept (Ullmann and Krasner, 1965). Consequently, the notions of independent determinants of illness tend to persist in the present day practice of medicine and continue to invade present day thought. This is the "either/or" model. Illness is viewed as being caused either by disease, or ... something else - generally something caused or created by the "mind". A symptom is "either" caused by a "real" disease "or" is the direct result of some other cause; hysteria for example (figure 1).

With the concept of "independent additive determinants", a given response is viewed as being influenced by more than one determinant and that the effects of various determinants are additive; that is, that a given response is the sum of the effects of various determinants (figure 1). The additive determinants notion also appears to have had a significant influence on current practice and thought in medicine and the approach to illness behaviour in general. This would appear to be the fundamental principle underlying the notion of "functional overlay" in medicine. In this case, the response, ILLNESS, is the sum of the effects of various determinants - disease plus the "other" non-disease factors. Rather than "... which one", the question now becomes "... how much" of illness is caused by "real" disease and how much by "other" factors.

Both the isolated (which one?) and additive (how much?) determinants of human behaviour concepts have essentially been discarded because they have not proven useful from an experimental point of view in providing meaningful formulations to account for observed events (Anastasi, 1976).

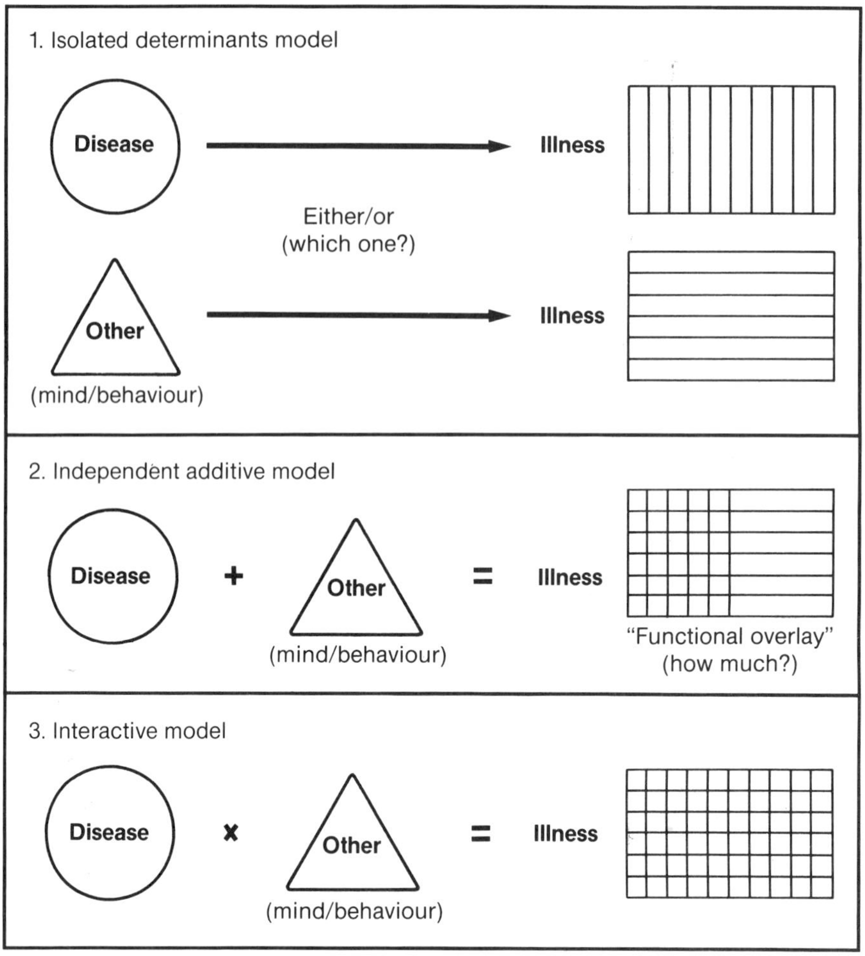


**FIGURE 1.** Contemporary models of disease/illness relationships

DISEASE-ILLNESS DISTINCTION MODEL

With the contemporary interactive models used in experimental behavioural sciences (Estes, 1978; Hearst, 1979; Keefe and Blumenthal, 1982), the dependent variable is the response variable (R) - the behaviour of the organism from which the various constructs of illness, wellness, etc., are inferred. The response variable includes any and all responses of the organism. The overt, directly observable behaviour includes autonomic and skeletal, as well as involuntary and voluntary responses (respondents and operants). The indirectly inferred responses include the entire range of subjective states - simple and complex sensory perceptions (eg., vision, pain), motivational and emotional states (eg., hunger, fear), and complex cognitive responses (beliefs and thoughts).

The potential independent variables are the internal and external stimulus (S) variable (including such things as blood chemistry, drug states, etc.); organismic (O) variable (including variables such as age, physical, structural, and chemical characteristics of the individual); and response (R)

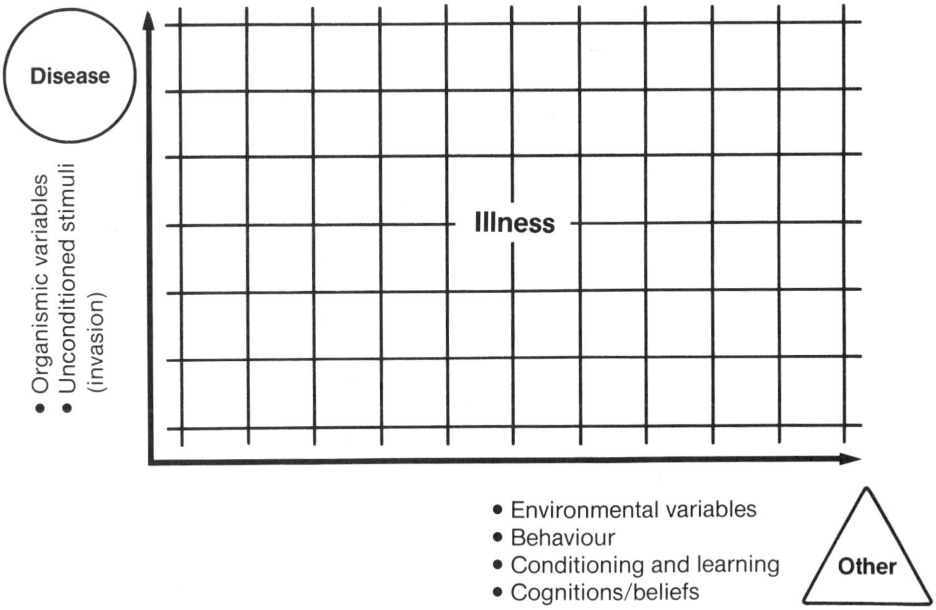


**FIGURE 2.** The disease-illness distinction model (interactive model)

variables involving all forms of other behaviour including cognitions and beliefs.

All behaviour of the organism, from the simplest involuntary autonomic reflexive responses to the highest order complex cognitive activities of human responding is viewed as being determined by a complex interaction of these stimuli, organismic, and response variables. There exists a substantial body of knowledge which describes such lawful relationships with regard to various developmental, behavioural and psychological processes of the organism. Such knowledge involves each of the different classes of responses within the many relevant areas of experimental psychology, such as learning and conditioning, physiological, developmental, memory, motivation, sensation and perception, and cognitive (Baddeley, 1976; Estes, 1978; Hearst, 1979; Mussen, 1979; Anderson, 1981; Bower, 1981; [figures 1 and 2]. Arising from each are the operational procedures, techniques, and relevant intervention strategies and formulations which can be used clinically. This basic interactive model (see Figure 2) is an excellent vehicle for integrating medical and behavioural concepts, principles, and techniques as well as operationally defining disease and illness.

## Disease

From a behavioural sciences standpoint, disease is either an organismic variable (some physical dysfunction of the organism) [R=f(O)], or it is a stimulus variable, a physical invader of the organism (such as a virus or bacterium) which results in a reflexive set of responses of the organism [R=f(S)].

Disease as an organismic variable. In order to incorporate meaningfully the concept of disease into the model as an organismic variable it is important to distinguish between disease as a discrete versus continuous variable. For the most part, the dichotomous nature of the concept of disease (ordered vs. disordered) makes it necessary to treat disease as a discrete variable. Since a set of stimulus-response laws is understood to exist only for a given intact organism, it follows that if that organism (the black box) is altered, the laws for the "normal" intact organism no longer apply but that another set do. It is for this reason that in the applied process described below, the initial essential step is that of a definitive diagnosis of disease in a manner sufficient to provide the clear operating parameters of irreducible limitations, conditions of optimal therapy (conditions for holding the new order constant), and contraindications necessary for behavioural analysis and intervention. In other words, the absence or presence of specific diseases which are discrete organismic states, each with its own set of operating principles unique to it.

In some cases it is possible to view disease as a continuous variable, as in cases such as rheumatoid arthritis in which it is possible, and perhaps meaningful, to quantify degree of disease. In such cases it may be possible and, therefore, useful to identify relationships between disease and responses such as reported subjective magnitudes of fatigue and pain. This should be carefully distinguished from the continuum of "normal" variations of an intact organism - something which behaviourally is viewed as an internal stimulus variable. Some examples of such internal stimuli include blood chemistry (osmolality, tonicity, volume, glucose levels, etc.), and neurochemistry (neurochemical balances and levels).

Disease as a stimulus variable. The invader aspect of the disease definition from a behavioural sciences standpoint is that of an unconditional stimulus which will result in a relatively well defined set of predictable responses (unconditional responses). The infection is a stimulus which results in an unlearned reflexive response (signs and symptoms).

Operational definition of disease: The utility requirement for defining disease. What distinguishes disease from other organismic and stimulus variables? What are the conditions necessary and sufficient for labelling an organismic or stimulus variable as a disease? For example, is so-called "degenerative disc disease", which is a natural continuous aging process observed in most people, best viewed as a disease process? What distinguishes that particular continuous organismic variable from the greying of hair, the wearing of teeth, and changes in the skin (Hall, 1980)? It seems that there has been a growing tendency to view the aging process, a natural continuous phenomenon, in disease entity terms as though it were a dysfunction.

From a utilitarian perspective, a condition necessary for clinically defining a variable as a "disease" is whether there exists a "cure" for that disease. That is, whether there exists some methodology for preventing, eliminating, reducing, or otherwise controlling that variable and its effects through physiological and corrective interventions (see below). From a research point of view, it is whether the disease formulation leads to methods for furthering knowledge and understanding of the phenomenon. Otherwise, there is limited benefit in labelling such phenomena as disease and, as will be discussed in detail further, there are great risks and costs to doing so.

## Illness

Illness is behaviour. From a behavioural point of view, therefore, illness is the response or effect of which disease is only one possible determinant.

Illness as a response variable. Illness can involve and encompass all classes of responses including: (a) "involuntary", reflexive, physiological responses such as cardiac responses (rate and arrhythmias, blood pressure, palpitations), body temperature (fevers), muscle spasms, gastric and intestinal motility, vasodilation, and sweating. Medically, this class of responses are called "symptoms" and "signs"; (b) "voluntary" or operant responses such as limping, crying, and complaining; and, (c) complex "cognitive" responses involving sensations and perceptions, motivational and emotional states such as fear, anxiety, and pain, and the complex belief and attributional cognitions and related social and cultural phenomena regarding the causes, cures, and meaning of various discriminable responses.

Illness as an interactive effect. Disease is a cause or determinant. Illness is response or effect. Illness is the result of an interaction between disease (the organismic or unconditional stimulus variable) and environmental (both internal and external) variables, other responses (behaviour), conditioning and learning, and the intervening variables of cognitions and beliefs (Fordyce, 1976; Mechanic, 1978; Melzack and Wall, 1982). The degree of illness which exists as a result of underlying disease is affected by factors such as conditioning, learning, beliefs, culture and social norms.

Using the basic interactive model described above, illness, like all other behaviours, is viewed as being determined by an "interaction" between disease (organismic and unconditional stimulus variables) and the other independent variables. It is, therefore, not a matter of asking "how much" illness is caused by disease and how much by other factors, but rather "how" the disease determinants and these other factors interact to produce illness.

For example, a person with a cancerous tumour and no symptoms has significant disease but no illness. The individual does not experience any symptoms or limitations and is unaware that the cancer exists. A paraplegic who is confined to a wheelchair but who leads an active social life, works steadily, never complains of feeling or being "ill", who has little notion of being particularly limited, and does not look to medicine for a solution or assistance, has by definition very little illness but does have profound disease. At the other extreme, there is the individual who has minimal disease with profound illness. A typical example is the individual with a minor "soft tissue injury" who has been off work for a year, has a very limited social life, and who stays home consuming analgesics. Most cases, of course, fall between these two extremes. Learning and conditioning, culture, beliefs and past experience, immediate circumstances and environmental factors in the home and work place, influence everyone. If a person has the "flu" and has to attend a particularly boring and/or difficult meeting at work, he may feel too "ill" to attend. However, if tickets to a significant sports or entertainment event are suddenly made available, the degree of illness may not be sufficient to prevent attendance! In other words, the degree of illness can vary considerably for a given disease determinant.

Operational definition of illness: The disease attribution requirement. Note that the definition of "illness" in this model involves the necessary condition of a cognitive causal attribution component. That is, a necessary condition to be defined as "Illness" is the requirement that the individual "attribute" the problem to a disease and/or look to medicine for a solution. A jogger who develops a muscular injury is unlikely to use the terminology of "illness", "health", and "disease" to describe or conceptualize the perceived problem. Such a person might use self-appraisals such as "out of shape" or "bruised" but not terms such as "unhealthy", "ill" or "disease". The person does not look to medicine for a solution to the problem and, therefore, by definition is not ill. Another individual with the same muscular problem but with different attributions (perhaps because of culture or recent experience with profound disease such as cancer) might tend to use labels such as "ill" and "disease" and immediately look to the medical profession for a solution to the problem. By definition, this individual is "Ill". Note that illness is defined by the subject's attributions, not those of others.

In the data presented in the following sections, various traditional measures of illness behaviour have been employed including subjective magnitude reports of symptoms (e.g., pain), of limitations with regard to specific activities, and use of medical facilities; self-monitoring data of actual activity (work, daily living, active and passive leisure), ingestion of medication, and use of medical facilities; as well as standard psychometric tools. Additional related outcome measures are also reported including actual work status (job change, partial disability placement, absentee rates), disability benefits status, and physician reports.

## Jurisdictions of the Medical and Behavioural Sciences

The Disease-Illness distinction model provides a framework that helps define more clearly the relevant clinical and research roles of medicine and behavioural science. Medicine deals with the disease determinant of illness. The various behavioural sciences deal with the other factors which influence "illness" - the conditioned, learned, and cognitive responses to disease, both voluntary and involuntary.

*The role of medicine.* Clinically, the primary objective of medical science is to identify and then control, reduce, or eliminate "disease". The degree to which medicine can do this is the degree to which it can effect illness state and, consequently, illness behaviour.

Conceptually, and from a practical research point of view, the medical model is best suited for studying organic and physical dysfunction; that is, disease process. The "corrective" and "reactive" focus of the medical model does not lend itself well to a meaningful formulation and understanding of the acquired components of human behaviour (learning, conditioning, cognitions), and consequently, has limited utility in the analysis and conceptualization of these non-disease determinants of illness behaviour.

*The role of behavioural science.* Behavioural science deals with, or at least has the body of knowledge, models, principles and techniques, for potentially dealing with the non-disease determinants of illness. This includes the entire spectrum of the behavioural sciences.

Conditioning and learning are particularly relevant to many common aspects of illness which cannot be accounted for on the basis of identifiable organicity and with which traditional medicine has difficulty (Fordyce, 1976; Fordyce et al, 1985). Pavlovian or Classical Conditioning, for example, is particularly relevant to pain problems which persist long after original injuries have healed, to continued irritable bowel symptoms, to various cardiac responses, and to both skeletal and smooth muscle spasms.

Operant or instrumental conditioning is particularly relevant to the types of "illness behaviour" referred to in sociological and anthropological studies: responses to injuries, the development of compensatory behaviours, and the evolution of invalid-like postures and role changes.

There are other well established conditioning and learning principles which are particularly relevant to medicine and illness behaviour, but are even less familiar and known in medicine and to practitioners in general. State dependent learning is a prime example of this and is particularly relevant when employing both drug and behavioural treatments simultaneously. Learning acquired under one drug state, may not readily transfer to another or non-drug state (Kumar, Stolerman, and Sternberg, 1970).

Cognitive restructuring principles are particularly relevant to altering causal attributions and other beliefs which have profound effects on determining the nature and extent of illness behaviour (Turk et al., 1983). Most physicians fail to appreciate that simple reassurance has little if any effect on altering patients' cognitions and behaviour.

## CONTEMPORARY HEALTH PROBLEMS AND THE DISEASE-ILLNESS DISTINCTION

### Illness is the Problem

In the context of the disease-illness model described above, a major aspect of modern day health problems has less to do with disease than with illness. In other words, the problem is illness rather than disease! The problem is illness which has no disease determinant or is discrepant with that which can be accounted for on the basis of disease alone. The incidence and prevalence of disease(s) have generally been declining, primarily as a result of prevention (hygienics and sanitation, immunization, and nutrition) and advancements in early detection, elimination and control of disease process (Turk et al, 1983). Yet, there appears to be a paradoxical increase in illness behaviour and related disability. Utilization of health care facilities and services continues to increase as does the cost of providing them. Many frequently used medications merely treat illness (e.g., valium, analgesics, etc.) rather than disease.

Results from a number of studies clearly suggest that significant numbers of patients with no evidence of having any disease process remain or become unnecessarily disabled with respect to employment and routine daily activities despite receiving reassurance (Waxler, Kimbiris, and Dreifus, 1971; Bemiller, Pepine, and Rogers, 1973; Kemp, Vokonas, Cohn, and Gorlin, 1973; Haynes, Sackett, Taylor, Gibson, and Johnson, 1978; Lavey and Winkle, 1979; Isner, Salem, Banas, and Levine, 1981). Ockene et al. (1980), for example, reported that approximately 50% of patients having chest pain and normal coronary arteries (as indicated by catheterization) and who were carefully reassured regarding their cardiac status, continued at a 16 month follow-up to report being unable to work and limiting their activities. Similarly, the author's own research has shown that unnecessary levels of disability exist in a significant number of patients who have no organic disease and have received optimal medical treatment (Cott, 1986, in press). For example, a cohort of 134 subjects derived from 2,083 consecutive hospital coronary care admissions were concluded to have chest pain of unknown etiology. Despite cardiac and other medical causes having been carefully excluded, half the sample continued to take cardiac medications and half of these subjects believed the cause of ongoing chest symptoms to be cardiac in origin. Further, there were significantly greater restrictions in work-related activities, and physical, recreational and social activities in those subjects continuing on cardiac medications.

The fact that only one individual in the entire population died with undiagnosed cardiac disease illustrates how effective and accurate medical assessment and screening procedures of cardiac disease are: there is evidence of only one failure to diagnose existing disease in 2,083 cases!

However, many of those without disease became or remained disabled! Excellent medical intervention failed to prevent and may have contributed to illness.

## SOURCES OF INAPPROPRIATE ILLNESS

The aspects of illness behaviour for which the label "inappropriate" is justified include any problems which are causally attributed to disease but for which no disease determinant has been demonstrated to exist. Also inappropriate are problems for which solutions are sought through medicine but for which medicine has no demonstrated solution or effective cure. There are two categories of such problems: those with an identifiable disease determinant and, therefore, a relevant medical component; and those with no disease determinant with inappropriate medical involvement.

### Inappropriate Illness with Medical Components

Disease-illness discrepancies. Major problems arise in medicine when the degree of illness is discrepant with that which can be accounted for on the basis of disease alone (the organismic dysfunction or the unconditional response to an invasion stimulus). The type of discrepancies can involve any of the response categories discussed previously including involuntary responses mediated by the autonomic nervous system (e.g., gastric motility and intestinal responses), reports of pain and pain behaviour, and all of the more complex voluntary behaviours and cognitions related to invalid-like postures in general.

Medicine by itself cannot deal adequately with the acquired (learned) components of illness or any responses which are discrepant with that which can be accounted for on the basis of organicity alone.

Medical involvement confounds the non-medical issues of problems. The involvement of a medical component in any human problem tends to have inadvertent adverse effects on all other aspects of the problem. The non-medical issues tend to become confused with the medical aspects of the problem. As a result, the various non-health related participants often become intimidated by the involvement of medicine and, consequently, relinquish ownership and responsibilities. Aspects of problems which are clearly not medical become "medicalized". People look to physicians for solutions and direction and physicians become inappropriately burdened with issues unrelated to medicine and disease. In other words, when any human behaviour or performance problem involves a medical component, the customary methods for dealing with personal and interpersonal problems are at risk of breaking down.

Inappropriate illness without medical components - the inappropriate "MEDICALIZATION" of problems. Ironically, it is the medical profession which has increasingly been looked to for solutions to many complex and important human problems that are clearly not disease related and, consequently, not particularly relevant to medicine (Zola, this volume). The range of problems which have become "medicalized" - for which solutions are sought in medicine - have broadened. The problems range from those for which the relationship to medicine is obvious and relevant, such as the problems of pain, sleep disorders, fatigue, and weight and eating disorders, to those with no related disease or organic determinants whatsoever, such as the inability to cope and so-called "stress" problems, and even "addictions" to gambling. It is noteworthy that none of the above problems have identifiable disease determinants. Most, however, are generally accepted unequivocally as being

TABLE 1. DISABILTY DATA (1978 - 1984)

Benefits Available

| TREATED SUBJECTS NOT WORKING DUE TO DISABILITY | NONE | | 70% OF PAY | | EQUAL TO PAY | |
|---|---|---|---|---|---|---|
| Outcomes: | | | | | | |
| Return to work | ( 73) | 66% | ( 28) | 36% | ( 3) | 33% |
| Job change/retrain | ( 25) | 23% | ( 8) | 12% | ( 0) | 0% |
| Early retirement | ( 3) | 3% | ( 5) | 6% | ( 1) | 11% |
| Dismissed by employer | ( 4) | 4% | ( 1) | 1% | ( 0) | 0% |
| Continued disability without benefits | ( 5) | 4% | ( 1) | 1% | ( 0) | 0% |
| Continued disability with benefits | ( 0) | 0% | ( 34) | 44% | ( 5) | 56% |
| TOTAL NUMBER: | 110 | 100% | 77 | 100% | 9 | 100% |

Job Income Available

| TREATED SUBJECTS NOT WORKING DUE TO DISABILITY | NONE | | LESS THAN JOB RATE | | EQUAL TO JOB RATE | |
|---|---|---|---|---|---|---|
| Outcomes: | | | | | | |
| Return to work | ( 0) | 0% | ( 14) | 47% | ( 90) | 71% |
| Job change/retrain | ( 22) | 56% | ( 3) | 10% | ( 8) | 6% |
| Early retirement | ( 0) | 0% | ( 1) | 3% | ( 8) | 6% |
| Dismissed by employer | ( 0) | 0% | ( 1) | 3% | ( 4) | 3% |
| Continued disability without benefits | ( 5) | 13% | ( 0) | 0% | ( 1) | 1% |
| Continued disability with benefits | ( 12) | 31% | ( 11) | 37% | ( 16) | 13% |
| TOTAL NUMBER: | 39 | 100% | 30 | 100% | 127 | 100% |

"medical" problems, although there appears to be no evidence that effective solutions to these problems exist in medicine.

On the surface, there would appear to be few risks and enormous potential benefits in attempting to use medical formulations and solutions to these problems. However, major risks for such medical formulations do exist. The danger is that there is strong tendency to confuse disease with illness, cause with effect, and stimulus with response. For example, it is not uncommon for "stress" to be treated as though it were a disease. Patients come to believe that they are stricken with a case of "stress" and that this "disease" is the cause of their inability to cope and function, when in fact it is the effect. Inability to cope - a behavioural skills problem - is the cause. The patient is often given valium (which treats illness and not disease) and is subtly lead to develop illness behaviour and unnecessary invalidism.

The solution - "DEMEDICALIZATION" - delineating the medical from non-medical issues. The obvious solution to the problems of inappropriate illness is a methodology which provides a clear definition and, consequently, effective separation of medical and non-medical issues. With the problems of disease-illness discrepancies and the confounding of medical and non-medical issues when there is a major medical component, a clinical methodology of "demedicalization" is required. The delineation of medical from non-medical issues is based on the empirical demonstration that the particular discipline does in fact have an effective solution to that aspect of the problem, rather than on traditional and historical jurisdictions.

Finally, with regard to problems which have no true disease or medically-related component and which have become inappropriately "medicalized", as is commonly the case with eating and weight control problems and coping skills problems, the effective solution to these problems is also "demedicalization". This process focuses on education rather than treatment, de-emphasizing the clinical and medical notions and stressing the educative and skill acquisition concepts. In such cases, a clinical procedure is not required and should not be utilized as with cases involving a valid disease and medical component.

## PRACTICAL APPLICATIONS: CLINICAL AND EDUCATIONAL STRATEGIES

### The Process: A Model for Interdisciplinary Intervention and Complex Case Management

The disease-illness model provides a conceptual framework for a clinical process which permits the systematic integration of interdisciplinary activities and, consequently, the management of complex cases. The principles of the process can also be usefully and meaningfully applied in the management of even the simplest of medical cases. The disease-illness distinction model drives the process and the activities of the various participants. The following are the principle elements of the process. (1)

(a) Simultaneous versus sequential assessment. An essential element of the process is that each of the assessments performed by the various disciplines must occur simultaneously rather than sequentially as is traditionally and commonly the case with interdisciplinary clinical activity. Often, medical problems are approached in hierarchical manner; that is, specific hypotheses and specific areas of concern are addressed and eliminated before other issues are addressed or even considered. Issues of physical organic disease are usually addressed first - assessed, treated and evaluated - before the next step in the assessment/treatment occurs.

In this process, it is very important that representatives from the relevant disciplines all assess the patient at the same time, in the same interview. This permits each specialist to observe the same data as the others and prevents ambiguity with regard to later interpretation of relevant data and possible communication problems. Everyone witnesses the same event, observes the same data collected by others, and when future discussions occur, there is no confusion with regard to whether differences in opinion are based on different data or different interpretations of the same data.

The various disciplines involved in a particular case can vary depending on the nature of the problem. However, there are at least three "managing" disciplines required: medical (ideally a general internist), psychiatric (primarily to help "eliminate" specific possibilities), and behavioural psychology (for behavioural analysis and for the "project" management of the case). Alternative or additional specialities can be involved initially, depending on the nature of the case, including neurology, neuropsychology, orthopedics, physiatry and rheumatology. These, however, are not essential at initial assessment so long as the three managing disciplines are represented.

The initial assessment must be conducted by senior members of the team. This is a "top down" process. Traditionally, initial screenings are conducted by a variety of non-senior personnel before being assessed by the "specialists". While such traditional methods may be less costly in the short run, they are generally much less cost effective in the long run.

This overall procedure, therefore, is heavily "front end loaded". That is, assessment occurs simultaneously by the senior specialists on the team. This ensures accurate communication and permits the optimal development of rationale and design of treatment programs which can be directed by the senior team. There is a greatly reduced risk of "mixed messages" to the patient and other relevant parties, as well as among the multidisciplinary treatment team itself.

The simultaneous interview requires some practice in order to avoid undue discomfort of the patient and inefficient data collection by the principles.

(b) Co-ordinative/integrative intervention. The focus of the management process is the co-ordination and integration of the treatment activities of

---

1. (previous page) The model, procedures and data presented in this paper were developed and collected over a ten-year period at the Behavioural Medicine Unit, St. Joseph's Hospital, Hamilton, Ontario, Canada. During this time, we have had the unique opportunity of developing a true interdisciplinary clinical research unit within a Department of Medicine in a teaching hospital of a university medical school - McMaster University. The effort evolved from an initial research project involving experimental behavioural psychology, psychiatry, and general internal medicine into a major service, research and educational facility. In addition to formal experimental studies, we have collected detailed data including a wide variety of treatment, non-treatment, demographic, and outcome variables on over 500 complex disability cases. An operational model for simultaneous interdisciplinary intervention and the management of complex disability cases based on the disease-illness model was developed and refined. The formal set of procedures for integrating and co-ordinating the interdisciplinary activities of medical and behavioural sciences in the treatment of complex disability cases developed is outlined in detail in this paper.

the various disciplines. This is accomplished by means of two critical elements: (a) a case conference management procedure, and (b) a senior case co-ordinator.

The case conference management procedure provides the vehicle by which the various professional disciplines contribute to the design and implementation of treatment, and are professionally and clinically held accountable. This involves a great deal more than the traditional use of a case conference for the sole purpose of discussion and communication among the various professional participants. In this process the case conference is actually used to "manage" the case and, in particular, the actions of the participants, so that once agreement and a concrete strategy are achieved with a specific set of time-targeted tasks and related responsibilities, each professional is accountable to the group for meeting defined responsibilities. Such accountability is quite foreign to the usual professional independence which is characteristic of the practice of most health professionals. Consequently, some discomfort can initially be expected.

For each case, the conference is chaired by the senior co-ordinator assigned to the case (see below). Each of the three or more initial senior assessors prepares a written independent assessment of the patient based on the initial simultaneous interview and provides these reports to the co-ordinator who presents the case at conference. The standard process described in detail in the following section is followed and a specific plan is developed, to be tracked by the case conference group.

The senior case co-ordinator or "senior case manager" acts as project manager outside of conference to ensure that all prescribed activities occur and are co-ordinated, and that the professionals from each of the participating disciplines are kept informed and held accountable for their areas of responsibility. The senior case co-ordinator is a senior member of the group, usually the behavioural psychologist, who merely manages the other professionals. Clinical judgements and responsibilities continue to rest with each relevant professional participant.

(c) "Demedicalization" process: Separating medical from non-medical components. The clinical "demedicalization" process is the method by which medical factors are separated from the non-medical factors of a clinical problem. The procedures described below provide the framework by which "medical" and "non-medical" issues are defined and delineated in a practical manner for clinical applications. It should be noted that this process necessitates the participation of a physician; that is, it is the physician who must separate the medical from the non-medical factors.

Medical Delineation

(a) Definitive medical diagnosis. An essential early step in the process is that of arriving at a clear and unequivocal diagnosis of organic dysfunction or disease process. Is there a clearly definable disease? The answer to this question should be definitive and unambiguous. In the great majority of cases, the answer to this question is straightforward. There either exists a physical condition known to modern medicine or there does not. Further, in most cases, there is a finite period of time within which a definitive decision regarding diagnosis should be reached.

Problems tend to arise when there are multiple and complex organic dysfunctions and disease process, or when no true identifiable organic cause or disease can be specified. To obtain a clear definitive diagnosis with potentially rare and complex diseases, an opinion with regard to the existence of an identifiable disease process or organic dysfunction should be sought early from a recognized authority in the field.

The term disease should not be employed to describe observed responses (symptoms and signs) which cannot be accounted for on the basis of identifiable organic causes or disease process. Poorly defined "syndromes", such as "fibrositis", which have no consistent physiological correlates and which do not lead to effective treatment or predictable outcomes and prognosis, do not meet the conditions necessary to be defined as a disease as discussed above. Simply, the question is: Does the patient have a disease - yes, or no? If so, what exactly is it?

(b) Optimal medical management. Once a definitive decision has been made with regard to diagnosis of disease, the next step is that of determining and arranging the conditions of optimal medical management. The conditions of optimal medical management define the limits in which the concurrent behavioural analysis and resulting intervention strategies can be applied. Optimal medical management involves not only providing optimal medical therapy for the disease, but also integrating and co-ordinating this with the delivery of all aspects of medical treatment being received by the patient.

Optimal medical therapy means that all procedures known to modern medical science which are appropriate for the (a) elimination or (b) control - reversal, reduction, and/or retardation - of the particular disease have been identified and employed. The specifications of optimal medical therapy should be and generally are straightforward. Either a known, effective intervention(s) for a particular disease exists or it does not!

For the most part, medical interventions for disease are either chemical: replacement, suppression, curatives - for repairing or correcting organismic disorder and homeostatic imbalance, or destroying or controlling a stimulus (invader); or structural: surgery, prosthesis - for repair and replacement.

The problems associated with integrating and co-ordinating the entire sphere of an individual's medical management tend often to be more political than technical in nature, particularly with complex cases involving multi-disciplinary intervention. This principle management role has traditionally been relegated to the family physician. While this is appropriate and desirable for the great majority of cases in which patients have well delineated medical problems and minimal disease-illness discrepancies, for the more complex cases involving many physicians and interdisciplinary health professionals, this has become an increasingly difficult and less appropriate function for family physicians. The management task requires great time and effort as well as specialized skills. Patients often find themselves receiving varied and frequently conflicting advice and directions from the many different people involved in their health care.

In this process, the senior case co-ordinator is given the responsibility to ensure that there is understanding and concurrence with the formulation and treatment plan among all of the patient's health professionals. This often necessitates rapid and frequent communication and negotiations.

It is critical that the conditions of optimal medical therapy be specified clearly and in detail to all relevant participants. This provides clear definitions for such important things as the parameters of behavioural formulations and intervention, and the therapeutic conditions required for reducing risks related to the disease. Unnecessary loss of access to employment and other activities and opportunities can thereby be avoided. Optimal medical therapy with such conditions as psychomotor epilepsy, for example, will reduce any risks associated with the disease to normal limits and thus prevent loss of access to employment by stating the conditions of optimal medical therapy as a "condition of employment".

Specification of irreducible limitations. This is another critical factor which sets the limits of the behavioural analysis. It is obviously important that the response limitations defined by the disease be clearly identified and specified. From a behavioural perspective, there are two concerns. First, it is important to specify those behaviours which are unconditional, unlearned, and reflexive and hence, can be accounted for solely on the basis of the disease. Since such responses are not acquired, it is unlikely that behavioural formulations aimed at eliminating learned responses will be effective. Second, it is equally important to understand the limitations imposed by the organic condition with regard to the nature and types of responses that are reasonable to be considered as potential target activities. This is particularly important in cases with neurological disorders and brain damage. It is obviously important to balance the dangers of setting unrealistic behavioural objectives with failing to test ability to acquire and alter responses through empirical procedures.

"Contraindications": "hurt" versus "harm". One of the most frequent, serious, and major causes of unnecessary invalidism, disability and other illness behaviour is the inadequate transfer of relevant information and understanding about the various issues for which the term "contraindicated" is used in medicine. The misunderstanding and confusion which can arise from the innocent and seemingly simple use of this term by a physician can have profound and long range effects on a patient's life and livelihood.

These potential problems can be avoided through use of a simple distinction between "hurt": (discomfort) and "harm" (threat of physical damage). Physicians often fail to communicate such distinctions when recommending or indicating "contraindicated" activities to patients and other relevant parties such as employers.

The distinction between "hurt" and "harm" is the distinction between the discomfort and pain associated with organic conditions and behaviours which are non-threatening physically (i.e., "hurt"), from that associated with diseases and activities which are physically threatening and can lead to further or more rapid physical deterioration, progression or additional damage (i.e., "harm"). Interpretations of pain and discomfort with regard to these issues will have obvious and significant effects on patients' behaviour. Discomfort with "harm" interpretations may lead to fear and be characterized by avoidance behaviour, while pain and other subjective states associated with "hurt" issues may be more characterized by escape behaviour. Consequently, confusing "hurt" with "harm" can lead to unnecessary invalidism and disability. Physicians often fail to make this distinction for patients who are understandably unable to do so on their own.

Two common contemporary illness behaviour problems which serve as excellent examples to illustrate the relevance of this confusion are (a) low back pain, presumably related to degenerative disc disease, and (b) chest discomfort associated with various cardiac-related diseases. With both these problems, the correlation between disease and illness is low (Nachemson, 1982; Eichner, 1983). In many cases, the disability related to the organic conditions is discrepant and directly related to the confusion between "hurt" and "harm".

Most cardiac-related problems such as mitral valve prolapse and coronary artery disease, rarely result in reports of excruciating intractable pain. It is rarely the pain and discomfort per se which is disabling! It is more likely the voluntary restriction and avoidance of activity resulting from beliefs and fears related to "harm" interpretations of the discomfort. The fear is associated with the incorrect belief that specific activities are harmful and that pain is necessarily indicative of "harm" - a destructive process of one's physical condition. It has been suggested that such anticipatory cognitive events may themselves elicit conditioned emotional responses which contribute to discomfort and pain and would, therefore, require therapeutic procedures directed at extinction (Cassel, 1982; Fordyce, Brockway, Bergman and Spengler, 1986). In fact, the nature and extent of people's physical activities has for the most part little if any effect on their organic condition or long-term risks (Eichner, 1983). Some individuals with coronary artery disease remain active and productive and even run marathons, while others avoid activity, become sedentary and totally disabled: same disease, different response. The confusion between "hurt" and "harm" issues is not trivial in such cases.

The disability associated with so-called degenerative disc disease is also primarily of this nature. In many such cases, it is not the pain per se which is disabling but rather the fear of what the pain indicates. Some people who report being disabled by "low back problems" may rarely suffer pain because they are so successful at avoiding activities believed to cause it. In such cases, pain is believed to indicate "harm". There is little evidence that such is the case (Nachemson, 1979, 1982; Hall 1980; Flor and Turk, 1984).

The tradition in medical practice appears to be toward erring on the side of "safety" and it is not unlikely that physicians will recommend "taking it easy" to such patients. This has the potential of being interpreted by patients as suggesting risk of physical threat associated with activity and, hence, possible "harm" issues. As a result, many self-imposed limitations in work-related and leisure activities can occur, not because the level of discomfort is intolerable or even uncomfortable, but rather because of mistaken beliefs and related unnecessary fear about what that pain indicates. In addition, the natural healing processes of the body are retarded by disuse and promoted by use (Bortz, 1984).

Understanding the distinction between "hurt" and "harm" issues could have significant beneficial effects on behaviours which influence levels of disability. With "hurt" issues, for example, the emphasis may be less on means of avoidance, and more on empirical problem solving strategies for increasing tolerance. With conditions such as rheumatoid arthritis, for example, in which the discomfort is popularly understood and accepted as not being associated with issues of "harm", it is not uncommon to observe cases with significant disease and no discrepant illness or disproportionate disability. In such cases, behaviour is characterized by "escape" rather than "avoidance"; that is, limitations in activity occur only when pain and discomfort reach intolerable levels. Without the concern of "doing oneself harm", the reduction and avoidance of activities associated with pain and discomfort can be markedly reduced. People need not be afraid to engage in activity.

From a cognitive-behavioural standpoint, engaging in activities which are incompatible with the belief and self-appraisal of "frailty" is significant with regard to altering general invalid-like beliefs and related illness behaviour.

Ambiguity and confusion about the issues related to the "hurt" vs. "harm" distinction can also have profound adverse effects on an individual's livelihood by unnecessarily limiting eligibility and accessibility to gainful employment by causing employers to prevent access to employment for fear of risks.

The use of the simple distinction and terminology of "hurt" and "harm" can avoid some of the unnecessary problems which might arise from ambiguity or confusion between the variety of issues associated with the general topic of "contraindications". As will be discussed in detail below, the delineation of these issues is particularly useful in providing a non-prejudicial methodology for dealing with issues of disability and access to employment opportunities for handicapped or impaired individuals.

Behavioural Analysis: Delineation of Non-Medical Issues

(a) Operating parameters. The medical delineation process described above provides the parameters for the behavioural analysis. The definitive diagnosis and the irreducible limitations define the new "black box", the new organism, for which a set of behavioural formulations must be derived.

The conditions of optimal medical therapy provide the limits and guidelines within which behavioural formulations and treatment can take place. For example, specific acquisition (learning) strategies may be influenced by types of medications. Responses learned under specific states of the organism (state dependent learning) may not transfer from non-drug to drug states and vice versa.

Contraindications define critical operating parameters of behavioural intervention. "Harm" related issues prevent certain activities from being considered as possible targets, while "hurt" related issues merely require systematic methodologies for testing response and performance limitations empirically.

In summary, the behavioural formulations and interventions must take place within well defined parameters dictated by the medical delineation process: (a) Which and to what degree can specific responses be accounted for on the basis of the disease determinant alone and, therefore, not likely to be amenable to any form of behavioural intervention; (b) What specific responses and response categories should not be considered as realistic potential target possibilities because the organic limits preclude their existence; (c) What activities can realistically be included as possible target behaviours; (d) What are the specific medical treatment conditions which must be maintained; (e) What specific activities must be excluded from any formulation because of risk (harm) and what are the costs and benefits; and (f) What are the realistic target boundaries (e.g., frequency, duration, magnitude) which can be expected for specific responses with a given disease.

(b) Obtaining valid relevant data. A prerequisite for behavioural analysis is valid and relevant data. This invariably involves direct observation of behaviour in the "real world" - in the home, workplace and other relevant environments by trained, skilled field observers.

It is well understood and universally accepted as a basic principle of behavioural analysis that people are not objective about their own behaviour and cannot be relied upon to provide accurate, unbiased, objective descriptions of their behaviour outside of the clinic, no matter how genuine the attempt to provide accurate data (Nelson, 1977; Bakal, 1979; Haynes and Wilson, 1979; Nisbett and Ross, 1980; Blackwell, this volume; Leventhal, this volume). Yet, this is usually the only source of information available to and used by most clinicians. Even in treatment programs which involve a major behavioural component, rarely does there appear to be direct field observation or intervention. Most behavioural medicine and pain clinics involve intervention in a clinic or on a ward or on an out-patient basis with instructions to patients regarding required environmental manipulations (Fordyce, 1976). From a learning perspective, there is no reason to expect that responses learned in a specific and controlled environment should generalize to the "natural" environment where very different stimuli and contingencies are in place. Self-appraisal tools such as self-monitoring techniques and minor environmental appraisals such as home or workplace assessments are employed as the closest approximation to detailed field observations and interventions.

For a truly valid and effective behavioural analysis, these behavioural and environmental data are critical. The importance of ensuring accurate communication of relevant therapeutic concepts and techniques to certain populations of patients as well as the difficulty in obtaining accurate objective measures of behaviour and environmental factors, led us to develop a behavioural medicine field consultant, trained in behavioural principles, to implement these strategies in the field as well as help gather relevant data through direct observations.

Additional important issues for which relevant data need to be obtained include vocational (physical, performance, skill, and knowledge requirements), financial and compensation contingencies (liabilities, eligibilities, accessibility) and cultural, family and psychosocial influences, and performance capabilities.

Psychometric data including personality inventories, intelligence, interest and aptitude batteries, and, when appropriate, extensive neuropsychological batteries, are very important and useful particularly to provide realistic guidelines for setting long range skill, educational and vocational goals and target behaviours.

Direct, "real world" observations and interventions are essential for the implementation of an ideal, comprehensive, integrated medical/behavioural treatment process. The appropriate professional must be highly trained in behavioural analysis (behavioural observation, behavioural principles, and behaviour therapy) as well as in medically-related issues. In addition, field consultants must have a good working knowledge of the other vocational, governmental, social service, and health care systems with which the patient is involved, in order to design and implement a therapeutic programme that is tailored to the individual and utilizes the services of all these agencies in a complementary and constructive way.

For assessment purposes field consultants can often provide invaluable data on an individual's level of functioning, as well as identify significant behavioural and psychosocial variables in the patient's home and work environments. In many cases these data alone are instrumental in forming a rational and effective treatment programme for the individual. Another function performed by field consultants is the implementation of treatment strategies and related environmental engineering in the relevant environments. A common problem with difficult illness behaviour cases is the complaint by practitioners of lack of compliance. Such field intervention increases the probability of accurate compliance with prescribed programmes. Lack of compliance is often a result of poor comprehension or need for simple modelling or prompting.

Finally, field consultants can ensure that treatment and communication among other health professionals is co-ordinated and accurate. By accompanying patients and dealing directly with any "significant others", misunderstandings and "mixed messages" to patients can be avoided and controlled.

Proper management of the above described functions of observation, intervention, communication, and effective co-ordination and case management in the field is extremely labour intensive and involves more than simple and frequent home and work-site visits. With difficult cases, field consultants

TABLE 2. COMPARISON OF BEHAVIOURAL MEDICINE UNIT OUTCOME DATA (1978 - 1984) FOR COMPLETED TREATMENT CASES BETWEEN "PROCESS" VERSUS "NO PROCESS"

| OUTCOMES: | PROCESS (EVALUATED AND TREATED) | | NO PROCESS (EVALUATED) | |
|---|---|---|---|---|
| Returned to work | 69 | (68%) | 35 | (37%) |
| Job change/retraining | 5 | ( 5%) | 28 | (29%) |
| Early retirement | 9 | ( 9%) | 0 | ( 0%) |
| Dismissed by employer | 3 | ( 2%) | 2 | ( 3%) |
| Continues disability without benefits | 0 | ( 0%) | 6 | ( 6%) |
| Continued disability | 16 | (16%) | 24 | (25%) |
| TOTAL NUMBER | 102 | (100%) | 95 | (100%) |

* Includes only cases of people who were (1) treated; (2) completed treatment (3) were not working when assessed; and (4) had been working before disability.

may be required to spend entire days on a continuous basis with patients at various times throughout treatment.

The field consultant reports to the senior case co-ordinator for case management, attends and reports to the managing case conference, and takes clinical direction from each of the managing clinical disciplines who have clinical responsibility and liability.

(c) <u>Formulation</u>. The behavioural formulation is the key integrating element in the process. It is essential that an overall interactive conceptual model is employed to tie together any and all models which might be relevant to the particular case. The emphasis at this stage must be on conceptual formulations rather than techniques and operations.

The behavioural formulation must be comprehensive and integrative, and use an overall behavioural analysis which incorporates principles and concepts from any areas which are relevant - from simple respondent and operant learning to more complex cognitive and social learning concepts, to issues of role and culture. All such formulations are compatible within the interactive model and should be employed concurrently.

Respondent formulations are relevant and effective with a wide variety of illness responses, particularly those generally viewed as being involuntary and/or mediated by the autonomic nervous system. These include respondent pain responses, skeletal and smooth muscle spasms, cardiac and cardiac-related responses including hypertension, vascular and related responses such as Raynaud's Disease and migraine, gastrointestinal responses including irritable bowel syndrome, and even drug-related responses including tolerance and addiction (Fordyce, 1976; Siegel, 1976; Bakal, 1982; Latimer, 1983; Fordyce et al, 1985; Leventhal, this volume).

Operant formulations are relevant for an equally wide range of responses: those for which biofeedback interventions may be effective (e.g., rectal sphincter dysfunction, specific central nervous system dysfunctions including epilepsy, headache, specific skeletal muscle control); operant pain behaviour and complex avoidance and escape responses related to conditioned emotional responses and fear (e.g., medication ingestion, invalid-like guarding responses); culturally specific sick role behaviours; and behaviours such as frequent attempts at fecal voiding and cyclic fasting and binging (Parsons, 1951; Fordyce, 1976; Black, Cott, and Pavloski, 1977; Mechanic, 1978; Cott, Pavloski, and Black, 1979; Latimer, 1983; Fordyce et al, 1985; Blackwell, this volume).

Cognitive formulations are useful in dealing with illness behaviour related to complex psychosocial issues, beliefs, culturally specific issues and coping and problem solving strategies (Parsons, 1951; Fordyce, 1976; Meichenbaum, 1977; Turk et al, 1983; Nisbett and Ross, 1980; Lazarus, this volume). Within this context, constructs such as Locus of Control and Self-Efficacy (Rotter, 1966, 1972; Bandura, 1977) are particularly relevant. Often clinical strategies within a medical model context lead to external locus of control and victim-like responses in patients. Clinical strategies which emphasize education rather than treatment (see below) often have the added advantage of enhancing effective problem solving and coping strategies. Within the context of a global behavioural formulation which may require respondent (desensitization and counter conditioning using increased physical activity), operant (extinction of avoidance responses associated with pain), as well as a cognitive component calling for incompatible response strategies to alter pain attributions and related external locus of control and self-efficacy issues, the required respondent and operant procedures could be implemented in a gymnasium or fitness facility rather than a physiotherapy clinic in order to meet the cognitive reattribution demands of therapy; that is, to treat the patient as a "jock" getting back into shape rather than as a patient getting healed.

(d) Design and implementation. Once data collection and formulation is complete, the entire treatment programme, including both medical and non-medical components, is designed and implemented in an integrated, co-ordinated manner. The entire programme is monitored and managed through the case conference managing procedure and case co-ordinator. The essential features of the treatment programme are:

The emphasis is on education as opposed to treatment for the non-disease, non-medical issues; the behavioural formulation is aimed at "demedicalizing" issues which are not medical and focussing on cognitive reattribution related to more relevant and effective coping and problem solving strategies; and, since the strength of any programme depends upon the degree to which the significant "real world" environmental factors can in fact be controlled, considerable effort must be made to deal effectively with vocational and family environments.

## Controlling the Work Environment

Two significant factors which contribute to illness behaviour and, consequently, to disability, are (i) access to employment opportunities and (ii) access to income protection and financial benefits (Cott and Gandz,

TABLE 3. PATIENT POPULATION BEHAVIOURAL MEDICINE UNIT (1978 - 1984)

A. DEMOGRAPHIC DATA

| | | |
|---|---|---|
| Total number assessed | 572 | |
| Sex: A) Males | 397 | (69%) |
| B) Females | 175 | (31%) |
| Age: Mean +/- SD (years) | 42 | +/-12 |
| Presenting complaints * Mean number | 3 | (range 1 - 4) |

B. EMPLOYMENT STATUS: (At time of referral)

| | | |
|---|---|---|
| Not working due to disability: | 402 | (70%) |
| Duration of disability Mean +/- SD (months) | 23 | +/-19 |
| Never worked: | | |
| Duration of disability | 51 | ( 9%) |
| Mean +/- SD (months) | 55 | +/-79 |
| Working: | 106 | (19%) |
| On modified work | 13 | ( 2%) |

* Typical complaints: low back pain, fatigue, other chronic pain, chest pain, G.I. complaints, memory - concentration, cognitive difficulties, work performance.

1984; Cott and Goldberg, 1985; Cott and Pavloski, 1985). A dramatic demonstration of this is provided in Table 1 which clearly shows the relationship between return to work and access to gainful employment, and (Table 2) access to disability benefits, independent of disease.

Patients often find themselves unnecessarily barred from access to gainful employment by employers who are not well educated and/or informed about issues of risk, hurt and harm, and prognosis (see below). This can easily be rectified through precise communication by the treatment team using simple, common language, and clearly addressing issues of risk and other concerns of the employer. When such issues are addressed, and if they can be addressed in a more systematic way, through formal management education and training programmes in a corporation, the results can be very dramatic in reducing the degree of unnecessary disability.

Results of our own work at the Behavioural Medicine Unit in this regard are presented in Table 2 which illustrates the difference in effective rehabilitation in corporations in which such formal training ("process") was implemented. The demographic data on these patients are presented in Table 3.

## DISABILITY, HANDICAP, AND HUMAN RIGHTS

With the ever expanding political complexities and overlapping jurisdictions of modern health care and other social welfare, legal and governmental systems and institutions, there is a growing need for a method of balancing such issues as non-prejudicial access to work (in which the focus is on ability to perform and not on physical handicap), with fair accommodation for injured or impaired people, (in which the focus tends to be on "justified impairment" and not on ability to perform).

The "hurt/harm" distinction provides an excellent framework for an empirical definition of disability with a simple non-prejudicial basis for dealing with issues of disability; namely, access to employment opportunities for handicapped or impaired individuals, conditions of employment, safety and risk, and performance limitations. The empirical formulation is ideal in that the focus is neither the individual nor the impairment or physical condition, but solely the empirical demonstration of safe, adequate performance. The organic condition or disease process is relevant only with regard to the "harm" aspects of safety and risk. Otherwise, the onus is on the employer to provide the employment opportunity if the patient/employee is able to perform adequately and safely. The "handicap" or disease is otherwise irrelevant.

If "harm" is the issue restrictions of activity and, consequently, access to employment is imposed. It is appropriate that the activities and risks are avoided. If "hurt" is the issue and associated discomfort can be controlled and/or tolerated, the question of ability to perform adequately is strictly empirical. That is, there is no reason to prevent the individual from having the opportunity to try and test empirically the ability to perform adequately. In addition, the opportunity to succeed can be made optimal by employing learning and other relevant behavioural principles systematically with appropriate environmental control and optimal medical therapy. From a clinical point of view, "trying" alone is unlikely to be sufficient in cases involving conditioned components. Therapeutic assistance or the "how To's" (e.g., extinction procedures), would be essential (Cassel, 1982; Fordyce, et al, 1986). If adequate safe performance can be demonstrated, there is no reason to prevent access to employment.

TABLE 4. EMPIRICAL DEFINITION OF DISABILITY

| ISSUE | CONSTRAINT | OUTCOME |
|---|---|---|
| "HARM": | Imposed | Prevention<br>"Avoidance" |
| "HURT": | Empirical | Opportunity (Try!)<br>Education<br>"Escape" |

The onus is on the employer to provide the job and reasonable assistance and accommodation. The onus is on the employee to demonstrate adequate, safe performance!

## AN EDUCATIVE APPROACH TO ILLNESS

While the medical components of illness require a treatment focus for correcting disorders, many aspects of the non-medical components require more of an educative than a treatment approach. The focus of many behavioural strategies as well as the natural outcome of the demedicalization procedure is away from the patient role and more on individual ownership and responsibility for problem solving and decision making. This educative focus is a major and critical portion of the non-medical component of the treatment described above. Such clinical applications with individuals is labour intensive and thus costly. Consequently, a major focus of our current research at the Behavioural Medicine Unit is testing specific group education procedures for altering unnecessary disability and illness for specific populations. The group intervention educative approach uses the disease-illness framework and demedicalization process as a basis for curriculum. Practical strategies are based on regular behavioural strategies for changing both invalid behaviours, and cognitions and beliefs. On a population of individuals with mitral valve prolapse (MVP) and unnecessary levels of disability some early data indicate promising trends in the effectiveness of these strategies.

This is part of a larger study currently underway, designed to examine optimal interventions in reducing disability related to chest discomfort associated with either MVP or no known cardiac disease. As with the previous study, individuals screened for this intervention study reported significant levels of disability and limitations on both activities for gainful employment and for daily living. The cognitions of MVP patients are consistent with their avoidance behaviours as well as illness behaviours, such as seeking further medical intervention. Preliminary trends indicate that cognitive-behavioural intervention administered in a group education format or by individual treatment produce very similar outcomes. Post intervention, subjects reported decreases in limitations in work and routine daily activities, leisure exercise and rest, and on sleep. Following intervention, subjects also reported decreases in frequency of chest discomfort.

These results strongly support the contention that the disease-illness distinction model and the demedicalization process can provide an effective foundation for corrective and preventive education programmes. Such educative rather than treatment strategies are conceptually and practically more appropriate and useful for minimizing and preventing illness behaviour.

## CONCLUSION

This chapter has attempted to illustrate three main points. First, that illness, as opposed to disease, is a significant health-care problem and that often illness remains even following optimal medical therapy. Second, the disease-illness distinction model provides for an optimal interdisciplinary intervention process for complex (and simple) cases involving both disease and illness. Finally, there exists a significant potential for a group educative focus for such interdisciplinary intervention and represents a powerful cost-effective mode of health-care delivery.

ACKNOWLEDGEMENT

The research reported in this chapter was supported by Health and Welfare Canada Grant 6606-2250-5 and 6606-1949-48 and by the St. Joseph's Hospital Foundation 81-410.

REFERENCES

Agras, W. S. (1982). Behavioural Medicine in the 1980's: Nonrandom connections. Journal of Consulting and Clinical Psychology, 50, 797-803.
Anastasi, A. (1976). Psychological testing (4th ed.). New York: MacMillan Publishing.
Anderson, J. R. (Ed.). (1981). Cognitive skills and their acquisition. Hillsdale, NJ: Lawrence Erlbaum.
Baddeley, A. (1976). The psychology of memory. New York: Basic Books.
Bailey, D. B. (1984). A triaxial model of the interdisciplinary team and group process. Exceptional Children, 51, 17-25.
Bakal, D. A. (1979). Psychology & medicine: Psychobiological dimensions of health and illness. New York: Springer Publishing.
Bakal, D. A. (1982). The psychobiology of chronic headache. New York: Springer Publishing.
Bandura, A. (1977). Self-efficacy: Toward a unifying of behavioural change. Psychological Review, 84, 191-215.
Baron, R. J. (1985). An introduction to medical phenomenology: I can't hear you while I'm listening. Annals of Internal Medicine, 103, 606-611.
Barondess, J. A. (1979). Disease and illness - a crucial distinction. The American Journal of Medicine, 66, 375-376.
Bemiller, C. R., Pepine, C. J., and Rogers, A. K. (1973). Long-term observations in patients with angina and normal coronary arteriograms. Circulation, 47, 36-43.
Black, A. H., Cott, A., & Pavloski, R. P. (1977). The operant learning theory approach to biofeedback. In G. E. Schwartz, & J. Beatty (Eds.), Biofeedback: Theory and research (pp. 89-127). New York: Academic Press.
Bortz, W. M. (1984). The disuse syndrome. The Western Journal of Medicine, 141, 691-694.
Bower, G. H., & Hilgard, E. R. (1981). Theories of learning. Englewood Cliffs, NJ: Prentice-Hall.
Cassel, E. J. (1982). The nature of suffering and the goals of medicine. The New England Journal of Medicine, 306, 639-645.
Cott, A. (in press). Practical applications of the disease-illness distinction model: New concepts in health-care delivery through the optimal integration of medical and behavioural sciences. Canadian Journal of Public Health.
Cott, A., & Gandz, J. (1984). Behavioural medicine: A new approach to managing performance problems. Business Quarterly, 49, 29-37.
Cott, A., & Goldberg, W. M. (1985). Doctors' notes to employers and insurers. Canadian Family Physician, 31, 1919-1925.
Cott, A., & Pavloski, R. P. (1985). Behavioural medicine: A process for managing performance problems. Canadian Psychology, 26, 160-167.
Cott, A., Pavloski, R. P., & Black, A. H. (1979). Reducing epileptic seizures through operant conditioning of central nervous system activity: Procedural variables. Science, 203, 73-75.
Eichner, E. R. (1983). Exercise and heart disease: Epidemiology of the exercise hypothesis. The American Journal of Medicine, 75, 1008-1023.
Estes, W. K. (Ed.). (1978). Handbook of learning and cognitive processes (Vol. 5). Hillsdale, NJ: Lawrence Erlbaum.
Fabrega, M., & Van Egeren, L. (1976). A behavioural framework for the study of human disease. Annals of Internal Medicine, 84, 200-208.
Fedoravicius, A. S. (1981). Chronic illness behaviour: A new model,

behavioural treatment, and future directions. Behavioural Medicine Update, 2, 18-22.
Flor, H. & Turk, D. C. (1984). Etiological theories and treatments for chronic back pain. I. Somatic models and interventions. Pain, 19, 105-121.
Fordyce, W. E. (1976). Behavioural methods for chronic pain and illness. St. Louis: Mosby.
Fordyce, W. E. (1981). On interdisciplinary peers. Archives of Physical Medicine, 62, 51-53.
Fordyce, W. E. (1982). Interdisciplinary process: Implications for rehabilitation psychology. Rehabilitation Psychology, 27, 5-11.
Fordyce, W. E., Roberts, A. H., Sternbach, R. A. (1985). The behavioural management of chronic pain: A response to critics. Pain, 22, 113-125.
Fordyce, W. E., Brockway, J. A., Bergman, J. A., and Spengler, D. (1986). Acute back pain: A control-group comparison of behavioural vs. traditional management methods. Journal of Behavioural Medicine, 9, 127-140.
Garfield, S. L. (Ed.). (1982). Behavioural Medicine [Special Issue]. Journal of Consulting and Clinical Psychology, 50.
Hall, H. (1980). The back doctor. Toronto: Gage Publishing Ltd.
Haynes, R. B, Sackett, D. L., Taylor, D. W., Gibson, E. S., & Johnson, A. L. (1978). Increased absenteeism from work after detection and labelling of hypertensive patients. New England Journal of Medicine, 299, 741-744.
Haynes, S. N., & Wilson, C. C. (1979). Self-Monitoring. In S. N. Haynes & C. C. Wilson (Eds.), Behavioural assessment, (pp. 206-240). San Francisco: Jossey-Bass.
Hearst, E. (Ed.). (1979). The first century of experimental psychology. Hillsdale, NJ: Lawrence Erlbaum.
Isner, J. M., Salem, D. N., Banas, J. S., & Levine, H. J. (1981). Long-term clinical course of patients with normal coronary arteriography: Follow-up study of 121 patients with normal or nearly normal coronary arteriograms. American Heart Journal, 102, 645-653.
Keefe, F. J., & Blumenthal, J. A. (1982). Behavioural medicine: Basic principles and theoretical foundations. In F. J. Keefe, & J. A. Blumenthal, (Eds.), Assessment strategies in behavioural medicine, (pp. 3-16). New York: Grune & Straton.
Kemp, H. G., Vokonas, P. S., Cohn, P. F., & Gorlin, R. (1973). The anginal syndrome associated with normal coronary arteriograms. American Journal of Medicine, 34, 735-742.
Kumar, R., Stolerman, I. P., Sternberg, H. (1970). Psychopharmocology. Annual Review of Psychology, 21, 595-628.
Latimer, P. R. (1983). Functional gastrointestinal disorders: A behavioural medicine approach. New York: Springer Publishing.
Lavey, E. B., & Winkle, R. A. (1979). Continuing disability of patients with chest pain and normal coronary arteriograms. Journal of Chronic Disease, 32, 191-196.
Lipkin, J. O. (1981). Understanding illness behaviour and its importance in the practice of medicine. Behavioural Medicine Update, 2, 15-18.
Mackintosh, N. J. (1974). The psychology of animal learning. London: Academic Press.
McWhinney, I. R. (1972). Beyond diagnosis: An approach to the integration of behavioural science and clinical medicine. New England Journal of Medicine, 287, 384-387.
Mechanic, D. (1962). The concept of illness behaviour. Journal of Chronic Disease, 15, 189-194.
Mechanic, D. (1978). Medical sociology (2nd ed.). New York: The Free Press.
Meichenbaum, D. (1977). Cognitive-behaviour modification: An integrative approach. New York: Plenum Press.
Melvin, J. L. (1980). Interdisciplinary multidisciplinary activities and ACRM. Archives of Physical Medicine Rehabilitation, 61, 379-380.

Melzack, R., & Wall, P. (1982). The challenge of pain. New York: Penguin Books.
Mussen, P. H., Conger, J. J., & Kagan, J. (1979). Child development and personality (5th ed.). New York: Harper & Row Publishers.
Nachemson, A. (1979). A critical look at the treatment for low back pain. Scandinavian Journal of Rehabilitation Medicine, 11, 143-149.
Nachemson, A. (1982). The natural course of low back pain. In A. A. White & S. L. Gordon, (Eds.), Idiopathic low back pain (pp. 46-51). St. Louis: C. V. Mosby.
Nelson, R. O. (1977). Assessment and therapeutic functions of self-monitoring. In M. Hersen, R. M. Eisler, & P. M. Miller (Eds.), Progress in behaviour modification. New York: Academic Press.
Nisbett, R., & Ross, L. (1980). Human inference: Strategies and short-comings of social judgement. Englewood Cliffs, NJ: Prentice-Hall.
Ockene, J. S., Shay, M. J., Alpert, J. S., Weiner, B. H., & Dalen, J. E. (1980). Unexplained chest pain in patients with normal coronary arteriograms. New England Journal of Medicine, 303, 1249-1252.
Parsons, T. (1951). The social system. New York: Free Press.
Rotter, J. B. (1966). Generalized expentancies for internal vs. external control of reinforcement. Psychological Monographs, 80, (Whole No.609).
Rotter, J. B., Chance, J. E., & Phares, E. J. (1972). Application of a social learning theory of personality. New York: Holt, Rinehart & Winston.
Schwartz, G. E. (1982). Testing the biopsychosocial model: The ultimate challenge facing behavioural medicine. Journal of Consulting and Clinical Psychology, 50, 1040-1053.
Siegel, S. (1976). Morphine analgesic tolerance: Its situation specificity supports a Pavlovian conditioning model. Science, 193, 323-325.
Siegel, S. (1983). Classical conditioning, drug tolerance, and drug dependence. In Y. Israel, F. B. Glaser, H. Kalant, R. E. Popham, W. Schmidt, R. G. Smart (Eds.), Research advances in alcohol and drug problems (Vol. 7, pp. 207-246). New York: Plenum Press.
Szasz, T. S. (1961). The myth of mental illness. New York: Hoeber.
Turk, D. C., Meichenbaum, D., & Genest, M. (1983). Pain and behavioural medicine. New York: Guildford Press.
Ullmann, L., & Krasner, L. (Eds.). (1965). Case studies in behaviour modification. New York: Holt, Rinehart, and Winston.
Waxler, E. B., Kimbiris, D., & Dreifus, L. S. (1971). The fate of women with normal coronary arteriograms and chest pain resembling angina pectoris. American Journal of Cardiology, 28, 25-32.
Wooley, S. C., Blackwell, B., & Winget, C. (1978). A learning theory model of chronic illness behaviour: Theory, treatment, and research. Psychosomatic Medicine, 40, 373-401.

# PART II THE SOCIOPSYCHOLOGICAL BASIS OF ILLNESS BEHAVIOUR

# ILLNESS BEHAVIOUR: AN OVERVIEW

David Mechanic

Institute for Health, Health Care Policy and Aging Research
Rutgers University

The concept of illness or disease refers to limited scientific models for characterizing constellations of symptoms and the conditions underlying them. The concept of illness behaviour, in contrast, describes the ways persons respond to bodily indications and the conditions under which they come to view them as abnormal. Illness behaviour thus involves the manner in which persons monitor their bodies, define and interpret their symptoms, take remedial action, and utilize various sources of help as well as the more formal health-care system. It also is concerned with how people monitor and respond to symptoms and symptom change over the course of an illness and how this affects behaviour, remedial actions taken, and response to treatment. The different perceptions, evaluations and responses to illness have, at times, dramatic impact on the extent to which symptoms interfere with usual life routines, chronicity, attainment of appropriate care and co-operation of the patient in treatment. Variables affecting illness behaviour usually come into play well before any medical scrutiny and treatment (Mechanic, 1978a).

A crucial premise in the study of illness behaviour is that illness, as well as illness experience, is shaped by sociocultural and social-psychological factors irrespective of their genetic, physiological, and other biological bases. Illness is often used to achieve a variety of social and personal objectives having little to do with biological systems or the pathogenesis of disease. The boundaries of illness and its definitions are extraordinarily broad, and the illness process can be used to negotiate a range of cultural, social, and personal tensions.

Cultural definitions, social development, and personal needs shape the experience of illness and meanings attributed to physical factors that serve as its basis. While magnitude, severity, persistence and character of symptoms all effect and establish limits for personal and social definitions, there is great variability in what is perceived, how it is defined, the interventions that are considered and used, requests for support and special consideration and illness outcomes.

---

Physicians and patients tend to view health status in fundamentally different ways. Physicians are trained to identify discrete illnesses to the extent possible and have no adequate measures of holistic functioning, vitality or well-being. Patients, in contrast, tend to view health more globally and experientially. Although they may become concerned about specific symptoms, they tend to view their health in terms of an overall sense of well-being, and the extent to which the symptoms they experience disrupt their ability to function or interfere in some significant fashion with their life activities. A variety of studies indicate that people's feeling states influence their sense of physical well-being (Apple, 1960; Baumann, 1961). Persons reporting poor physical health are frequently depressed, feel neglected, have low morale, suffer from alienation, and are less satisfied with life (Maddox, 1962).

## FOUR APPROACHES TO UNDERSTANDING ILLNESS BEHAVIOUR

There are at least four ways in which illness behaviour can be viewed: as a disposition of the person; as a result of an interaction between personal and environmental factors in populations; as a decision-making process, or as a response to the health-care services system.

### The Study of Dispositions

The dispositional approach assumes that persons have a fairly stable orientation to respond to illness in particular ways. While some persons tend to be stoical in the face of illness, others are matter-of-fact or hypochondriacal. While some patients seek care readily for even minor symptoms, others are reluctant to seek care for even life-threatening illnesses. There is also considerable variability in people's responses from one situation to another and over time.

Most dispositional studies are efforts to understand the development of the behaviour pattern. For example, most studies of illness show that women report symptoms more frequently than men do and that they use physicians and psychiatrists more frequently as well (Lewis and Lewis, 1977). One interpretation is that women more than men develop a learned predisposition to define and respond to symptoms. Other interpretations are: that there are real differences in the prevalence of disorder; that sex differences reflect the characteristics of the measures used and the judgements made that involve sex biases; that women have lower thresholds to perceive symptoms; that women are more willing to acknowledge symptoms and seek care; that women have greater knowledge and interest in health matters and, thus, are more attentive to symptoms; and, that the different role responsibilities between the sexes affect the use of services. Although each of these interpretations is given from time to time, few studies successfully compare competing explanations (Mechanic, 1978b), but there are growing efforts toward the testing of competing hypotheses (Cleary and Mechanic, 1983). Within this general approach, the focus of the investigator is the manner in which varying types of dispositions develop and how they can be modified to improve health and induce more appropriate and effective behaviour.

### Person-Environment Interactions: The Epidemiological Survey

A typical approach to studying illness behaviour is the epidemiological survey which identifies those using or not using certain types of care or those who engage in particular health and illness practices. Other data from the survey are then used to account for these differences. Such surveys typically examine sociodemographic factors, access to medical care, distress, life-change events, social supports, coping and attitudes toward medical care. Among factors commonly found to be associated with utilization of medical care are the quality and severity of symptoms, insurance status and barriers to care such as deductibles and co-insurance, levels of distress, social networks, sex, inclination to use medical facilities, skepticism of medical care and faith in doctors (Mechanic, 1982).

Patients' Perceptions and Interpretations - The Decision-Making Process

A third approach to illness behaviour is to focus on the processes through which persons identify and evaluate symptoms, make interpretations of their causes and implications, and decide on the types of help to seek. Persons experiencing changes in their feeling states and physical functioning attempt to make sense of what is happening, and they tend to examine different intuitive hypotheses about the seriousness of their problems and the need for assistance (Leventhal, 1983; Leventhal, Prochaska, and Hirschman, 1985). A major dimension of this process is the way people evaluate the causes of a problem and its seriousness. An important function of health education is to shape such processes of evaluation and attribution so that they result in an effective pattern of care. Understanding attribution processes and the ways to modify them has many rehabilitative implications.

Much attention is now being devoted to patients' appraisals of their symptoms, the assumptions they make about causes, and how responses to medical advice are conditioned by the "naive" theories that patients use to understand their bodily responses. Studies consistently demonstrate major inconsistencies between physicians' expectations and assumptions and patients' responses resulting in poor communication and difficulties in treatment. Leventhal and his colleagues (1980, 1985) find, for example, that while physicians assume that patients with hypertension cannot make judgements of their blood pressure, many patients feel confident in their abilities to assess when their blood pressure is high or low, and they adjust their treatment regimens accordingly. Knowing the physician's view they withhold communicating their assumptions or information about modifications of regimen. Understanding illness theories used by patients thus offers potential for improved communication and more appropriate therapeutic instruction.

One of the most persistent observations in the epidemiologic literature concerns the substantial relationships among reports of physical morbidity, psychological symptoms and self-assessments of health. In one sense these relationships may be a result of dualism in our language and conceptualizations; there is only a single body but we talk in parallel languages about it (Graham, 1967). At least three central hypotheses have emerged about the relationship between physical and psychological symptoms, each correct to some degree. First, the enormity of serious physical illness causes psychological distress and perhaps some psychiatric illnesses as well among vulnerable persons. Second, it has been known for decades that major and persistent psychological stress predisposes individuals to physical illness (Dohrenwend and Dohrenwend, 1974, 1981). While there has been active controversy as to whether these effects are specific to a limited set of diagnoses (Graham, 1967), or relevant to all diagnoses and bodily systems, few seriously doubt that the "psychosomatic hypothesis" is in some sense valid. The problem consists less in the validity of the insight and more in our ability to conceptualize such relationships in a manner promoting increased understanding and improved interventions. A third hypothesis is that certain predispositions of the individual, whether shaped by biology, culture or particular psychological histories, increase the sensitivity or vulnerability of individuals to both physical and psychological symptoms. In our current work we focus on one such predisposition - the tendency to introspect, e.g., to be particularly concerned with one's thoughts and feelings in a diffuse way. This predisposition is shaped by both culture and social relations and interacts with varying aspects of social situations.

### Effects of Health Service Organization

A fourth approach to illness behaviour is to examine how varying features of the health-care system influence the responses of a patient. One crucial determinant of help-seeking among patients is the accessibility of medical care (Lewis, Fein, and Mechanic, 1976), and barriers to care may develop because of location, financial requirements, bureaucratic responses to the patient, social distance between client and professional, and stigma in seeking assistance (Mechanic, 1976). The point is that the problem can often be attacked more effectively by modifying the way agencies and professionals organize to deal with the problem than by attempting to change patient behaviour. Cost-sharing requirements, distance to the site of care, waiting time, and a personal and continuing relationship with the practitioner - all may have different significance to varying population groups, and these must be understood for effective organization of medical services.

## VOCABULARIES OF DISTRESS

It is apparent that social learning affects the vocabularies that people use to describe their problems and complaints. It is reasonable to anticipate that persons from origins in which the expression of symptoms and a desire for help are permissible will be more likely to voice such feelings than those who are socialized in cultural settings that encourage denial of such feelings. Moreover, social groups differ in the extent to which they use and accept psychological vocabularies, and these are likely to shape the way people conceptualize and deal with their distress (Kleinman, 1982). Kadushin (1969) found, for example, that persons who were receptive to psychotherapy were part of a loose social network of friends and supporters of psychotherapy. They shared the same life styles, liked the same music, and had in common many social and political ideas. Such networks tend to support and encourage psychological conceptualizations of problems just as certain families do. In contrast, other families and subgroups disapprove of such patterns of expression and tend to discourage them.

The vocabularies used to describe illness have great practical importance because much psychosocial distress and psychological disorder may be perceived or defined as somatic conditions by the patient not only resulting in unnecessary financial cost, but also in an increased risk from use of inappropriate and possibly dangerous diagnostic and treatment procedures. It is particularly important in primary medical care to identify somatic complaints that are related to psychosocial difficulties and to help patients better understand the source of their distress. Many studies have examined whether attention to psychosocial concerns and mental health care reduce the demand for general medical care among patients with such difficulties. The issues are complex and the processes not well understood, but there is evidence that psychosocial care is related to a reduction in both inpatient and outpatient utilization (Jones and Vischi, 1979; Jones, 1982).

### Determinants of Alternative Expression Patterns

People experience many troubles and tensions that culminate in a variety of adaptations including physical illness, psychological disorder, and a wide range of attack, escape, and risk-taking behaviours. Biology and culture are clearly major limiting factors on how such internal states are expressed, but a large proportion of what is viewed as illness in modern society appears to be an end point of a process that had a variety of alternative pathways. It is estimated that as many as 50 percent of patients entering medical care have symptoms and complaints that do not fit the International Classification of Disease, and many others are motivated in seeking care by problems and symptoms other than those they present (White, 1970). This suggests the limitations of medical knowledge to some extent, but it also reflects the fact that going to a doctor is part of a process of illness behaviour that involves such factors as felt need, perception, appraisal, definition, attribution of cause, motive and decision-making.

To the epidemiologist, who begins with a medical definition of a case and not with the processes that lead to its social definition, there are many anomalous findings. Why, for example, are rates of depression, neurotic disturbance, demoralization, and use of prescription and over-the-counter medication relatively high among women, and alcoholism, hard drug use, and violence particularly high among men? Are these independent observations, or is there an underlying process leading to alternative pathways of expression? Why, among populations such as the Chinese are affective expressions of depression uncommon but the somatic components relatively frequent? Why are rates of suicide among Blacks in the United States relatively low, but rates of homicide so high? Understanding such questions requires inquiries into culture, social situations and personal predispositions.

## Sociocultural Influences

The extraordinary differences among cultures and characterizations of illness, conceptions of causation, and modes of treatment are substantially documented in the anthropological literature (Harwood, 1981). Even in modern populations one finds a blend of sophisticated scientific ideas and folk wisdom. Such cultural content affects the recognition and conceptualization of symptoms, the vocabularies for communication, modes and content of expression, and the range of remedial efforts attempted. Even limited historical study reveals how substantially expressions of distress and illness are transformed from one era to another.

The expression of illness through psychological and social vocabularies is a relatively modern phenomenon co-existent with a growth of personal self-awareness and broad self-expression. Female hysteria, for example, characterized by fainting, conversion reactions and "kicking about" have virtually disappeared in the urban modern environment although vestiges of the disorder are still occasionally seen in isolated rural cultures that are relatively psychologically unsophisticated and repressive. One interpretation of the disappearance of hysteria is that it no longer brings a sympathetic response from the social environment and is suspect not only among physicians but among sophisticated persons more generally (Veith, 1970). But while the dramatic histrionics of hysteria are rarely seen, more mundane expressions of the somatization of distress are ubiquitous and constitute a major load on the medical care system in all nations.

In any historical period the prevailing norms and ideologies encourage or constrain the selection among alternative modes of tension reduction. People facing personal troubles draw on existing sociocultural conceptions of the nature of these troubles and what one might do about them. At any point in time there may be more or less social concensus surrounding the definition of the problem, beliefs about cause, and conceptions of possible remedies. These shape how people view their troubles and what actions they contemplate.

## Personal Predispositions

The variability in patient behaviour in a given subculture despite similarity of symptoms also reflects major differences in psychological orientations and predispositions. At a simple level, people vary in their tolerance for discomfort, the knowledge, information and understanding they have about the illness process, and the specific ways bodily indications affect needs and ongoing social roles. People seem to vary a great deal in their subjective response to pain and discomfort, although there appears to be much less difference in physical thresholds. Much research has demonstrated that pain has an important subjective component, and there is no clear relationship between the amount of tissue damage and the degree of discomfort reported by the patient (Beecher, 1959; Melzack, 1973). What people know, believe, and think about illness, of course, affects what symptoms they think are important, what is viewed as more or less serious, and what one should do.

One specific predisposition which is believed to be fundamental to understanding appraisal and illness behaviour (Mechanic, 1983) is introspectiveness (a tendency to think about oneself, and one's motivations and feelings). Over the years there have been numerous efforts to measure personal traits that characterize individuals who display an exaggerated illness dependency. During the height of dominance of psychodynamic ideas in psychiatry, such persons were commonly characterized as "neurotic", and more recently as "worried wells", but neither concept provides an adequate conceptualization of such personal traits or the processes by which exaggerated illness patterns develop.

The concept of enduring personal traits has increasingly been called into question. There was little evidence that personal characteristics were stable across situations or over time. While the difficulty of demonstrating stability may be in part methodological (Epstein, 1979), current data suggest that it is more appropriate to speak of predispositions or orientations which may be operative only under certain conditions.

Introspection appears to be an important orientation in the illness behaviour process. Results from research programs investigating such varied issues as self-esteem, objective self-awareness, pain response, behaviour and health, private self-consciousness, and ego defense processes all support the hypothesis that attention to self increases the prevalence of reported psychological and physical symptoms and negative self-evaluations (Mechanic, 1983).

I first made this observation more than 20 years ago, but did not fully appreciate its significance. Mothers of young children were asked to keep detailed illness diaries for themselves and other family members, requiring responses to a specific symptom inventory each day. There was some difficulty in gaining co-operation and when we queried mothers who were reluctant, some indicated that the attention to symptoms required by completing the diary made them feel sicker. What was so evident phenomenologically to the persons involved has now been clearly established in a variety of laboratory studies under controlled conditions.

In a variety of studies examining introspection it has been found that persons with such an orientation report more physical and psychological distress, are more upset by stressful life events, and use more medical, psychiatric and other helping services (Mechanic, 1979, 1980). This orientation is believed to be conditioned by sociocultural factors and childhood socialization, and it may be triggered by particular situational events (Mechanic, 1972).

The fact that people cope much of the time without awareness is a central point in understanding personal and social adaptation. To become aware, to become self-conscious, is an indication of more than a routine problem, a greater challenge, a break in the flow of normal activity. People can at any time be confronted with serious illness or personal tragedy, but it is not psychologically economical to worry about what one cannot predict or control, and individuals maintain a sense of invulnerability by inattention to potential threat (Mechanic, 1972; Janis, 1951). Too much inattention or denial distracts attention from essential information acquisition and planning, but we maintain our comfort by considerable filtering of potentially threatening information.

Persons who are more introspective probably know themselves better, and perhaps have better understanding of the influences that affect them, but they also appear more uncomfortable with themselves and their life situations. They are more prone to react to threatening situations and are more likely to define many common, self-limited bodily sensations as symptoms. While introspectiveness, properly guided, may be associated with valued consequences such as creativity, sensitivity and empathy with others, and artistic expression, it also appears to exaggerate the experience of distress and illness.

Introspectiveness is only one of many possible personal inclinations or traits that may interact with perceptions of threat, coping, and the illness experience. Such traits may profoundly affect perceptions and response, the course of the illness experience, and the quality of adaptation. They also may affect the propensity to view oneself as ill, the degree of personal suffering experienced, and the degree to which common bodily signals are defined in a threatening way.

## IMPLICATIONS FOR PREVENTIVE MEDICINE AND PUBLIC HEALTH

Illness behaviour is a dynamic process through which the person defines problems, struggles with them, and attempts to achieve a comfortable accommodation. Such processes of adaptation are partly learned and partly shaped by the social situation and influences in the immediate environment. The health professional thus can help guide the process by suggesting constructive alternatives for the patient and by avoiding the reinforcement of distorted meanings and maladaptive responses. Treatment personnel similarly have considerable choice as to whether they encourage realistic understanding and coping efforts among patients or whether they encourage dependence and helplessness. Much of medical care has encouraged the patient to assume a dependent stance relative to the professional and has failed to support the patient's ability to struggle for mastery over problems. This is particularly evident in chronic illness where the degree of social disability characterizing many patients far exceeds that required by the physical condition of the patient.

From a more theoretical standpoint, illness behaviour reflects the person's needs and competence in coping. Much of the use of medical care is a product of failures in behavioural adaptation and not the occurrence of physical morbidity. Extreme patterns of illness behaviour, thus, can be a substitute for social competence and environmental mastery and frequently is indicative of socially maladaptive behaviour. From a public health perspective, it is extraordinarily important to promote more effective coping and a sense of efficacy (Mechanic, 1974). Various studies suggest that self-esteem and a personal sense of environmental control are essential not only for a feeling of physical vitality and enjoyment of life, but also are linked with a wide a variety of promotive health responses. While we know too little about such important patterns and ways to encourage them, a prudent public health policy would do whatever possible to promote a sense of personal mastery and to prevent syndromes of helplessness (Seligman, 1975).

In the area of chronic disease, and with the increasing proportion of aged in the population, it becomes essential to develop a public health policy approach that encourages continued functioning and environmental mastery and that discourages unnecessary dependency on health personnel and the health-care system. The curative health-care system often encourages patterns of illness behaviour that limit personal responsibility and a sense of control over one's own fate, but there is perhaps no principle more important in the care of the long-term chronic patient or in the functioning of the aged than that they retain a sense of activity, participation, and personal efficacy. The health professional can make a large contribution in preventing unnecessary or premature loss of social function.

## REFERENCES


Apple, D. (1960). How laymen define illness. Journal of Health and Human Behavior, I, 219-225.

Baumann, B. (1961). Diversities in conceptions of health and physical fitness. Journal of Health and Human Behavior, 2, 39-46.

Beecher, H. K. (1959). Measurement of subjective responses: Quantitative effects of drugs. New York: Oxford University Press.

Cleary, P. D., & Mechanic, D. (1983). Sex differences in psychological distress among married people. Journal of Health and Social Behavior, 24, 111-121.

Dohrenwend, B. S., & Dohrenwend, B. P. (Eds.). (1974). Stressful life events: Their nature and effects. New York: Wiley-Interscience.

Dohrenwend, B. S., & Dohrenwend, B. P. (Eds.). (1981). Stressful life events and their contexts. New Brunswick, NJ: Rutgers University Press.

Epstein, S. (1979). The stability of behavior I: On predicting most of the people much of the time. Journal of Personality and Social Psychology, 37, 1097-1126.

Graham, D. T. (1967). Health, disease, and the mind-body problem: Linguistic parallelism. Psychosomatic Medicine, 29, 52-71.

Harwood, A. (Ed.). (1981). Ethnicity and medical care. Cambridge: Harvard University Press.

Janis, I. L. (1951). Air war and emotional stress: Psychological studies of bombing and civilian defense. New York: McGraw-Hill.

Jones, K. (Ed.). (1982). Report on a conference on the impact of alcohol, drug abuse, and mental health on medical care utilization, ADAMHA. (DHHS Publication No. ADM 81-1180).

Jones, K. R., & Vischi, T. R. (1979). Impact of alcohol, drug abuse, and mental health treatment of medical care utilization, a review of the research literature. Medical Care, (Suppl. 2), Vol. 17, No. 12.

Kadushin, C. (1969). Why people go to psychiatrists. New York: Atherton.

Kleinman, A. M. (1982). Neurasthenia and depression: A study of somatization and culture in China. Culture, Medicine and Psychiatry, 6, 117-190.

Leventhal, H. (1983). Behavioral medicine: Psychology in health care. In D. Mechanic (Ed.), Handbook of health, health care, and the health professions (pp. 709-743). New York: Free Press.

Leventhal, H., Meyer, & D., Nerenz, D. (1980). The common-sense representation of illness danger. In S. Rachman (Ed.), Medical Psychology, 2. New York: Pergamon.

Leventhal, H., Prochaska, T. R., & Hirschman, R. S. (1985). In J. C. Rosen & L. J. Solomon (Eds.), Preventing health risk behaviors and promoting coping with illness. Vol. 8. Hanover, NH: University of New England.

Lewis, C. E., Fein, R., & Mechanic, D. (1976). A right to health: The problem of access to primary medical care. New York: Wiley-Interscience.

Lewis, C. E., & Lewis, M. A. (1977). The potential impact of sexual equality on health. New England Journal of Medicine, 297, 863-869.

Maddox, G. L. (1962). Some correlates of differences in self-assessment of health status among the elderly. Journal of Gerontology, 17, 180-185.

Mechanic, D. (1972). Social psychologic factors affecting the presentation of bodily complaints. New England Journal of Medicine, 286, 1132-1139.

Mechanic, D. (1974). Social structure and personal adaptation: Some neglected dimensions. In G. V. Coelho, D. A. Hamburg, & J. E. Adams (Eds.), Coping and adaptation. New York: Basic Books.

Mechanic, D. (1976). The growth of bureaucratic medicine: An inquiry into the dynamics of patient behavior and the organization of medical care. (pp. 83-98). New York: Wiley-Interscience.

Mechanic, D. (1978a). Medical Sociology (2nd ed.). New York: Free Press.

Mechanic, D. (1978b). Sex, illness, illness behavior, and the use of health services. Journal of Human stress, 2, 29-40.

Mechanic, D. (1979). Development of psychological distress among young adults. Archives of General Psychiatry, 36, 1233-1239.

Mechanic, D. (1980). The experience and reporting of common physical complaints. Journal of Health and Social Behavior, 21, 146-155.

Mechanic, D. (Ed.). (1982). Symptoms, illness behavior, and help-seeking. New Brunswick, NJ: Rutgers University Press.

Mechanic, D. (1983). Adolescent health and illness behavior: Hypotheses for the study of distress in youth. Journal of Human Stress, 9, 4-13.

Melzack, R. (1973). The puzzle of pain: Revolution in theory and treatment. New York: Basic Books.

Seligman, M. E. P. (1975). Helplessness: On depression, development, and death. San Francisco: W. H. Freeman.

Veith, I. (1970). Hysteria: The history of a disease. Chicago: Univeristy of Chicago Press.

White, K. L. (1970). Evaluation of medical education and health care. In W. Lathem, & A. Newbery (Eds.), Community medicine: Teaching, research, and health care. New York: Appleton-Century-Crofts.

# SOMATIZATION AND THE SOCIAL CONSTRUCTION OF ILLNESS EXPERIENCE

Laurence Kirmayer

Department of Psychiatry
McGill University

Somatization has been defined as the tendency to experience or express psychological states as somatic symptoms (Lipowski, 1968) or the use of somatic symptoms for psychological purposes (Ford, 1983). People who might be expected to complain of depression, anxiety or marital conflict are found instead to suffer from headaches, fatigue, indigestion and a myriad of other physical symptoms. The assumption that physical symptoms can be caused by social difficulties and amplified by attention is basic to psychological medicine. What somatization adds to this picture is a focus on the discrepancy between patients' experiences of their problems as somatic, and the belief of health-care providers that the problem is psychological or social in nature.

This chapter will address current concepts of somatization and the pragmatics of deciding that an individual is somatizing. Somatization is neither a discrete clinical entity nor the result of a single pathological process. Consideration of clinical examples suggests that somatization cuts across diagnostic categories and is best considered the result of processes that shape the experience and expression of every illness episode. A model that incorporates some of the possible mechanisms for somatization will be outlined. This chapter concludes with a brief discussion of the role of social processes and bodily experience in the construction of the sense of self in health and illness.

## VARIETIES OF SOMATIZATION

The term somatization is currently used in at least four different clinical situations resulting in much conceptual confusion. Somatization refers variously to a style of symptom presentation, a tendency to attribute problems to somatic causes, a distinct psychiatric disorder, and a presumed etiology for functional somatic symptoms. We shall consider each of these in turn.

### Somatization as the Somatic Presentation of Affective Disorders

The clearest use of the term somatization concerns people who present to health-care providers complaining primarily of somatic symptoms and who are subsequently found to have an affective disorder or other psychological or social problem that the clinician believes accounts for the somatic symptoms. Major depression presenting as somatic symptoms is the most commonly studied example (Katon, Kleinman, and Rosen, 1982, Kleinman, 1977).

Case 1. Mrs. A., a 37-year-old secretary, is the mother of three teenage children and married to a 40-year-old former truck driver, himself disabled by chronic intractable low-back pain. Mrs. A. presented to a university primary care medicine clinic with chief complaints of headache and backache. The internist found no organic lesions but noted several tender points - anatomical regions where moderate finger pressure caused a disproportionately strong pain. He diagnosed "fibrositis syndrome" (Bennett, 1981) and referred her to the behavioural medicine clinic. Psychiatric examination revealed a recent history of increasing anxiety, sporadic diarrhea and constipation, patchy alopecia, several months of sleep disturbance with early morning wakening, anorexia with 3-4 kilograms weight loss, and frequent crying spells. Her family history was positive for depression in her mother and alcoholism in her father. Although, when asked directly, Mrs. A. acknowledged she was feeling sad, anxious and irritable, she did not describe her problem as psychological and was reluctant to accept a diagnosis of depression as an explanation for her symptoms. She thought her somatic symptoms were more significant than her emotional distress and sought somatic treatment. This was despite having had a previous episode of depression one year earlier, which was acknowledged as such by her and successfully treated with antidepressant medication and six months of psychotherapy. Although she had readily spoken of past traumas and current interpersonal conflicts during her psychotherapy, Mrs. A. was embarrassed by her recurrent depression. It meant to her that she had failed to cope with her life, to support her family and that she was somehow "weak".

Somatic symptoms are a prominent part of affective disorders and may be the first indication of a major depression (Cadoret, Widmer and Troughton, 1980; Widmer and Cadoret, 1978). Even after medical labelling and treatment as a psychological disorder, recurrent episodes of depression can present as somatic illness (Widmer and Cadoret, 1979). Anorexia, weight loss, early morning wakening and diurnal mood variation are considered core vegetative signs of depression and are predictive of a good response to tricyclic antidepressants (Nelson and Charney, 1981). Patients with major depression or anxiety may present with localized or generalized pain, shortness of breath, tinnitus, subjective loss or alterations of sensory function, nausea, gastrointestinal complaints, dizziness, weakness, fatigue, and malaise (Jefferson and Marshall, 1981; Mathew, Weinman, and Mirabi, 1981; Whybrown, Akiskal and McKinney, 1983). Depression can cause elevated muscle tension (Greden, Genero, and Price, 1985) and may be associated with the muscular pains of fibrositis, a functional rheumatologic syndrome (Hudson, Hudson, Pliner, Goldenberg, and Pope, 1985).

Cross-cultural studies report a high incidence of somatic symptoms in depressed and anxious patients in non-Western cultures (Kirmayer, 1984). Reports of low incidences of affective disorders have been attributed to somatic presentations (Marsella, 1981). For example, a common presentation of both depression and anxiety disorders in Nigeria is the syndrome of brain fag, symptoms of a burning or crawling feeling in the head attributed to the exhausting effects on the brain of mental work (Morakinyo, 1980, 1985; Prince, 1960). This is not unlike the syndrome of neurasthenia, a popular diagnosis in the West around the turn of the century that still enjoys currency in some psychiatric systems (Kleinman, 1982; Sicherman, 1977).

Some authors have suggested that somatic symptoms in the complete absence of discernable cognitive or affective symptoms of depression can be considered a form of "masked depression" (Lesse, 1974). If cognitive-affective complaints were entirely absent it would be hard to know what to make of such an open-ended definition of depression. Neurological studies of brain damaged patients suggest the possibility of an anatomical dissociaton between some somatic and affective aspects of depression (Ross and Rush, 1981). If an independent biological marker for depression could be found, then cases in which the marker was present, but psychological symptoms of depression absent, might be construed as "non-affective depression". The dexamethasone suppression test was initially thought to provide a specific marker for major depression but appears to have little more specificity than early morning wakening and other such vegetative symptoms (Shapiro and Lehman, 1983). Response to tricyclic antidepressant medication, thought by some to confirm the diagnosis of non-affective depression, is inadequate because these medications have peripheral and central affects on pain and are not specific for depression (Turk and Salovey, 1984).

Somatization as the Misattribution of Psychophysiological Symptoms

Patients who declare both emotional and physical problems but who are preoccupied with their physical symptoms or who attribute their emotional distress entirely to their physical problems may also be said to somatize.

Case 2. Mr. B., a 35-year-old self-employed house painter is married and has three adolescent children. He was referred by his surgeon to the behavioural medicine clinic for treatment of gastrointestinal symptoms including "stomach pain and bloating" after eating. His symptoms began three years prior following partial gastrectomy with vagotomy for duodenal ulcers. He stated that after every meal he experiences bloating of his stomach "to the point where I can't get my pants on." Gastric function studies did not document any problem with motility or emptying. Mr. B. volunteered that he was an anxious, tense and dependent person. He had divorced and remarried the same woman after a one-year separation and feared that the marriage was failing again. Despite his awareness of social and psychological difficulties, Mr. B. was reluctant to focus on them in treatment. He arrived for sessions complaining of feeling bloated and focused on sensations of physical discomfort during discussions of both emotionally distressing and apparently neutral topics. When encouraged to bring his wife into sessions of couple therapy, Mr. B. found it impossible. He seemed to feel powerless to enlist her aid in what he defined as his own problem.

Patients with somatic symptoms exacerbated by psychological events may be said to somatize when the clinician has reason to believe that the emotional distress is in some sense primary. This primacy of psychological distress can be temporal, as when emotional distress is thought to give rise to psychophysiological disorders such as tension headaches or irritable bowel syndrome, or it may reflect relative severity, as when a somatic problem seems minor in comparison to the person's psychosocial difficulties. But what is primary for the observer need not be so for the patient. Mr. B.'s somatic symptoms were compelling to him. Although he was able to identify major life difficulties, he did not feel they could account for the severity of his physical distress.

In many ways this notion of somatization is a generalization of the first use. If the severe and sustained affective disturbances of major depression or panic disorder can give rise to persistent somatic symptoms that occlude the affective component of distress, then milder but no less persistent emotional disturbances engendered by problems of everyday life could give rise to somatic symptoms as well. If these symptoms are sufficiently painful or worrying to the individual, they may also eclipse the psychosocial problems. Somatization is here applied in two situations: (1) patients who completely reject psychosocial causes for their distress; and (2) patients who accept a psychosocial cause but who continue to be preoccupied with their somatic symptoms and seek physical solutions. This broad use of the term somatization encompasses almost the whole territory of psychosomatic medicine, limiting the precision and utility of the term for clinical and research purposes.

Somatization as Somatoform Disorder

Certain patients with somatic symptoms without organic pathology (functional somatic symptoms: Kellner, 1985) come to psychiatric attention because the persistence of their anxious help-seeking or the urgency of their complaints constitutes a special problem for health-care providers. The current nosology of the American Psychiatric Association (DSM-III) describes several "somatoform disorders" including hypochondriasis, conversion disorder, somatization disorder and psychogenic pain disorder.

Hypochondriasis, in this nomenclature, refers to a syndrome of fear or belief of illness despite medical reassurance, which may occur in the absence of somatic symptoms (American Psychiatric Association, 1980). Hypochondriasis may be a primary syndrome but more often it accompanies other psychiatric disorders including depression, anxiety, obsessive-compulsive disorder, schizophrenia and personality disorders (Kenyon, 1976). Transient hypochondriacal fears are often seen as part of a stress response syndrome.

Conversion disorder is a syndrome of functional somatic symptoms involving alterations or losses of sensory and somatomotor function that resemble neurological disorders (APA, 1980). Most isolated conversion symptoms are transient and resolve spontaneously within hours to days (Nemiah, 1985). They are commonly seen in medical practice, reported by 25 percent of psychiatric patients, 30 percent of medically ill women and about 20 percent of normal postpartum women. Conversion symptoms are more common in women and lower socioeconomic status patients (Goodwin and Guze, 1983).

Hypochondriasis and conversion disorder are best viewed as symptoms or states rather than discrete clinical syndromes. Their natural history reflects that of the underlying or concomitant psychiatric disorder and social problem. The strongest justification for viewing a somatoform disorder as a distinct psychiatric entity comes from work on somatization disorder (Briquet's syndrome). These patients, formerly called "hysteric", have a longstanding history of many functional somatic symptoms involving multiple organ systems.

Case 3. Mr. C., a 31-year-old computer programmer, is married and has a seven-year-old child. He was referred to psychiatry from an internal medicine clinic, where he was undergoing investigation for abdominal cramps and constipation. He had attended medical clinics frequently for several years along with many visits to other physicians and alternative health-care providers. He presented a multitude of symptoms and worries affecting almost every part of the body. These included, in order of seriousness to him (and in his own words): "constant ringing in ears; dizziness-lightheadedness; headaches with numbness in the face, squeezing at the temples with bands of pressure, 'fuzzy head'; pain in lower right abdomen; jerking sensation in throat, chest and stomach; rapid-steady throbbing throughout the entire body; pains in middle back, left shoulder and arm; numbness in left forearm and hand (right forearm and hand less often); spots before eyes - occasionally; hard-to-breathe feeling; rapid irregular heartbeat and pounding slow heartbeat, both usually accompanied by nausea and lasting several hours." He worried that his symptoms were caused by some as yet undiscovered grave illness, perhaps cancer, although many of these symptoms had begun in early adolescence. Fear of his symptoms prevented Mr. C. from visiting with friends, and he and his wife had greatly restricted their social life from the start of their marriage. Mr. C. blandly denied any personal, marital or family conflicts. He felt his wife and daughter were frustrated that his symptoms restricted family activities, but that their attitude toward him was one of unwavering support and concern.

Somatization disorder is a chronic but fluctuating condition which begins early in life and is characterized by multiple recurrent somatic complaints without apparent physical disease. Somatization disorder achieves better diagnostic reliability than the other somatoform diagnoses due to stringent diagnostic criteria that select for a chronically highly symptomatic group. To reach criterion level, symptoms must have begun before the age of 30 and patients must report at least 14 symptoms (12 for males) of the 37 listed (APA, 1980). The most common reports are of varied pains, headaches, faints, nausea and vomiting, abdominal pains with irritable bowel symptoms, anxiety and fatigue (Goodwin and Guze, 1983). Conversion symptoms are common as are sexual difficulties including dysmenorrhea, dyspareunia, and frigidity. Patients have been clinically described as dramatic, exhibitionistic, narcissistic, emotional, seductive, dependent, and manipulative (Nemiah, 1985). However, empirical studies tend not to support this characterization (Kaminsky and Slavney, 1983). More than 60 percent of these patients report feeling depressed and virtually all state they are "nervous" (Perley and Guze, 1962). These patients are at markedly increased risk for unnecessary surgery and invasive medical procedures (Goodwin and Guze, 1983).

The criterion symptom level for the diagnosis of somatization disorder has been set arbitrarily (Sigvardsson, von Knorring, 1984). It remains unclear whether there is a discontinuous process that would justify labelling somatization disorder a distinct entity rather than viewing it as an exaggeration of normal processes of symptom reporting brought about by enduring situational factors. Women judged to be somatizers on the basis of greater than two work absences per year for minor illnesses were found to be distinguishable from other psychiatric groups. Two patterns of somatization were found (Cloninger, Sigvardsson, and von Knorring, 1984): Type I, "high frequency somatizers" had predominately abdominal distress and low-back pain accompanied by psychiatric disability resulting in many days of sick leave from work. Type II, "diversiform somatizers" had more varied symptoms from one illness episode to the next but less frequent psychiatric and work disability than Type I. Diversiform somatization was associated with a history of alcoholism in biological or adoptive fathers while high-frequency somatization subjects' biological fathers had an increased incidence of petty criminal behaviour (Bohman, Cloninger, von Knorring, and Sigvardsson, 1984). The finding of different genetic and environmental antecedents in these two somatizing groups suggests the possibility that separate processes are contributing in each case.

## Somatization as an Explanation for Idiopathic Symptoms

Finally, patients with somatic symptoms of unknown origin are often presumed to be "somatizing". The determination that a symptom of obscure origin is primarily functional is fraught with difficulty. Psychologically oriented clinicians may feel pressured to offer a functional explanation in the absence of direct evidence when they and their colleagues face the ambiguity and uncertainty of persistent illness. The labelling of chronic pain of obscure origin as "psychogenic" provides an important example of this problematic use of the concept of somatization.

Case 4. Mrs. D., a 38-year-old married housewife and mother of two adolescent boys, was employed as a part-time school teacher. She had a history of two episodes of major depression, one before college graduation and the other in her late twenties after the birth of her first child. Chronic pain in her right lower jaw and gum began at age 33 following routine dental surgery. Extensive dental and medical investigations revealed no organic pathology. Non-narcotic analgesics afforded her little relief. After two years of pain she had a third episode of major depression with worsening of the pain and thoughts of suicide. The depression responded to tricyclic antidepressant medication but her pain continued largely unabated. Having survived this harrowing time, Mrs. D. felt more frightened of her pain and less certain of her ability to live with it. She renewed her efforts to find a cure, visiting dental surgeons, neurologists, and pain clinics in succession. Each consultant gave her a slightly different explanation and she dwelt on the at times subtle differences, amplifying her anxiety and confusion. Most treatments gave her temporary relief but after a few weeks the pain returned to its previous level. After three years she quit her job as a teacher and greatly restricted her social activities. After about four years her pain began to spread to involve the other side of her face. Transcutaneous nerve stimulation relieved this "secondary" pain but was only slightly effective at the original site. One year later an oral surgeon found "a spot" on X-ray near the base of a tooth in the region of her pain and "opened it up and cleaned it out". (The surgeon reported no organic pathology). She experienced qualitatively different pain during recovery which gave her renewed hope. Subsequently, her pain diminished to its lowest level in five years. It was still present but bearable. She began to go out more often and contemplate family gatherings and vacations with some enthusiasm.

In an influential paper, Engel (1959) suggested that patients with chronic intractable benign pain may have a "pain-prone personality". Recently, this concept has been revised to suggest that chronic pain results from a "pain prone disorder" consisting of certain personality characteristics (workaholism or "ergomania", denial of conflict with idealization of self and family, hypochondriacal preoccupation) in combination with a "masked" depression (Blumer and Heilbronn, 1982). Evidence for this view is equivocal and has been ably reviewed and critiqued (Romano and Turner, 1985; Turk and Salovey, 1984). Psychological conflict and depression can exacerbate pain of any origin. Our present state of knowledge suggests that somatization may be one factor in the adaptation to pain but should not be construed as an explanation for chronic idiopathic pain.

## CLINICAL RECOGNITION OF SOMATIZATION

These four examples of the clinical use of somatization make it clear that no single entity or process is involved. While some authors suggest that somatizing people constitute a distinct class of patients who are somehow different in pathobiology, psychology or sociocultural circumstances, their clinical diversity suggests that it makes little sense to speak of "the somatizer" as though a particular type of person or specific pathology is being addressed. What brings these disparate examples together is the common assumption that the somatic symptoms that are in the foreground of the patient's suffering are somehow caused by or stand in place of other psychological or social problems that the patient could - but does not - express.

People who are "somatizing" perceive their problem as physical or bodily in nature. One has to ask who is it that decides that the source or nature of their distress is best described as psychosocial? The conventional answer is that the clinician, grounded in scientific empiricism and armed with observational expertise, is able to discover the true cause of distress. (2)

This cause then defines the nature of the distress. But one consequence of categorizing distress on the basis of its biomedical cause is to subordinate the quality of the patient's experience to an abstract explanatory model (Eisenberg, 1977).

---

2. How clinicians draw inferences about the "true" cause of the patient's suffering constitutes a problem in clinical epistemology and is beyond the scope of the present discussion. It is worth noting that cross-cultural studies show there are other ways than mind and body to categorize distress and different conceptual models, appositional rather than causal, for generating medical explanations (Kleinman, 1980; Lock, 1980; Ohnuki-Tierney, 1984).

In practice clinicians operate with less than complete information and their judgements may be influenced by many extraneous factors. In the absence of any clear marker for a psychosocial influence in patients who fail to report such problems, clinicians tend to hypothesize psychosocial factors when: (1) another explanation is not available or explanations are insufficient to account for the quality or severity of symptoms; (2) another explanation did not lead to a successful intervention; (3) the patient displays obvious interpersonal difficulties in the clinical interview; (4) the patient is fractious, challenging of clinical authority, poorly adherent to the treatment regimen or otherwise unpleasant for the clinician (Kirmayer, in press).

For the physician who focuses primarily on organic disease such patients will be viewed as problematic but often not further characterized. In the absence of effective treatment they may be left to seek other sources of help or referred to psychiatric consultants. Somatization is a concept used only by practitioners who recognize the importance of psychosocial factors.

When there is evidence that important psychosocial stressors exist it is tempting to invoke them as an explanation for all that is puzzling in the patient's condition. The patient's protest that the psychosocial events are not severe enough to account for the symptom can be viewed as denial and, by the classical psychoanalytic inversion of negation, taken as further evidence in favour of a significant link.

Clinicians have a propensity for "either/or" thinking. If an organic problem is found, there is no need to search for psychological troubles. If a patient's psychological misery is apparent, it is easy to attribute all of their symptoms to this and curtail the search for an organic explanation (Tollefson, Straud, Hughes, and Garvey, 1984). There is no reason though, other than a misplaced hope for parsimony, why somatic symptoms with good physiological explanations cannot also be strongly influenced by psychological factors. Multicausality is the rule, not the exception, in medicine.

Numerous powerful influences of psychosocial events on physiological processes have been demonstrated in laboratory and epidemiological studies. However, it is very difficult to determine how important such influences are in a particular individual for a specific illness episode. Diffuseness or vagueness of a somatic symptom is no indicator that it is psychological in origin. Most symptoms in medicine are nonspecific in this sense. The inference that somatic symptoms are caused by psychosocial events is usually based on simple contiguity. However, both physicians and patients may over-estimate the significance of temporal contiguity. Chronic pain patients arrive at all sorts of hypothetical associations between the weather, foods, activities and their symptoms and it is hard to decide which are accurate observations and which are superstitions.

When a significant psychosocial event precedes a somatic symptom it is certainly reasonable to consider a causal link. But patients' acceptance of such an explanation does not confirm its truth. Further, the therapeutic utility and scientific truth of causal explanations are separate issues. An explanation can have therapeutic value, whether or not it is true, when it helps to make coherent meaning of suffering. Patients who do not report psychosocial stressors or are unsatisfied with psychosocial explanations still have the need to make meaning of their symptoms. Somatization and psychologization must be understood as outcomes of the active construction of illness meaning. The clinician's one-sided insistance on either organic or psychosocial causation reflects a bias that must be justified not only by appeal to theory but by its therapeutic consequences.

## SOMATIZATION AS PROCESS

Somatization represents the outcome of universal processes of illness behaviour. Somatic symptoms are very common in the general population. In any one week, about 75 percent of the population experiences at least one notable somatic symptom (Kellner and Sheffield, 1973). Pennebaker and Skelton (1978) found that 80 percent of their college student sample were currently experiencing some degree of at least one of 12 common physical symptoms when surveyed during class. Most of these symptoms are mild but estimates derived from British and American morbidity surveys suggest that in an average month, three out of four people take definite action for a somatic symptom, including the use of medication, bed rest, consulting a physician or limiting their activity (Mechanic, 1972).

Most measures of somatization are simply somatic symptom checklists. However, subjects reporting high levels of somatic symptoms cannot be assumed to be somatizing. People reporting the highest levels of unexplained somatic symptoms generally also report high levels of psychological symptoms (Wells and Strickland, 1982). In the absence of organic disease, somatic symptoms are presumed to be a result of psychological processes. But somatic symptoms may result from unrecognized organic illness that also gives rise to psychological distress (Hall, Garner, Stickney, et al., 1980). Such somato-psychic processes cannot be ruled out simply on the basis of symptomatology.

Various strategies have been tried to identify functional somatic symptoms in epidemiological surveys, but with limited success. Crandell and Dohrenwend (1967) had physicians classify symptoms on the Langner scale as psychogenic or physiogenic. They found that lower socioeconomic status (SES) subjects reported both psychophysiological and psychological symptoms more frequently than did higher SES subjects. The negative correlation of psychophysiological symptoms with SES was greater than the negative correlation of psychological symptoms and SES. The authors interpreted these relationships as support for the hypothesis that lower SES subjects are more likely than higher SES subjects to express psychosocial distress as somatic symptoms.

Recent studies have not supported the separation of the Langner scale into psychophysiological and physiological items (De Marco, 1984; Wheaton, 1982). Recognizing that identical symptoms may have different causes in different individuals, Wells and Strickland (1982) attempted to distinguish between physiogenic and psychogenic symptoms by refined data collection. Respondents acknowledging a symptom were asked whether they had received a medical diagnosis and whether the symptom had occurred either only in association with the diagnosed disease or only when they were taking medication, drugs or alcohol. Symptoms that could not be traced to organic disease or substance use were used to construct a psychogenic symptom score. Somatic symptoms without clear physiological cause were correlated just as strongly with the total psychogenic score as were psychological symptoms. This suggests that somatic symptoms without organic cause may be related to psychological distress. The somatization disorder section of the Diagnostic Interview Schedule (DIS: Robins, Helzer, Croughon, and Ratcliff, 1981) uses similar probe questions to identify functional organic symptoms. Because respondents may offer plausible medical explanations for symptoms which would not stand up to expert scrutiny, survey measures like the DIS may under-recognize functional somatic symptoms (Robins and Helzer, 1982).

It is not surprising that attempts to separate physical symptoms of organic disease from psychophysiological and psychological symptoms on a priori grounds have been largely unsuccessful. The current direction of research in psychosomatic medicine is to suggest that virtually any physical symptom may be exacerbated by psychosocial stress. This has led to the replacement in psychiatric nomenclature (DSM III) of a distinct class of

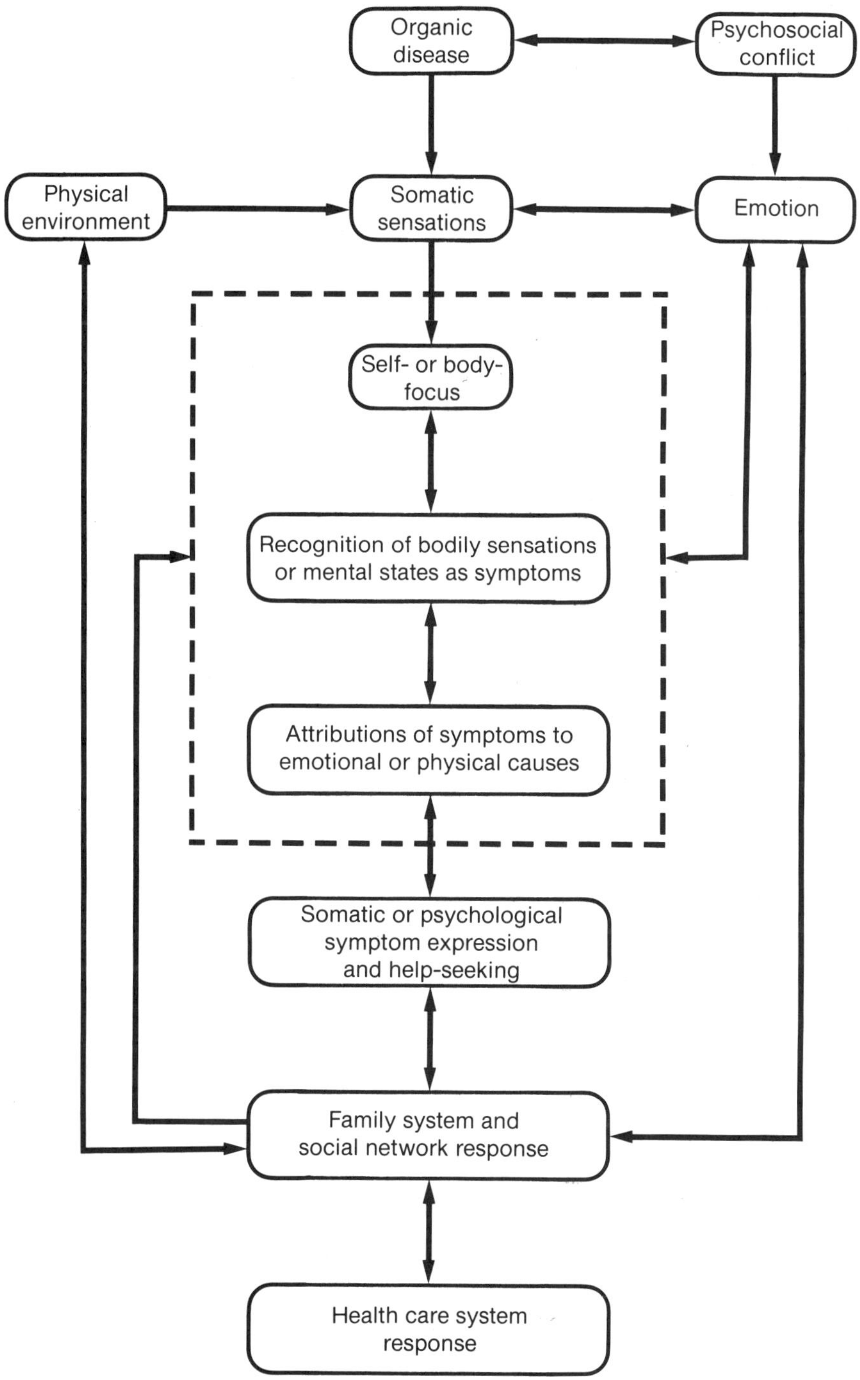


**FIGURE 1.** A model of somatization

psychophysiological disorders with the open-ended descriptor "psychological factors affecting physical condition".

## MODELS OF SOMATIZATION

Given that somatic symptoms are common and regularly accompany psychological distress and social difficulties, what makes somatizing patients who come to medical attention distinctive is not so much the nature of their symptoms but their frequency, severity and persistance. At present it is not possible to separate the experience of symptoms from the reporting of symptoms. The distress that somatizing patients present to a physician may reflect high levels of symptom experience or may be a result of their style of expression and help-seeking. Somatization is not simply a function of the transduction of emotional distress into somatic symptoms. Other psychological and social processes that bias perception and shape expression are crucial to the quality of the somatizing person's experience. A model of somatization that incorporates some likely mechanisms will be outlined. This model views somatization as resulting from: (a) somatic processes that give rise to physical symptoms both as the direct bodily concomitant of emotion and (b) through the inhibition of emotional expression; (c) attentional processes that focus perception on the self as psychological or bodily agent; (d) cognitive-affective processes that appraise sensations as threatening and hence symptoms of illness; (e) attributional processes that ascribe somatic, psychological or social causes to symptoms; (f) family and interpersonal processes that proscribe direct expression of psychological distress while reinforcing bodily expression; (g) cultural processes that elaborate bodily symptoms as an idiom of distress; (h) health-care systems that sanction bodily symptoms as a means of help-seeking while offering limited access to psychologically oriented services. As outlined in Figure 1, these processes may be viewed as hierarchically organized and linked by mutually amplifying feedback loops.

### Somatization as the Bodily-Felt Aspect of Emotion

Bodily changes regularly accompany emotions. Persistent bodily symptoms may result when emotions are sustained by intrapsychic conflict or relentless social problems. The vascular system and the muscles for facial expression are intimately involved in the experience and communication of affect (Buck, 1980; Zajonc, 1985). Back pain and other somatic symptoms may result from persistently high levels of muscle tension or imbalance (Dolce and Raczynski, 1985). Patients with chronic low back pain show elevations of muscle activity specifically in their paravertebral muscles when emotionally stressed (Flor, Turk and Birbaumer, 1985). Chronic somatic symptoms may result from emotional distress when a physical diathesis renders one region of the body vulnerable to changes in tension that accompany emotion.

Individuals vary in their sensitivity to visceral and somatic sensations (Buck, 1980; Grings and Dawson, 1978; Shields and Stern, 1979). However, more sensitive individuals are not necessarily more accurate reporters of their own visceral activity. People with high scores on self-report measures of autonomic perception have generally high levels of autonomic reactivity and variability and tend to over-estimate their autonomic levels relative to objective measures (Mandler, 1984; Pennebaker, 1982). Hypochondriasis may be viewed as the result of chronically elevated arousal or sensitivity to sensory stimuli (Hanback and Revelle, 1978). Thus, hypochondriacal patients may experience more intense bodily sensations of emotion and so report both elevated somatic and psychic symptoms in response to even mild stress. Increased sensitivity to bodily sensations that results in more intense emotion could further increase somatic symptoms by a positive feedback loop. In this model, somatizers are people with heightened states of emotional arousal and sensitivity to autonomic sensations. They readily report the intense and varied somatic symptoms that accompany all forms of distress, psychosocial or otherwise.

Figure 1 represents a model of some likely processes that contribute to the somatization and psychologization of distress. For clarity only a few representative pathways are drawn. The origins of distress include stressors in the physical environment, social problems, and psychological conflict. (A) These give rise to somatic sensations either directly, through emotions, or through the pathophysiology of disease. (B) Somatic sensations then compete for attention with the intrapsychic self or external social environment. (C) Once attended to, sensations must be recognized as abnormal, that is, as indicating a problem. (D) Abnormal sensations are then interpreted as symptoms of a disease, or an emotional or social problem. (E) The cognitive processes of focus, recognition and interpretation feedback to the experience of emotion. This may lead to an increase in somatic symptoms and a cycle of mutual amplification resulting in high levels of somatic symptoms and emotional distress. This type of feedback process may characterize hypochondriasis. (F) As symptoms are interpreted they are expressed as part of the help-seeking process. (G) Inhibition of emotional expression may prevent the resolution of emotional and social conflicts leading to sustained levels of arousal and increased somatic symptoms or organic disease. (H) The expression of symptoms is shaped by family process and the larger social network which dictate what forms of expression will be accepted and effective in mobilizing support. (I) The family system influences the development of the individual's style of cognitive evaluation of sensations, as well as (J) the style of expression of emotions and conflict resolution. (K) The health-care system, and wider social system, determine what forms of help are available and what economic and social costs they entail.

Somatization as Inability to Express Emotion

In contrast to the view that somatization is simply the amplification of the bodily aspect of emotion is the proposal that a lack or suppression of verbal emotional expression leads to physical symptoms.

Several lines of research support the hypothesis that individuals who are open and expressive about their emotions display reduced autonomic reactivity compared to individuals who deny or fail to report their feelings (Leventhal, Nerenz, and Straus, 1982; Pennebaker, 1985). Grings and Dawson's (1978, p. 62-63) summary work, utilizing the MMPI repression-sensitization scale, shows that repressors who report less emotional distress exhibit greater autonomic (electrodermal) response to laboratory stressors. Anderson (1981) found negative correlations between level of autonomic activity and subjective ratings of stressfulness in patients with migraine, tension headache, essential hypertension and rheumatoid arthritis. Several authors report a negative correlation between facial expression and autonomic responsivity to emotion (Vaughn and Lanzetta, 1980). Pennebaker (1985) reviewed other evidence that the inhibition of emotional expression results in elevated autonomic arousal.

When emotional expression is inhibited by social disapproval or punishment, situations that evoke emotion may elicit conditioned anxiety (Lanzetta, Cartwright, and Kleck, 1976). Pennebaker (1985) found an association between a history of childhood sexual abuse and elevated somatic symptom reporting. Social restrictions on the emotional expression of sexual trauma may leave individuals vulnerable to physical symptoms due to chronic physiological arousal.

The concept of alexithymia, a term coined from roots meaning "no words for feeling" (Sifneos, 1973), gains plausibility from these studies. Alexithymic individuals are said to display diminished capacity for affective and psychological expression, as well as a constricted fantasy-life. They are hypothesized to be more likely to develop psychophysiologic disorders (Sifneos, 1973).

DeGood and others (1985) used the Cognitive-Somatic Anxiety scale (Schwartz, Davison and Goleman, 1978) to study chronic pain patients. Compared to college students, the patients as a group reported dramatically less anxiety. Patients reported somatic expressions of anxiety more often than cognitive expressions while the reverse was true for students. The authors interpreted low cognitive symptoms of anxiety among the pain patients as evidence of alexithymia. They did not, however, control for substantial age and education differences between the groups. Spence, Pilowksy and Minniti (1985) found elevated levels of autonomic arousal among chronic pain patients who reported low levels of dysphoria and denied life problems when compared to chronic pain patients who acknowledged dysphoria and social problems.

Alexithymia is defined in terms of impaired verbal, expressive and symbolic affective functions but it has proved difficult to establish a reliable measure of alexithymia that goes beyond the denial of emotional distress. Despite agreement among clinicians that such patients exist, some have questioned alexithymia's construct validity (Lesser and Lesser, 1983). Research to date has been hampered by the arbitrary classification of disorders as "psychosomatic" and by inadequate or absent control groups. In a controlled comparison of patient's attending a psychosomatic medicine clinic and patients attending a traditional outpatient psychiatric clinic in a county general hospital, Lesser and others (1979) found no differences in the incidence of alexithymic traits between the two groups. Alexithymia was, however, more prevalent among the lower SES patients in both clinics. Alexithymic traits may thus reflect social class or cultural differences in the open expression of emotion.

In social groups that limit the display of certain emotions, individuals may not be able to express or resolve feeling states explicitly (Kleinman, 1980). They can, however, focus attention on the somatic concomitants of emotion and describe their bodily state provided it is divorced from other aspects of emotion like private fantasy and social context. Focussing on somatic symptoms may also lessen suffering by diverting attention from painful emotional and social circumstances that are percieved as unchangeable.

Alexithymia has been assumed to play a causal role in the development of psychophysiological disorders but it is equally possible that people with somatic disease become somatically preoccupied and change their style of communication. Alexithymia could represent a state not a trait. Patients who persist in talking about bodily symptoms without accepting the importance of psychosocial processes can frustrate the helper who values psychological insight. The tendency to view alexithymic patients as "deficient" would then reflect cross-purposes between psychotherapists' wish to talk about psychological experience and suffering individuals' need to express their more pressing somatic concerns.

## Somatization as Self- and Body-Consciousness

Awareness of one's internal state is a function of control processes that monitor the availability and urgency of internal compared to external information (Carver, 1979). A varied external environment will reduce attention to internal information and so decrease reporting of somatic sensations. This cue competition theory has received support in a variety of experimental and naturalistic studies performed by Pennebaker and colleagues (Pennebaker, 1982). Joggers running a novel course over complex terrain report fewer somatic symptoms of fatigue than those running a familiar track. Subjects watching a movie cough more often during boring parts than when they are enthralled. Such changes in focus of attention may help account for the observation that people who live alone report more symptoms than those who have more social contact (Pennebaker, 1982).

External information is not simply a distraction from internal sensations. A person who is focussed on somatic symptoms may direct the attention of others to similar sensations in their own bodies. People in a theatre audience tend to cough when others do perhaps because the sound of coughing focuses attention on throat sensations (Pennebaker, 1982). This is probably not the result of consciously waiting for an opportune time to cough because the effect occurs as well when subjects are asleep. Patients with chronic pain may focus the attention of their family members on their own corresponding body regions, evoking muscle tension. In concert with vicarious autonomic arousal due to witnessing a loved one in pain (Block, 1981), such attentional focus could give rise to similar somatic complaints. Such processes could account for the observation of symptoms of abdominal distress in husbands of pregnant women (Lipkin and Lamb, 1982) although recent studies have not confirmed this "couvade syndrome" (Quill, Lipkin, and Lamb, 1984).

People show stable differences in the tendency to be self-conscious and aware of their psychological state (Fenigstein, Scheier, and Buss, 1975). There are also individual differences in the tendency to be aware of one's body and bodily sensations (Miller, Murphy and Buss, 1981). Higher levels of both private self-consciousness and private body-consciousness are associated with elevated somatic symptom reporting (Pennebaker, 1982). (See Hansell and Mechanic, this volume.)

## Somatization as Symptom Appraisal

The evaluation of a bodily sensation as threatening and hence as an indication of illness can be viewed as the outcome of a process of cognitive appraisal. Cognitive schemata direct the search for bodily sensations and their translation into symptoms of disease. Burnham and Pennebaker (Pennebaker, 1982) asked students to fill out a list of the degree to which they were experiencing 12 common symptoms, half of which were flu-related. When given the prompt that this was flu season, students reported more symptoms and more flu-related symptoms than non-flu related symptoms. Thus, expectancy set can influence symptom reporting. In experimental paradigms where physiological arousal was increased by exercise prior to testing, this expectancy effect was even stronger (Pennebaker, 1982).

Such expectancy sets may form more or less enduring personality traits. Hypochondriasis can be understood as the tendency to evaluate ordinary sensations as symptoms of disease. Factorial studies of scales of hypochondriasis reveal three dimensions: bodily pre-occupation, worry or fear about disease, and a conviction that one is ill despite medical reassurance (Pilowsky, 1967). To these factors one might add the beliefs that one is vulnerable to illness and sensitive to pain or physical distress. All of these factors constitute expectancies that could bias the cognitive evaluative process toward higher symptom recognition and reporting. If individuals vary in their sense of vulnerability to emotional versus physical illness, similar processes could influence the reporting of somatic or affective symptoms (Robbins and Kirmayer, this volume). (3)

---

3. Some patients who insist on somatic explanations for all of their distress perceive themselves as highly vulnerable emotionally. It is the very fear of emotional disability that fuels their insistance on a somatic explanation.

The theory of cognitive appraisal in stress research suggests that the comparison of the perceived demands of the environment with available coping resources determines the extent of affective and somatic distress induced by an environmental event (Lazarus and Folkman, 1984). Similar processes of appraisal may govern individuals' responses to bodily changes. If coping resources are adequate, a bodily sensation may be dismissed or viewed as subsidiary to more challenging psychosocial difficulties. Hence, the use of different coping strategies should influence the experience of symptoms. Davidson and Schwartz (1976) have proposed that anxiety involves somatic and cognitive aspects that may be differentially affected by coping strategies. The relative preponderance of physical or cognitive symptoms that accompany an episode of anxiety may differ with the type of anxiety provoking situation as well as the individual's type of response. They review evidence that anxiety scales tend to measure two major subsets of response: awareness of somatic changes and conscious unpleasant thoughts. They devised a Cognitive-Somatic Anxiety scale that differentiated well between students who practiced cognitively based passive meditation and students who participated in regular physical exercise classes (Schwartz, Davidson, and Goleman, 1978). The meditators exhibited no significant difference between the modes of anxiety while the exercisers were significantly higher on cognitive anxiety and lower on somatic anxiety symptoms. This supported the idea that the method of coping influenced somatic or psychological symptom expression. As the authors noted, their retrospective study design did not preclude the possibility that the observed differences were the result of traits that led subjects to choose a specific means of relaxation (meditation versus exercise).

## Somatization as Causal Attribution

Part of making sense of a symptom is deciding what caused it. Causes may be as varied as the categories of a peoples' metaphysics. There is evidence that ideas of causation are based not simply on observing how one event follows another but on substantive ideas about how one event generates another (Shultz, 1982). Thus, attributing a symptom to a psychosocial cause depends not just on recognizing that a significant emotional event preceded the onset of a physical symptom but on having a model of how a psychosocial event could generate the observed symptom. In the absense of such models, it may be easier to explain a physical symptom by a corresponding physical process.

Work on cultural differences in causal attributions suggests that social groups have preferred modes of explanation for patterns of human behaviour (White, 1982). It is not known whether people have stable generalized biases in causal attribution nor what effect one illness episode has on subsequent symptom interpretation. In the first case described, Mrs. A.'s acceptance of the explanation of depression for her symptoms did not prevent her from attributing subsequent pains exclusively to physical disease. The bodily quality of symptomatology may overshadow psychosocial explanations unless there are strong personal or social reasons for preferring such an explanation.

Causal attribution involves building abstract models which may vary from elaborate generative schemes to simple classifications based on a single property. Many people have ill-formed, inconsistent and incomplete notions about the cause of their symptoms. The attempt to describe a person's explanatory model may impose an exaggerated coherence on fragmentary models (Young, 1981).

## Somatization as Communication in Family and Social Context

Once a symptom is expressed it becomes communication. Somatic symptoms are read as messages by others whether or not they are intended as such by the sufferer. In a tightly-knit social group like the family, symptoms may be involved in powerful contingencies that reinforce some types of expression while extinguishing others. In addition to determining the extent of social disability, the reinforcement of expressive behaviours may alter the experience of distress (Fordyce, 1978). Thus, families that ignore or punish emotional complaints or respond with more attention and nurturance to physical symptoms, will reinforce a somatic style of expression. Family process can shape symptom experience and expression, without the sufferer's awareness, toward a form that maintains the stability and function of the family system (Minuchin et al., 1975). While somatization can be viewed as a consequence of family process acting on the individual, in the circular causality of the family system somatic symptoms act in turn on family structure.

The ability to articulate interpersonal problems within the family or the wider social sphere depends on a measure of acceptance of social protest. In settings where power is maintained by a rigid hierarchy, the mere mention of psychosocial complaints can be perceived as a threat to authority and met with harsh sanctions. Somatic symptoms offer a way to express dissatisfaction obliquely without a direct challenge to authority. The sick person wields power through justified demands on the time and energies of others. Legitimate illness demands a care-giving response from family members. Somatic symptoms constitute a strong bid for legitimacy and provide a strategy for the weak to redress the inequities of power in social life.

Somatization as Idiom of Distress in Cultural Context

Somatization can be viewed as the use of an idiom for the expression of distress (Nichter, 1981). As an idiom of distress, somatization is shaped not only by the nature of bodily suffering but by a symbolic code given in, and constrained by, culture. Physical symptoms can communicate information about the intensity, source and meaning of personal and social distress through the use of the body as metaphor. It is this communicative value of somatic symptoms that supports their persistance when other modes of expression are restricted.

Ohnuki-Tierney (1984) has proposed a theory of somatization as "physiomorphism" - a term introduced by Levi-Strauss (1966) to refer to the process of giving bodily shape to something that may not be physical in the first place. Parts of the body and bodily processes which stand in metonymic relationship to physical illness are used as extended metaphors for the social imbalances thought to underlie illness. These metaphors can be extended to yield implication for social action. Physical symptoms can then be used to comment on and restructure social situations.

The language of emotion is replete with bodily metaphors (Good, 1977). Some of these are grounded in the somatic concomitants of emotion. A terrifying threat stands our hair on end. Anger makes the blood boil. We choke back tears and feel a lump in our throat. Although the correspondance between body parts and functions varies with culture, similar idioms have universal currency. While sophisticated speakers may be aware they are using a figure of speech, the metaphor supplies its own meanings, rules of use and implications. The way in which a bodily metaphor is extended depends on its relationship to ethnophysiological ideas, which are based in turn on metaphoric models.

Metaphor is not an exotic feature of language. Children are able to use metaphor long before they recognize it as a trope or figure of speech (Winner, Rosenstiel, and Gardner, 1976). Sophistication lies in knowing when one is using a metaphor and observing its limits. But metaphors underlie our most abstract conceptualizations (Lakoff and Johnson, 1980). Although we may be aware of idiosyncratic or newly invented tropes, the fabric of culture is woven of metaphors we take for literal descriptions.

Bodily metaphors should not be construed as primitive or concrete thinking. Metaphors drawn from the body have a special cogency and immediacy due to the salience of bodily experience. The individual who resorts to bodily metaphors to describe a social predicament is using a powerful and subtly articulated code for the expression of distress. Like all rhetoric, it must be judged in terms of its effect on its intended audience. Understood in family and cultural context, somatic metaphors can be an eloquent and effective expression of social distress.

## Somatization as Result of the Health-Care System

There is evidence that the use of self-report symptom checklists can dramatically increase the recognition of depression in primary care settings (Nielsen and Williams, 1981). If such a simple means of data collection increases the recognition of somatized depression, one ought to ask whether it is patients' somatic presentations or physicians' diagnostic methods that account for the clinical "masking" of depression (Carlson and Cantwell, 1980). Physicians somatize patient's distress when they ignore psychological symptoms in favour of organic pathology which they find more interesting or feel better able to treat (Tollefson, Straud, Hughes, and Garvey, 1984).

The very structure of the health-care system may result in the tendency to express distress in somatic terms because such problems are considered more serious and worthy of care. The physical nature of diagnostic procedures and therapeutic intervention maintains a focus on the body and encourages somatic attributions of symptoms.

Mental illness is highly stigmatized in North America and the benefits of the sick-role tend to accrue to physical illness rather than psychiatric or psychosomatic illness (Blackwell, 1967). People who emphasize their somatic distress are pursuing the most direct path to the ratification of the sick-role.

For the most part health-care workers share the layperson's negative view of psychiatric illness. Physicians who wish to spare their patients the pain of stigmatization may avoid recognizing psychological problems. Contemporary biological psychiatry has developed a view of affective disorders and other major psychiatric syndromes as physical disease. This perspective is offered to patients to encourage them to view depression as something happening to their bodies that can be described in somatic terms and treated with medication and other physical interventions. At times the somatic bias of biological psychiatry exceeds anything conceived of by laypeople. Faced with the somatic emphasis of medicine, people may psychologize their problems. Bursten (1985) reports on patients who are reluctant to take antidepressant medication because it implies their problem is not psychological but physical and hence beyond their personal control. They reject the somatic explanations of biomedicine in favour of a psychological or existential view of their distress that allows them greater autonomy and potential self-efficacy.

## Body and Emotion in the Social Construction of Illness Experience

Somatization and psychologization are not curious artifacts of the practice of medicine. They arise from basic processes in the social construction of the person (Kleinman and Kleinman, 1985). The sense of self is rooted in both bodily experience and social transaction. The details of socialization and, consequently, the way in which one experiences the self in health and illness must be understood in terms of the interaction of bodily and social processes. Emotional experience plays a special role in this interaction because emotions indicate what matters to individuals both as bodies and as social agents. Emotions bridge the body and the social situation in the construction of the self.

Despite efforts to develop purely cognitive accounts of emotion, it is clear that bodily sensations contribute to the essential meaning of emotion (Leventhal, 1979; Zajonc, 1982). The somatic concomitants of emotion are not accidental or arbitrary social constructions. Pennebaker (1982) asked subjects to produce a specific emotional state in themselves, then record the physical symptoms they were feeling. Consistent and specific patterns of bodily response to joy, anger, sadness, guilt, embarrassment and fear were reported. Given specific symptom clusters subjects could also consistently associate them with the corresponding emotion. While this might reflect associations based on linguistic convention, the physical responses to some emotions are developmentally earlier than learned associations between emotion words and bodily changes (Ekman, 1972; Hesse and Cichetti, 1982).

While bodily experience lends emotion its distinctive "hot" or "moving" quality, the cognitive aspects of emotion are fundamentally social (Harre, Clarke and De Carlo, 1985). This is clearly evident in the case of more complex emotional experiences. For example, Pennebaker's (1982) subjects could not discriminate pride from joy on physical grounds. Bodily reactions distinguish only a few universal emotions of basic adaptive significance (Cannon, 1929; Ekman, 1972)). Emotions that show important cross-cultural differences may be constructed out of sequences of interpersonal interaction. While some emotions are more closely tied to bodily experience and others are almost pure abstractions about social interaction, both bodily and social factors contribute to the meaning of emotional experience.

Since emotions partake of both the bodily and social aspects of self, somatization is not simply the misdirected expression of psychosocial distress but an emphasis on one aspect of all distress. It is symmetrical to psychologization - the emphasis on personal and social dimensions of suffering. Somatization and psychologization must be understood as contrasting methods of constructing illness meaning that assimilate emotional experience to either the bodily or the social realm.

Worldwide, somatization, along with other forms of illness experience that may be more morally charged, (e.g., possession), appears to be more common than psychologization (Kirmayer, 1984). Psychologization is something of a modern Western anomaly and, bearing in mind the problem of self-reflexivity, ought to receive closer study.

While the tension between body and society is not a unique creation of Western metaphysics, the location of the self in relation to body and society is culture-specific (Shweder and Bourne, 1982). The Western concept of person is based on the experience of an inner world. This inner world is a social construction that comes into being by subordinating the body to its willful plans. The Western norm for the psychological expression of distress follows from the need to give an account of the vagaries of the body that supports the central role of the inner world of the person.

Experiences of distress and illness have an exemplary role in the differentiation of bodily and social aspects of the self. Pain and strong emotion make one acutely aware of the body. Speaking of one's relationship to the body opens up a distance between the sensory quality of pain and psychological suffering. In that gap there is room for a self that imagines itself superordinate to the body. Thus, one can be more or less identified with one's body and may seek to dis-identify with the body to escape its pain.

Pain and emotion also alter the experience of interpersonal relationships. Chronically ill people, debilitated by physical suffering, may experience others as irritating and withdraw into themselves with an exaggerated sense of isolation and interiority. The self is taken up with the task of managing the unruly body and is unavailable for social intercourse. Preoccupation with the body can then become a shield against the continuing failure of relationships to succor and heal.

Western values of autonomy and self-efficacy imply psychological control of the social presentation of the body. Health is a sign of self-mastery. When illness supervenes, psychologization is a way to preserve the omnipotence of the social self. In this context, to somatize is to recognize the primacy of the body and declare the limits of self-control and social responsiblity. According to prevailing social norms one may then be judged as either sick or immoral.

The somatizing person's rejection of psychological explanation makes it uncertain whether they should be judged responsible for their illness. The moral confusion that surrounds somatization can be seen in sex-role differences in the diagnosis of somatoform disorders. Women with unexplained somatic symptoms are likely to be viewed as not responsible for their actions and hence psychologically ill, while men with similar symptoms are more likely to be viewed as willfully malingering for material gain (Winstead, 1984). In allowing that people with functional symptoms are ill we tend to deprive them of rationality and view them as morally weak (Kirmayer, in press). The somatizing patient claims the prerogatives of the sick role but achieves instead the role of psychiatric patient with its heavy weight of perjoration.

## CONCLUSIONS

The term somatization suffers from inflation. Extended over a broad territory that includes most of psychosomatic medicine, it would be better restricted to those processes that bias the experience and expression of distress toward an emphasis on somatic symptoms.

Most current research on somatization tends to evade basic epistemological and pragmatic issues, adopting the view that somatization is a process that resides entirely within the patient. But somatization is a concept of interest only to psychosocially oriented practitioners. The clinical recognition of somatization depends on a discrepancy between patients' illness experiences and clinicians' expectations for emotionally expressive behaviour. Somatization is thus rooted in a conflict between competing interpretations of illness. This can arise from difficulties in doctor-patient negotiation or a social organization of the sick role that compels people to adopt somatic styles for the expression of distress to legitimate their efforts to find help. Somatization is irreducibly social in nature.

In the explanation of human behaviour, reasons can be causes (Harre, Clarke and DeCarlo, 1985). Patients' own accounts of their problems are not simply data about illness behaviour - their idiosyncratic response to the univocal (biological) reality of their disease. The beliefs held by an individual influence every stage of illness experience from the perceptual organization of unusual bodily sensations, to their objectification as symptoms indicating illness, to the directed search for appropriate help.

The clinical reality is that when a person suffers from somatic symptoms and organizes his/her distress (social, psychic or existential) around these bodily concerns, one is in conflict with the person's mode of constructing illness meaning if one attempts to redirect their bodily suffering to some other realm (Good and Good, 1980). Reinterpreting somatic distress as psychosocial will prove helpful only if the person has the intrapsychic and social resources to utilize an alternate framework. In the absence of empirical demonstrations of such benefits, the effort to subjugate a person's bodily experience to a psychological or social preoccupation may be the imposition of an alien system of values. The analysis of the efficacy of psychological or social interpretation rests on demonstrations that such specific cognizing has beneficial psychological and/or physiological effects (e.g., denial versus confession). The analysis of its social efficacy rests on understanding the implications of situating distress in various locations. As psychic suffering, it is contained within the person who may consequently be invalidated and rendered still more powerless. As social suffering, it constitutes a challenge or threat to the established social order and is a tactic to be used only cautiously by the powerless and disenfranchised.

Suffering, inchoate at first, must be organized, named and categorized in ways that are intelligible to self and others. But misery does not respect the Cartesian categories of medical care. Physical pain invites fear and depression. The psychic conflicts of everyday life yield headaches and heavy hearts. Still, Western civilization is heavily invested in the psychologization of suffering - in the assimilation of all distress - bodily and social - into the inner arena of the person. It is our tacit acceptance of the psychological perspective that leads to a fascination with somatization as deviant.


## ACKNOWLEDGEMENTS

The author thanks Jim Robbins for his help at every stage of this work.


## REFERENCES


American Psychiatric Association. (1980). Diagnostic and statistical manual (3rd ed.). Washington: American Psychiatric Association.

Anderson, C. D. (1981). Expression of affect and physiological response in psychosomatic patients. Journal of Psychosomatic Research, 25, 143-149.

Bennett, R. M. (1981). Fibrositis: Misnomer for a common rheumatic disorder. Western Journal of Medicine, 134, 405-413.

Blackwell, B. (1967). Upper middle class adult expectations about entering the sick role for physical and psychiatric dysfunctions. Journal of Health and Social Behavior, 8, 83-95.

Block, A. (1981). An investigation of the response of the spouse to chronic pain behavior. Psychosomatic Medicine, 43, 415-422.

Blumer, D., & Heilbronn, M. (1982). Chronic pain as a variant of depressive disease. Journal of Nervous and Mental Disease, 170, 381-406.

Bohman, M., Cloninger, C. R., von Knorring, A. L., & Sigvardsson, S. (1984). An adoption study of somatoform disorders: III. Cross-fostering analysis and genetic relationship to alcoholism and criminality. Archives of General Psychiatry, 41, 863-871.

Buck, R. (1980). Nonverbal behavior and the theory of emotion: The facial feedback hypothesis. Journal of Personality and Social Psychology, 38, 811-824.

Bursten, B. (1985). Medication nonadherence due to feelings of loss of control in "biological depression". American Journal of Psychiatry, 142, 244-246.

Cadoret, R., Widmer, R. B., & Troughton, E. P. (1980). Somatic complaints: Harbinger of depression in primary care. Journal of Affective Disorders. 2, 61-70.

Cannon, W. B. (1929). Bodily changes in pain, hunger, fear and rage (2nd ed.). New York: Harper & Row.

Carlson, G. A., & Cantwell, D. P. (1980). Unmasking masked depression in children and adolescents. American Journal of Psychiatry, 137, 445-449.

Carver, C. S. (1979). A cybernetic model of self-attention processes. Journal of Personality and Social Psychology, 37, 1251-1281.

Cloninger, C. R., Sigvardsson, S., von Knorring, A. L., & Bohman, M. (1984). An adoption study of somatoform disorders: II. Identification of two discrete somatoform disorders. Archives of General Psychiatry, 41, 863-871.

Crandell, D. L., & Dohrenwend, B. P. (1967). Some relations among psychiatric symptoms, organic illness, and social class. American Journal of Psychiatry, 123, 1527-1537.
Davidson, R. J., & Schwartz, G. E. (1976). The psychophysiology of relaxation and related states: A multi-process theory. In D. I. Mostofsky (Ed.), Behavior control and modification of physiological activity (pp. 399-442). Englewood-Cliffs, NJ: Prentice-Hall.
DeGood, D. E., Buckelew, S. P., & Tait, R. C. (1985). Cognitive-somatic anxiety response patterning in chronic pain patients and nonpatients. Journal of Consulting and Clinical Psychology, 53, 137-138.
De Marco, R. (1984). Relationships between physical and psychological symptomatology in the 22-item Langner's scale. Social Science and Medicine, 19, 59-65.
Dolce, J. J., & Raczynski, J. M. (1985). Neuromuscular activity and electromyography in painful backs: Psychological and biomechanical models in assessment and treatment. Psychological Bulletin, 97, 502-520.
Eisenberg, L. (1977). Disease and illness: Distinctions between professional and popular ideas of sickness. Culture, Medicine and Psychiatry, 1, 9-23.
Ekman, P. (1972). Universals and cultural differences in facial expressions of emotion. Nebraska symposium on motivation. Lincoln: University of Nebraska Press.
Engel, G. L. (1959). "Psychogenic" pain and the pain-prone patient. American Journal of Medicine, 26, 899-918.
Fenigstein, A., Scheier, M. F., & Buss, A. H. (1975). Public and private self-consciousness: Assessment and theory. Journal of Consulting and Clinical Psychology, 43, 522-527.
Flor, H., Turk, D. C., & Birbaumer, N. (1985). Assessment of stress-related psychophysiological reactions in chronic back pain patients. Journal of Consulting and Clinical Psychology, 53, 354-364.
Ford, C. V. (1983). The somatizing disorders: Illness as a way of life. New York: Elsevier.
Fordyce, W. E. (1978). Learning processes in pain. In R. A. Sternbach (Ed.), The psychology of pain. New York : Raven Press.
Good, B. J. (1977). The heart of what's the matter: The semantics of illness in Iran. Culture, Medicine and Psychiatry, 1, 25-58.
Good, B. J., Good, M. J. (1980). The meaning of symptoms: A cultural-hermeneutic model for clinical practice. In L. Eisenberg, & A. Kleinman (Eds.), The relevance of social science for medicine (pp. 165-196). Dordrecht, Holland: Reidel.
Goodwin, D. W., & Guze, S. B. (1983). Psychiatric diagnosis (3rd ed.). Oxford University Press.
Greden, J. F., Genero, N., & Price, H. L. (1985). Agitation-increased electromyogram activity in the corrugator muscle region: A possible explanation of the "omega sign"? American Journal of Psychiatry, 142, 348-351.
Grings, W. W., & Dawson, M. E. (1978). Emotions and bodily responses: A psychophysiological approach. New York: Academic Press.
Hall, R. C. W., Gardner, E. R., Stickney, S. K., et al. (1980). Physical illness manifesting as psychiatric disease. Archives of General Psychiatry, 37, 985-989.
Hanback, J. W., & Revelle, W. (1978). Arousal and perceptual sensitivity in hypochondriasis. Journal of Abnormal Psychology, 87, 523-530.
Harre, R., Clarke, D., & De Carlo, N. (1985). Motives and mechanisms: An introduction to the psychology of action. London: Methuen.
Hesse, P., & Cichetti, D. (1982). Perspectives on an integrated theory of emotional development. In D. Ciccheti & P. Hesse (Eds.), Emotional development. San Francisco: Jossey Bass.
Hudson, J. I., Hudson, M. S., Pliner, L. F., Goldenberg, D. L., & Pope, H. J. Jr. (1985). Fibromyalgia and major affective disorder: A controlled phenomenology and family history study. American Journal of Psychiatry, 142, 441-446.

Jefferson, J. W., & Marshall, J. R. (1981). Neuropsychiatric features of medical disorders. New York: Plenum Press.

Kaminsky, M. J., & Slavney, P. R. (1983). Hysterical and obsessional features in patients with Briquet's syndrome (somatization disorder). Psychological Medicine, 13, 111-120.

Katon, W., Kleinman, A., & Rosen, G. (1982). Depression and somatization: A review. I & II. American Journal of Medicine, 72, 127-135 & 241-247.

Kellner, R. (1985). Functional somatic symptoms and hypochondriasis. Archives of General Psychiatry, 42, 821-833.

Kellner, R., & Sheffield, B. F. (1973). The one week prevalence of symptoms in neurotic patients and normals. American Journal of Psychiatry, 130, 102-105.

Kenyon, F. E. (1976). Hypochondriacal states. British Journal of Psychiatry, 129, 1-14.

Kirmayer, L. J. (1984). Culture, affect and somatization. I & II. Transcultural Psychiatric Research Review, 21, 159-188 & 21, 237-262.

Kirmayer, L. J. (in press). Mind and body as metaphors: Hidden values in biomedicine. In M. Lock & D. Gordon (Eds.), Knowledge and practice in medicine. Dordrecht, Holland: D. Reidel.

Kleinman, A. (1977). Depression, somatization and the "new cross-cultural psychiatry". Social Science and Medicine, 11, 3-10.

Kleinman, A. (1980). Patients and healers in the context of culture. Berkeley: University of California Press.

Kleinman, A. (1982). Neurasthenia and depression: A study of somatization and culture in China. Culture, Medicine and Psychiatry, 6, 117-190.

Kleinman, A., & Kleinman, J. (1985). Somatization: The interconnections among culture, depressive experiences, and the meanings of pain. A study in Chinese society. In A. Kleinman & B. Good (Eds.), Culture and depression. Berkeley: University of California Press.

Lakoff, G., & Johnson, M. (1980). Metaphors we live by. Chicago: University of Chicago Press.

Lanzetta, J. T., Cartwright-Smith, J., & Kleck, R. E. (1976). Effects of nonverbal dissimulation on emotional experience and autonomic arousal. Journal of Personality and Social Psychology, 33, 354-370.

Lazarus, R. S., & Folkman, S. (1984). Stress, appraisal, and coping. New York: Springer.

Lesse, S. (1974). Hypochondriasis and psychosomatic disorders masking depression. In S. Lesse (Ed.), Masked depression (pp. 53-74). New York: Aronson.

Lesser, I. M., Ford, C. V., & Friedmann, C. T. H. (1979). Alexithymia in somatizing patients. General Hospital Psychiatry, 1, 256-261.

Lesser, I. M., & Lesser, B. Z. (1983). Alexithymia: Examining the development of a psychological concept. American Journal of Psychiatry, 140, 1305-1308.

Leventhal, H. (1979). A perceptual-motor processing model of emotion. In P. Pliner, K. R. Blankstein, & I. M. Spigel (Eds.), Perception of emotion of self and others. New York: Plenum Press.

Leventhal, H., Nerenz, D. R., & Straus, A. (1982). Self-regulation and the mechanisms for symptom appraisal. In D. Mechanic (Ed.), Symptoms, illness behavior and help-seeking (pp. 55-86). New York: Watson.

Levi-Strauss, C. (1966). The savage mind. Chicago: University of Chicago Press.

Lipkin, M., & Lamb, G. (1982). The couvade syndrome: An epidemiologic study. Annals of Internal Medicine, 96, 509-511.

Lipowski, Z. J. (1968). Review of consultation psychiatry and psychosomatic medicine. III. Theoretical issues. Psychosomatic Medicine, 30, 395-422.

Lock, M. (1978). East Asian medicine in urban Japan. Berkeley: University of California Press.

Mandler, G. (1984). Mind and body. New York: Norton.

Marsella, A. (1981). Depressive experience and disorder across cultures. In H. C. Triandis, & J. W. Berry (Eds.), Handbook of cross-cultural psychology, Vol. 6. Boston: Allyn & Bacon.

Mathew, R. J., Weinman, M. L., & Mirabi, M. (1981). Physical symptoms of depression. British Journal of Psychiatry, 139, 293-296.
Mechanic, D. (1972). Social psychologic factors affecting the presentation of bodily complaints. New England Journal of Medicine, 286, 1132-1139.
Miller, L. C., Murphy, R., & Buss, A. H. (1981). Consciousness of body: Private and public. Journal of Personality and Social Psychology, 41, 397-406.
Minuchin, S., Baker, L., Rosman, B., Leibman, R., Milman, L., & Todd, T. A. (1975). Conceptual model of psychosomatic illness in children. Archives of General Psychiatry, 32, 1031-1038.
Morakinyo, O. (1980). A psychophysiological theory of a psychiatric illness (the brain fag syndrome) associated with study among Africans. Journal of Nervous and Mental Disease, 168, 84-89.
Morakinyo, O. (1985). Phobic states presenting as somatic complaint syndromes in Nigeria: Socio-cultural factors associated with diagnosis and psychotherapy. Acta Psychiatrica Scandinavia, 71, 356-365.
Nelson, J. C., Charney, D. S. (1981). The symptoms of major depressive illness. American Journal of Psychiatry, 138, 1-13.
Nemiah, H. (1985). Somatoform disorders. In H. I. Kaplan, & B. J. Sadock (Eds.), Comprehensive textbook of psychiatry (pp. 924-942). (4th ed.). Baltimore: Williams & Wilkins.
Nichter, M. (1981). Idioms of distress: Alternatives in the expression of psychosocial distress: A case study from South India. Culture, Medicine and Psychiatry, 5, 379-408.
Neilsen, A. C., & Williams, T. A. (1980). Depression in ambulatory medical patients: Prevalence by self-report questionnaire and recognition by nonpsychiatric physicians. Archives of General Psychiatry, 37, 999-1004.
Ohnuki-Tierney, E. (1984). Illness and culture in contemporary Japan: An anthropological view. Cambridge University Press.
Pennebaker, J. W. (1982). The psychology of physical symptoms. New York: Springer.
Pennebaker, J. W. (1985). Traumatic experience and psychosomatic disease: Exploring the roles of behavioural inhibition, obsession, and confiding. Canadian Psychology, 26, 82-95.
Pennebaker, J. W., & Skelton, J. A. (1978). Psychological parameters of physical symptoms. Personality and Social Psychology Bulletin, 4, 524-530.
Perley, & Guze, S. (1962). Hysteria - the stability and usefulness of clinical criteria. New England Journal of Medicine, 266, 421-426.
Pilowksy, I. (1967). Dimensions of hypochondriasis. British Journal of Psychiatry, 113, 89-93.
Prince, R. (1960). The "brain fag" syndrome in Nigerian students. Journal of Mental Science, 106, 559-570.
Quill, T. E., Lipkin, M., & Lamb, G. S. (1984). Health-care seeking by men in their spouse's pregnancy. Psychosomatic Medicine, 46, 277-283.
Robins, L. N., & Helzer, J. E. (1982). Diagnostic interview schedule. (Reply to a letter to the editor.) Archives of General Psychiatry, 39, 1443-1445.
Robins, L, N., Helzer, J. E., Croughon, J., & Ratcliff, K. W. (1981). National Institute of Mental Health diagnostic interview schedule. Archives of General Psychiatry, 38, 381-389.
Romano, J. M., & Turner, J. A. (1985). Chronic pain and depression: Does the evidence support a relationship? Psychological Bulletin, 97(1), 18-34.
Ross, E. D., & Rush, A. J. (1981). Diagnosis and neuroanatomical correlates of depression in brain damaged patients: Implications for a neurology of depression. Archives of General Psychiatry, 38, 1344-1354.
Schwartz, G. E., Davidson, R. J., & Goleman, D. J. (1978). Patterning of cognitive and somatic processes in the self-regulation of anxiety: Effects of meditation versus exercise. Psychosomatic Medicine, 40, 321-328.
Shapiro, M. F., & Lehman, A. F. (1983). The diagnosis of depression in different clinical settings: An analysis of the literature on the dexamethasone suppression test. Journal of Nervous and Mental Disease, 17, 714-720.
Shields, S. A., & Stern, R. M. (1979). The perception of bodily change. In

P. Pliner, K. R. Blankstein, & I. M. Spigel (Eds.), Perception of emotion in self and others (pp. 85-106). New York: Plenum Press.
Shultz, T. R. (1982). Rules of causal attribution. Monographs of the Society for Research in Child Development. 47, 1-51.
Shweder, R., & Bourne, E. (1982). Do conceptions of the person vary cross-culturally? In A. Marsella, & G. White (Eds.), Cultural conceptions of mental health and therapy (pp. 97-137). Dordrecht, Holland: Reidel.
Sicherman, B. (1977). The uses of a diagnosis: Doctors, patients and neurasthenia. Journal of the History of Medicine and Allied Sciences, 32, 33-54.
Sifneos, P. E. (1973). The prevalence of 'alexithymic' characteristics in psychosomatic patients. Psychotherapy and Psychosomatics, 22, 255-262.
Sigvardsson, S., von Knorring, A. L., Bohman, M., & Cloninger, C. R. (1984). An adoption study of somatoform disorders. Archives of General Psychiatry, 41, 853-859.
Spence, N. D., Pilowsky, I., & Minniti, R. (1985). The attribution of affect in pain clinic patients: A psychophysiological study of the conversion process. International Journal of Psychiatry in Medicine, 15, 1-11.
Tollefson, G., & Straud, L., Hughes, E., & Garvey, M. G. (1984). The functional-organic dichotomy in new patient evaluations by residents in family practice. Comprehensive Psychiatry, 25, 419-425.
Turk, D. C., & Salovey, P. (1984). "Chronic pain as a variant of depressive disease": A critical reappraisal. Journal of Nervous and Mental Disease, 172, 398-404.
Vaughn, K. B., Lanzetta, J. T. (1980). Vicarious instigation and conditioning of facial expressive and autonomic responses to a model's expressive display of pain. Journal of Personality and Social Psychology, 38, 909-923.
Wells, J. A., & Strickland, D. E. (1982). Physiogenic bias as invalidity in psychiatric symptom scales. Journal of Health and Social Behavior, 23, 235-252.
Wheaton, B. (1982). Uses and abuses of the Langner Index: A re-examination of findings on psychological and psychophysiological distress. In D. Mechanic (Ed.), Symptoms, illness behavior and help-seeking (pp. 25-54). New York: Prodist.
White, G. (1982). The role of cultural explanation in "psychologization" and "somatization". Social Science and Medicine, 16, 1519-1530.
Whybrow, P., Akiskal, H, & McKinney, W. T. (1983). Mood disorders. Plenum Press.
Widmer, R. B., & Cadoret, R. J. (1978). Depression in family practice: changes in pattern of patient visits and complaints during a developing depression. Journal of Family Practice, 7, 293-302.
Widmer, R. B., & Cadoret, R. J. (1979). Depression in family practice: Changes in pattern of patient visits and complaints during subsequent developing depression. Journal of Family Practice, 9, 1017-1021.
Winner, E., Rosenstiel, A., & Gardner, H. (1976). The development of metaphoric understanding. Developmental Psychology, 12, 289-297.
Winstead, B. A. (1984). Hysteria. In C. S. Widom (Ed.), Sex roles and psychopathology (pp. 73-100) New York: Plenum Press.
Young, A. (1981). When rational men fall sick. Culture, Medicine and Psychiatry, 5, 317-335.
Zajonc, R. (1982). On the primacy of feeling. American Psychologist, 39(2), 117-123.
Zajonc, R. B. (1985). Emotion and facial efference: A theory reclaimed. Science, 228, 15-21.

# SEX DIFFERENCES IN THE USE OF HEALTH SERVICES

Ronald Kessler

Institute for Social Research
The University of Michigan

It is widely known that women have much higher rates of physician utilization than men. This is true even when pregnancy-related visits are taken out of consideration (Nathanson, 1977). It might be that this difference accurately describes the higher rates of ill health experienced by women, but proponents of an illness behaviour perspective argue that it also reflects a more active female response to symptoms (Mechanic, 1976). This argument is consistent with the fact that women are much more likely than men to present with complaints of mild symptoms (Verbrugge, 1976). Discretion in seeking professional help for symptoms of this sort is high (Mechanic, 1978).

Until recently, there was little direct evidence about sex differences in response to illness. Indeed, as recently as 1979 a major review article concluded that such evidence was for the most part limited to mental symptoms and noncontemporary periods (Vergrugge, 1979). Despite the availability of relevant data in a number of health surveys, the implications of these data for the study of sex differences were largely unexplored.

The situation has changed in the past few years. A number of investigators have begun to explore the empirical evidence. A review of this work shows a number of consistent results, and a critical analysis shows that there are some much needed correctives which should be implemented if remaining uncertainties are to be resolved.

## BASIC ASSOCIATIONS

First, the basic association between sex and response to ill health will be considered. Theoretical discussions for over a decade have assumed that women more actively seek help for medical problems than men. The task of the theoretical work has been to account for this sex difference. Yet until recently there was no firm evidence that such a difference actually exists. Even now there is controversy. One recent review, for example, asserted that "women and men with comparable health problems and work roles seek out medical care and restrict their activities at the same pace. Thus, men are not delayers compared to women" (Vergrugge, 1985a). If this is true, then there is little reason to speculate about illness behaviour factors.

Three main types of empirical studies have been carried out to address this issue. The first, and most common, are general population surveys of self-reported health and physician contact. The second are similar surveys which use information obtained from medical examinations rather than self-reports to measure health. And the third are treatment population studies which focus on delay in treatment. Evidence from all three types of studies will be reviewed.

Self-report Surveys

A number of large-scale surveys have been conducted to analyze the determinants of physician utilization. Many of these were guided by a conceptual scheme developed by Andersen and his associates (1975), which looks on utilization as a joint function of predisposing, enabling and need variables. Predisposing variables provide motivation to seek care while enabling variables provide the resources to do so. The importance of these variables independent of actual need for services is a central focus of research using this framework.

Andersen and his colleagues have conducted several large-scale studies of physician utilization. For example, one of these surveys is based on a representative national sample of 3,880 families comprising nearly 12,000 individuals (Andersen, Kravits, and Anderson, 1975). Another is based on national data from almost 8,000 individuals (Andersen and Aday, 1978). These data have been extensively analyzed and show clearly that the main determinants of utilization are the measures of need. The overall effects of the predisposing and enabling factors are small when the need variables are controlled.

The same general result has been reported in a number of other large-scale self-report studies of physician utilization. Kohn and White's (1976) international study of utilization in seven countries found that variables other than need accounted for trivial variance in physician service use. The same result was found by Wolinsky (1978) in an analysis of the Health Interview Survey and by Wilensky and Cafferata (1983) in an analysis of the National Medical Care Expenditure Survey.

A problem with using the results of these large utilization surveys to make inferences about sex differences is that they have generally used analysis strategies which are biased against finding such differences. This fact can be documented indirectly by noting that the several investigations which have explicitly examined self-report survey data to see if sex differences in response to illness exist have all found such differences. The discrepancy in results might stem from the fact that these special studies of sex differences used inappropriate analysis methods. These studies include either prediction equations that allow for interactions between sex and self-reported health or analysis schemes which study the effect of sex separately within subsamples of respondents who report symptoms. The general purpose utilization studies, in contrast, never focus on detailed specifications of this sort.

One of the most persuasive self-report studies which examined sex differences explicitly was carried out by Marcus and Siegal (1982). They considered a subsample of respondents in a community health survey who reported either some chronic condition or recent acute symptoms. The authors found that women were more likely to have sought professional help than men among those with chronic conditions but not among those with acute conditions.

Kessler (1981) studied help-seeking for emotional problems. This study was conducted in a university community and focused on seeking help from the student psychiatric clinic. The analysis showed that a greater proportion of female than male students with self-reported emotional problems sought help at the clinic.

An analysis of four large-scale general population surveys found results consistent with these. Women in these studies sought psychiatric help more often than men with comparable levels of self-reported distress (Kessler, Brown, and Broman, 1981).

The psychiatric help-seeking surveys also showed sex differences in obtaining psychiatric help to be more pronounced among people with mild symptoms than among those whose symptoms were more extreme. This result is consistent with the notion that discretionary influences on help-seeking should be greatest when the symptoms are sufficiently benign that help is not definitely required. This specification appears in other studies that have examined symptom severity as will be seen below.

The critical feature of all these studies is that the analysis is confined to the subsample of respondents with self-defined illness. As noted, the standard approach in general purpose utilization surveys is to work with the total sample including those who report no symptoms, to use reports of symptoms as predictor variables in a multiple regression equation, and to assume additive effects between symptoms and other predictors. This approach, especially the assumption about additive effects, cannot be correct if there are systematic sex differences in response to perceived illness.

It is important to note that researchers who analyze general purpose utilization surveys are aware that non-additive effects are possible. They commonly check to see if the additivity assumption can be supported by the data. However, these omnibus tests fail to recognize the special importance of interactions involving the measures of perceived illness. The typical search for interaction, not guided by theory, (Andersen et al., 1975) and global evaluations of multiple interactions concurrently (Wolinsky, 1978) are both hopelessly inadequate. These strategies have extremely low statistical power, virtually no precision in their ability to evaluate the existence of specific interactions, and consequently can be expected to yield negative evidence for overall nonadditivity.

A much better understanding of sex differences in response to perceived illness could be obtained if these general purpose utilization surveys were reanalyzed with sensitive methods that searched systematically for subgroup effects among respondents who reported symptoms. There is a massive amount of relevant information available in these surveys which remains almost entirely unexamined in this critical way.

## Health Examination Studies

Concerns have been raised about the comparative validity of self-report illness measures among men and women (Mechanic, 1979). This concern is resolved in surveys which measure illness with medical examinations and biomedical tests assessed blind to the sex and self-reported health status of the respondent.

Surprisingly, almost no attempt has been made to carry out analyses of this sort. By far the most extensive survey available for this type of analysis is the National Health and Nutrition Examination Survey (NHANES) which provides information about self-reported health and recent doctor visits along with information obtained in physician examinations and a variety of biomedical tests (Miller, 1973).

One investigation which used NHANES to study sex differences in this way focused on osteoarthrosis (Davis, 1981). The NHANES included radiographic examinations which were rated independently by two rheumatologists who were blind to the respondents' sex and self-reported symptoms. A measure of osteoarthrosis was generated from the combined ratings and compared to the respondents' self-reports about knee pain.

Davis' study is generally cited as providing evidence that the relationship between "true" pain and self-reports is the same for men and women (Gove, 1984; Verbrugge, 1985a). However, a very substantial sex difference is apparent in Davis' data which neither she nor the subsequent reviewers of her paper have noted. Nearly twice as many women as men (21 percent versus 12 percent) with objective evidence of osteoarthrosis reported recent physician contact for this problem.

Furthermore, there is an intriguing interaction in the data between self-reported knee pain and service utilization. Among those who reported recent knee pain the sex difference in service utilization is considerably smaller than among those who did not report such pain. (1) In other words, the overall sex difference in the likelihood of seeking professional help for this objectively defined medical problem is most pronounced among people with the most benign symptoms. This result is consistent with the specification reported by Kessler (1981) and Kessler et al. (1981) in self-report studies of psychiatric help-seeking.

The National Institute of Mental Health has recently completed a series of Epidemiologic Catchment Area (ECA) studies which provide comparable information about psychiatric help-seeking. A structured psychiatric interview schedule was developed for this set of surveys (Robins, Helzer, Croughan, and Ratcliff, 1981) and administered to nearly 20,000 adult respondents across five separate community sample sites (Regier et al., 1984). These data show quite convincingly that there are sex differences in help-seeking for major psychiatric disorders. In each of the three ECA sites currently available for analysis, women with recent psychiatric disorders were consistently more likely than men to report some type of recent treatment (Shapiro et al., 1984).

The ECA data also show that women with psychiatric impairments are much more likely than comparable men to seek help from the general medical sector rather than from a mental health professional. This fact almost certainly compounds the already formidable difficulties faced by researchers who seek to determine whether primary care visits made by men and women are equally linked to genuine medical disorders.

The ECA evidence on sex differences in location of treatment might also reflect physician differences in handling complaints presented by men and women. A recent analysis of data obtained in the National Ambulatory Medical Care Survey found that primary care physicians who are confronted with a patient whose main complaint is mental distress are likely to refer the patient to a mental health specialist if the patient is male but to treat her with mild tranqilizers if she is a female (Verbrugge, 1984). This type of differential physician response to male and female patients makes it even more difficult to study the patient's response to illness.

### Delay in Treatment Studies

A third group of studies focus on samples of patients under treatment for a particular medical problem. In general, studies of this sort find that men and women do not differ in the speed with which they seek treatment for life-threatening or serious acute conditions. Among people in treatment, however, women take more time off for the problem and are more likely to quit

---

1. Among the former, 38 percent of women and 23 percent of men sought physician services for the knee problems - a female:male ratio of 1.65. Among those respondents without recent pain, eight percent of women and two percent of men with objective evidence of impairment sought professional care - a female:male ration of 4.00.

employment outside the home (Brown and Rawlinson, 1977; Chirikos and Nestel, 1985; Chirikos and Nickel, 1984; Marshall, Gregorio, and Walsh, 1982).

It is important to note that this type of study is confined to conditions which are so serious that all people who truly have the condition eventually come into contact with the medical care system. It is consistent with the illness behaviour perspective that sex differences in speed of seeking initial help would be minimal for conditions of this sort (Mechanic, 1978).

### An Overview of Basic Associations

Two tentative conclusions can be made from the data reviewed above. First, there is no evidence that men and women with life-threatening or serious acute health problems differ in the speed with which they seek professional help. Second, there is evidence that women with less dramatic health problems are more likely than their male counterparts to seek professional help. This has been documented for two objectively measured conditions - chronic osteoarthrosis and major psychiatric disorder. It has also been documented in self-report studies of psychiatric distress and perceived physical illness.

The evidence for differential response to perceived physical illness has been more strongly documented for chronic than acute symptoms (Marcus and Siegel, 1982). Further, treatment population studies have shown that women more persistently care for their conditions than men even though they do not differ in speed of initial contact. These results raise the issue of whether evidence about sex differences in response reflect differences in the likelihood of making an inital contact, a follow-up visit, or both. General population studies of self-reported utilization do not distinguish these types of contact even though the theorectical and policy importance of the two differ greatly.

## HYPOTHESES ABOUT SEX DIFFERENCES IN HELP-SEEKING

A great many hypotheses have been advanced to account for sex differences in physician utilization. The hypotheses having to do with illness behaviour can be conveniently organized into four categories (Verbrugge, 1985a). Men and women could differ in their (1) recognition of symptoms, (2) interpretation of symptoms as sufficiently serious to warrant medical attention, (3) psychological readiness to seek professional help, and (4) ability to do so. Some evidence is available about each of these hypotheses.

### Recognition/Reporting of Symptoms

The main argument here is that women might be more sensitive than men to bodily symptoms and thereby more likely to recognize and seek help for a symptom. Mechanic (1979) has argued that differences of this sort could explain why self-report studies of perceived illness sometimes fail to find sex differences in response, because the self-reports of women capture their more sensitive recognition of symptoms and give the appearance that women have more illness when they actually differ from men more in their recognition of symptoms.

To test this possibility empirically, Mechanic and his associates have developed a scale to measure introspectiveness. Their research shows clearly that among adolescents, girls are more likely than boys to introspect (Hansell and Mechanic, in press). There is as yet no evidence, though, as to whether this helps explain sex differences in symptom reporting.

There is reason to believe that introspectiveness, or some related psychological characteristic, is an important determinant of symptom recognition and reporting. Pennebaker (1982) has demonstrated that experimental manipulation of symptom sensitivity can affect symptom reporting. Hansell and Mechanic's work may be able to demonstrate that introspectiveness is associated with more stable differences of this sort.

There is some indirect evidence that the perception of symptoms is affected by factors other than true health status and that these influences could affect women more than men. Tessler and Mechanic (1978) reported data from four surveys which showed that self-reported perceptions of physical health are affected by psychological well-being. Women have considerably lower rates of well being than men (Gove, 1978) and this means that sex differences in self-reported physical illness might be distorted by this influence.

A direct evaluation of this potential bias would require us to obtain information about true health independent of self-reports. As noted earlier, Davis (1981) conducted an investigation of this sort using data from the NHANES. She found that symptom recognition for osteoarthrosis was similar for men and women. The NHANES contains information which could be used to provide a more broad-based assessment than this, but these data have not yet been used for this purpose.

Other types of validation studies are also possible if the focus of attention is shifted to the comparative validity of self-reported illness measures. The most detailed work on this issue has been done by Cannell and his associates. In one of their studies, health plan enrollees were interviewed in a household survey to determine how accurately they reported chronic conditions which were recorded in their medical records. Respondents did not know that the interviewer had access to these records nor that any attempt was being made to validate their reports. No evidence was found for a sex difference in the accuracy of self-reports (Cannell, 1967). (2)

On a related point, there is no evidence that men and women differ in their willingness to disclose symptoms which might be embarrassing. Gove and his associates (Gove and Geerken, 1977; Gove, McCorkel, and Hughes, 1976) carried out extensive internal validity analyses of various response scales in relation to self-report measures of psychological distress and found no meaningful sex differences.

Furthermore, there is no evidence that men and women differ in the accuracy of retrospective reports about doctor visits. Cannell and Fowler (1965) investigated this issue by interviewing a sample of people known to have made recent doctor visits. The comparison of self-reports showed that men and women do not differ in the accuracy of their retrospective reports about doctor visits.

However, an important caution is in order. In their most recent work, Cannell and his associates have conducted experimental investigations in which respondents to the Health Interview Survey were randomly assigned either to face-to-face or telephone interviews. Analysis showed that self-reports about health as well as about doctor visits are influenced by mode of administration among women but not among men (Cannell, Groves, Magilavy, Mathiowetz, and Miller, 1982). Sex differences are significantly larger when data are collected over the phone than when they are collected face-to-face. This means that the comparability of male and female report accuracy

---

2. Cleary and Jette (1984) present independent data consistent with this conclusion.

documented in validation studies of face-to-face interviews would not be maintained in telephone interviews. Fortunately most utilization surveys have been conducted in face-to-face interviews so far, so this problem is presently more potential than real.

More detailed information about symptom recognition would be very helpful. The evidence reviewed actually describes more about the relationship between validated reports and self-reports than about recognition itself. The effects of selective recall, differential willingness to disclose private information to interviewers, or some other factors unrelated to symptom recognition might be operating here.

Unfortunately, accurate information about the complex perceptions people have about their bodily sensations is too subtle to be obtained with the conventional methods of survey analysis. A serious effort to study sex differences in recognition will almost certainly require more highly specialized methods of validation and data collection.

## Interpretation of Symptoms

The argument here is that women are more likely than men to interpret perceived symptoms as sufficiently serious to warrant medical intervention. Several reasons for this putative difference have been isolated, including that women have more knowledge about signs and symptoms, are more willing to confront the implications of symptoms, and are more concerned about their health (Verbrugge, 1985a).

This set of hypotheses is considerably easier to study than hypotheses about symptom recognition. Yet there is virtually no evidence about sex differences in symptom interpretation. One study focused on symptoms of psychological distress and psychiatric help-seeking. In each of four large-scale surveys the analysis documented that the perception of needing help strongly mediated the relationship between distress and professional help-seeking (Kessler et al., 1981).

Further analysis of these data showed that women in distress are more likely than men to perceive themselves as needing help. Furthermore, this sex difference is most pronounced among people experiencing moderate or mild rather than extreme levels of distress.

This specification is consistent with the interaction found by Davis (1981) between severity of knee pain and sex differences in doctor visits for osteoarthrosis. Patterns of this sort support the idea that discretion in the interpretation of symptoms is greatest in situations where symptoms are most benign.

## Psychological Readiness

The argument here is that women are socialized in such a way that they more readily adopt the sick role than men. Numerous beliefs and attitudes have been cited as instances of such sex differences (Mechanic, 1976; Nathanson, 1977).

A great deal of inferential evidence consistent with this hypothesis has been found in health surveys. There have been several investigations of children which show that willingness to adopt the sick role is more common among girls than boys even at early ages (Campbell, 1978; Lewis, Lewis and Lorimer, 1977; Mechanic, 1965; Nader and Brink, 1981). Studies among adults have documented similar results. Women report a greater tendency to consult physicians for hypothetical physical health problems (Cleary, Mechanic, and Greenley, 1982), and they are more likely to believe in the efficacy of medical intervention (Depner, 1981).

Despite this consistency, there is no firm evidence that psychological readiness plays a part in the more active physician utilization by women. Unfortunately, all of the research which has examined this issue has used additive multiple regression analysis, which is an insensitive procedure unlikely to yield strong evidence of an effect. This is so because additive regression analysis makes the unrealistic assumption that psychological propensity is equally important in predicting utilization no matter what level of perceived symptoms the person has. It is little surprise, then, that the major investigations of the predictive power of psychological readiness have concluded that beliefs and attitudes of this sort do not help explain sex differences in the use of physician services (Cleary et al., 1982).

A recent investigation by Leaf and others (1985) demonstrates that a more sensitive analysis can yield evidence for an effect of psychological readiness. This analysis studied psychiatric help-seeking in the New Haven Epidemiological Catchment Area study. The prediction equation in this analysis included an interaction term between a clinical diagnosis of psychiatric disorder and the respondent's self-reported receptivity to psychiatric help. This interaction was significant in the sample as a whole and more pronounced among women than men. The greater effect of receptivity among women helped importantly to explain their greater likelihood of seeking professional treatment. Interestingly, this was true even though mean levels of receptivity were not higher among women than men.

Ability to Obtain Care

The final set of hypotheses asserts that women might have more ready access to medical care than men. Women have a regular physician more often than men because of the need to obtain periodic gynecological examinations. This reduces an important barrier to seeking care. In addition, women often have more flexible work schedules than men, which makes it easier to make doctor visits. On the other side of the issue, many more women than men live in poverty and this creates a barrier to care.

Some research has been done on each of these issues. In general, it appears that financial barriers operate to reduce the utilization of women more than men (Wilensky and Cafferata, 1983). It also appears that having a personal physician operates to increase the utilization of women relative to men. By implication, other barriers that remain unexamined operate differently to affect the utilization rates of men and women.

The most carefully examined influence of this sort involves role flexibility. The main argument here is that medical care utilization and subsequent compliance with medical advice require a flexible set of role obligations. Indirect evidence for this position has been available for some time in retrospective reports by people who delayed seeking medical care or who failed to do so even though they were ill. These people commonly report that they are too busy to see a doctor or unable to give up their normal duties (Suchman, 1965).

More objective data are available as well. One study found that part of the higher female utilization rate can be traced to their lower rate of full-time employment outside the home (Marcus and Siegel, 1982). Women with the same self-reported levels of chronic physical health problems were more likely to seek medical attention if they were not employed full time.

This line of reasoning is not convincing for two reasons. The first is specific to the particular measures of role flexibility used so far, which have not included information on the numbers and ages of children. This is a serious omission. Children represent fixed demands for homemakers that are in many ways more demanding than jobs outside the home. In fact, Gove (1985) has recently argued that the demands placed on women by their children and spouses for nurturant role activities make it less easy for women than men to take time off for illness. While this view may not be correct, it is clear that consideration of a more comprehensive set of role demands is important to make a clear assessment of the part played by role flexibility in accounting for the illness behaviours of men and women.

Second, this research has failed to consider that health affects role incumbancy. In particular, women with chronic health problems are more likely to quit their jobs than men with similar problems (Brown and Rawlinson, 1977; Chirikos and Nestel, 1985). It is likely, then, that the relationship between physician utilization and employment status at least partly reflects selection on the basis of prior health status or health care orientation. Indeed, this interpretation makes sense of the otherwise unexplained result that employment status is associated with help-seeking for chronic but not for acute medical problems in the data of Marcus and his associates. The opposite would be expected if role flexibility were acting as a causal factor, consistent with prior evidence that illness behaviour influences should be strongest when the medical condition is transient and mild.

An Overview of the Hypotheses

The review has shown mixed support for the four hypotheses. The importance of symptom recognition is largely unexamined and is likely to remain so. It is simply too difficult to obtain valid information on true medical problems of a minor sort to allow this issue to be studied systematically with survey data.

There is little evidence about whether psychological propensity to obtain medical care is an important determinant of sex differences. As noted earlier, limitations in the analysis methods used to assess this association could be responsible for the negative evidence found in most previous research. The single study which estimated an interactive model between need and propensity found the latter to have a significant effect. More work is needed before a firm conclusion can be drawn here.

There is evidence that access to care is associated with utilization, but there are limitations in this work which raise doubts about whether access is of great importance. Once again, sensitive interactive models have not been widely used to assess this hypothesis, and more work will be required before a reasonable assessment can be made. In work on role flexibility as a determinant of utilization some adjustment must be made for the possibility that chronic illness and an active help-seeking style are associated with abandoning employment. The evidence shows that this selection process is particularly pronounced among women. Failure to adjust for this will almost certainly bias any attempt to assess the fixed role hypothesis.

The fourth hypothesis concerns symptom interpretation. From the available evidence, sex differences in utilization might be importantly affected by such interpretations. In research on psychiatric help-seeking, it has been established that women are substantially more likely than men to interpret symptoms as sufficiently serious to warrant medical intervention. This is particularly true at mild and moderate symptom levels. Furthermore, it has been documented that there is no sex difference in the likelihood of seeking professional help for an emotional problem among people who define themselves as needing it (Kessler et al., 1981). This evidence from several different surveys argues that interpretation is a core determinant of psychiatric help-seeking. It is conceivable that this might be equally true of help-seeking for physical health problems, but empirical research on this issue is lacking.

## CONCLUSION

Much of the theoretical writing about sex differences in illness behaviour over the past decade has assumed that men and women differ in their responses to perceived health problems. Yet this assumption has not been firmly based on data. As well, to the extent that this assumption has been demonstrated, it is unclear whether it applies equally to chronic and acute conditions or to conditions which differ in severity and symptom clarity.

The very first requirement for future research must be to resolve this uncertainty about basic associations. To do this one must determine if men and women who have identical levels of ill health differ in their utilization behaviour. Only a fraction of the data available to study such associations has been used. The NHANES provides an extraordinary opportunity to do analysis of this sort with objectively defined information on a wide variety of medical conditions. There are many other health surveys that contain information which can be used in a similar way to study the relationship between self-reported health and medical care utilization.

This work must proceed by increasing the precision of measures and by using more appropriate analysis procedures than in the past. On the side of measurement, it is important to distinguish between acute and chronic conditions. The most desirable situation would be to conduct separate studies for a large number of different symptom clusters in order to determine the range over which sex differences in utilization exist.

An effort should be made to distinguish initial contact from follow-up in measuring physician utilization. Women are more consistent in their compliance with medical regimens than men (Verbrugge, 1985a). This could mean that the higher number of visits reported by women in health surveys are confined to follow-up visits. The fact that sex differences in doctor visits are greater for self-reported chronic conditions than acute conditions is consistent with this possibility but cannot be established unequivocally unless initial and follow-up visits are distinguished in future studies of utilization.

Analysis strategies must also be improved. Most analyses of health survey data utilize linear additive regression models in which need for services is treated as simply one variable among many. This is an entirely inappropriate approach. Such analyses should begin by documenting that symptoms are associated with utilization and should then move on to study the other variables which help determine patterns of utilization among people with symptoms.

Even conventional interaction analysis is insufficiently precise to allow accurate assessment of basic associations. This is true because we can expect sex differences in response to symptoms to vary inversely with the magnitude of symptoms, which means that at the extremes - both when symptoms are severe and when they are totally absent - sex differences in response will be small. This nonmonotonic interaction is not captured in conventional multiplicative interaction analyses. (3)

In summary, the documentation of basic associations between sex and response to illness requires rigorous replicated analyses of subgroup relationships between validated measures of morbidity or disaggregated measures of self-reported symptoms on one side and information about

---

3. This could well explain why at least one recent study failed to detect an interaction between sex and symptoms in predicting physician utilization (Cleary et al., 1982).

physician visits on the other. The utilization data should distinguish initial contacts for a particular symptom cluster from follow-up visits. The interpretation of these associations should distinguish as many subtypes of illness as possible, in an attempt to separate chronic from acute and serious from mild. The goal here is to document as carefully as possible the range of illness conditions over which sex differences in response exist and the relative contributions of initial physician visits and follow-up visits.

Once basic associations have been established and a decision has been made to focus on particular measures of ill health as anchors from which to study sex differences in response, a great deal of work will need to be done on the determinants of such differences.

It was noted earlier that almost nothing is known about sex differences in the translation of diffuse bodily feelings into symptoms recognition. This association is too complex to be studied with conventional survey methods. Therefore, until some workable method for carrying out this analysis is available, illness behaviour research should abandon the study of symptom recognition and concentrate instead on the relationship between self-reported illness and medical care utilization. It has been noted that a sex difference in physician visits can be documented among men and women who are alike in their self-reported levels of ill health. The magnitude of this difference is substantial. In the Marcus and Siegel (1982) study, for example, women were 35 percent more likely than men to seek professional help for a self-reported chronic health problem. This is nearly as high as the overall sex difference in rates of doctor visits in the United States (Nathanson, 1977). Therefore, a major component of the overall sex difference in service use can be studied even when we limit ourselves to the analysis of self-reported health.

The other hypotheses about the determinants of greater female response involving interpretations, psychological propensity and access are all plausible. Some evidence for each of them has been reported in the literature. The evidence in favour of symptom interpretation is considerably stronger than for the others at this time, but it could well be that this varies depending on the type of health problem considered. All of the research on symptom interpretation so far has involved seeking help for psychiatric problems. A more broadbased assessment of this and the other hypotheses is needed, using appropriate measures and analysis methods.

Finally, the complexity of the questions raised about sex and illness behaviour requires some research that is more fine-grained than the health surveys conducted so far. There is one study which meets the main requirements cited, namely Verbrugge's (1985a) general population sample of men and women interviewed about their health perceptions and attitudes, general perceived health status, and access to health care. Following this interview, each respondent was asked to complete a daily health diary for a period of six weeks.

These data have been used so far to study triggers of health actions in response to daily symptoms (Verbrugge, 1985b). The detailed records available in the daily diaries minimize the problem of recall bias. The existence of continuous daily records over a substantial period of time makes it possible to study spells of symptomatic days in which health actions can differ in frequency or timing. Also the detail available in symptom reports and profiles across many observations for each individual respondent allows separate analysis of particular symptom profiles. Data as detailed as these, collected on large samples of respondents and used to study the probablility and timing of initial contacts and follow-up visits, are required to resolve unequivocally the complex web of associations which chracterize sex differences in response to ill health.

ACKNOWLEDGEMENTS

The research for this paper was supported by an NIMH Research Scientist Development Awared 1 K02 MH00507. I would like to thank Duane Alwin, Paul Cleary, Steve Hansell, Philip Leaf and Lois Verbrugge for helpful discussions and for commenting on an earlier draft of the paper.

REFERENCES

Andersen, R., & Aday, L. A. (1978). Access to medical care in the U.S.: Realized and potential. Medical Care, 16, 533-546.

Andersen, R., Kravits, J., & Anderson, O. W. (Eds.). (1975). Equity in health services: Empirical analyses in social policy. Cambridge: Ballinger.

Brown, J. S., Rawlinson, M. E. (1977). Sex differences in sick role rejection and in work performance following cardiac surgery. Journal of Health and Social Behavior, 18, 276-292.

Campbell, J. D. (1978). The child in the sick role: Contributions of age, sex, parental status, and parental values. Journal of Health and Social Behavior, 19, 35-51.

Cannell, C. F. (1967). Interview data on chronic conditions compared with information derived from medical records. Vital and Health Statistics, Series 2, Number 23. Washington, D.C.: National Center for Health Statistics.

Cannell, C. F., & Fowler, F. (1965). Hospitalization reporting in three survey procedures. Vital and Health Statistics, Series 2, No. 8. Washington, D.C.: National Center for Health Statistics.

Cannell, C. F., Groves, R. M., Magilavy, L. J., Mathiowetz, N. A., & Miller P. V. (1982). An experimental comparison of telephone and personal health surveys. Final Report, Contract HEW 233-78-2034. Ann Arbor, MI: Institute for Social Research, The Univeristy of Michigan.

Chirikos, T. N., & Nestel, G. (1985). Further evidence on the economic effects of poor health. Review of Economics and Statistics, 67, 61-69.

Chirikos, T. N., & Nickel, J. L. (1984). Work disability from coronary heart disease in women. Women and Health, 9, 55-74.

Cleary, P. D., & Jette, A. M. (1984). The validity of self-reported physician utilization measures. Medical Care, 22, 796-803.

Cleary, P. D., Mechanic, D., & Greenley, J. R. (1982). Sex differences in medical care utilization: An empirical investigation. Journal of Health and Social Behavior, 23, 106-118.

Davis, M. (1981). Sex differences in reporting osteoarthritic symptoms: A sociomedical approach. Journal of Health and Social Behavior, 22, 298-309.

Depner, C. E. (1981). Predictor variables. Technical Report No. 2. Health in Detroit Study. Ann Arbor, MI: Institute for Social Research, The University of Michigan.

Gove, W. R. (1978). Sex differences in mental illness among adult men and women. Social Science and Medicine, 12B, 187-198.

Gove, W. R. (1984). Gender differences in mental and physical illness: The effects of fixed roles and nurturant roles. Social Science and Medicine, 19, 77-91.

Gove, W. R., & Geerken, M. R. (1977). Response bias in surveys of mental health: An empirical investigation. American Journal of Sociology, 82, 1289-1317.

Gove, W. R., McCorkel, J., Fain, T., & Hughes, M. (1976). Response bias in community studies of mental health: Systematic bias or random noise? Social Science and Medicine, 13, 55-67.

Hansell, S., & Mechanic, D. (in press). Introspectiveness and adolescent symptom reporting. Journal of Human Stress.

Kessler, R. C. (1981). Reply to Gove and Swafford. Social Forces, 59, 1219-1226.

Kessler, R. C., Brown, R. L., & Broman, C. L. (1981). Sex differences in psychiatric help-seeking: Evidence from four large-scale surveys. Journal of Health and Social Behavior, 22, 49-64.

Kohn, R., & White K. L. (1976). Health care - An international study. Report of the World Health Organization/International Collaborative Study of Medical Care Utilization. London: Oxford University Press.

Leaf, P. J., & Livingston, M. M. (1985). The effects of gender, clinical status and attitudes on the use of mental health services. Unpublished manuscript, Yale University, New Haven, CT.

Lewis, C. E., Lewis M. A., & Lorimer, A. (1977). Child-initiated care: The use of school nursing services by children in an 'adult-free' system. Pediatrics, 60, 499-507.

Marcus, A. C., and Siegel, J. M. (1982). Sex differences in the use of physician services: A preliminary test of the fixed role hypothesis. Journal of Health and Social Behavior, 23, 186-197.

Marshall, J. R., Gregorio, D. I., & Walsh, D. (1982). Sex differences in illness behaviour: Care seeking among cancer patients. Journal of Health and Social Behavior, 23, 197-204.

Mechanic, D. (1965). Perception of parental responses to illness. Journal of Health and Social Behavior, 6, 253-257.

Mechanic, D. (1976). Sex, illness, illness behaviour, and the use of health services. Journal of Human Stress, 2, 29-40.

Mechanic, D. (1978). Sex, illness, illness behaviour, and the use of health services. Social Science and Medicine, 12, 207-214.

Mechanic, D. (1979). Correlates of physicians utilization: Why do major multivariate studies of physician utilization find trivial psychosocial and organizational effects? Journal of Health and Social Behavior, 20, 387-398.

Miller, H. W. (1973). Plan and operation of the Health and Nutrition Examination survey: United States, 1971-1973. Vital Health Statistics, Series 1, No. 10a. Washington, D.C.: National Center for Health Statistics.

Nader, P. R., & Brink, S. G. (1981). Does visiting the school health room teach appropriate or inappropriate use of health services? Children's use of school health rooms. American Journal of Public Health, 71, 416-419.

Nathanson, C. A. (1977). Sex, illness, and medical care: A review of data, theory, and method. Social Science and Medicine, 11, 13-25.

Pennebaker, J. W. (1982). The psychology of physical symptoms. New York: Springer-Verlag.

Regier, D. A., Myers, J. K., Kramer, M., Robins, L. N., Blazer, D. G., Hough, R. L., Eaton, W. W., & Locke, B. Z. (1984). The epidemiologic catchment area program: Historical context, major objectives, and study population characteristics. Archives of General Psychiatry, 41, 934-941.

Robins, L. N., Helzer, J. E., Croughan, J., & Ratcliff, K. S. (1981). National institute of mental health diagnostic interview schedule: Its history, characteristics, and validity. Archives of General Psychiatry, 38, 381-389.

Suchman, E. A. (1965). Stages of illness and medical care. Journal of Health and Social Behavior, 6, 114-128.

Tessler, R. D., & Mechanic, D. (1978). Psychological distress and perceived health status. Journal of Health and Social Behavior, 19, 254-262.

Verbrugge, L. M. (1976). Sex differentials in morbidity and mortality in the United States. Social Biology, 23, 275-296.

Verbrugge, L. M. (1979). Female illness rates and illness behaviour: Testing hypotheses about sex differences in health. Women and Health, 4, 61-79.

Verbrugge, L. M. (1984). How physicians treat mentally distressed men and women. Social Science and Medicine, 18, 1-9.

Verbrugge, L. M. (1985a). Gender and health: An update on hypotheses and evidence. Journal of Health and Social Behavior, 26, 156-182.

Verbrugge, L. M. (1985b). Triggers of symptoms and health care. Social Science and Medicine, 20, 855-876.

Weissman, M., & Klerman, G. L. (1977). Sex differences and the epidemiology of depression. Archives of General Psychiatry, 34, 98-111.

Wilensky, G. R., & Cafferata, G. L. (1983). Women and the use of health services. Women and Health, 73, 128-133.

Wolinsky, F. C. (1978). Assessing the effects of predisposing, enabling, and illness-morbidity characteristics on health service utilization. Journal of Health and Social Behavior, 19, 384-396.

# PART III CONTEXT OF THE ILLNESS EXPERIENCE

# ILLNESS MEANINGS AND ILLNESS BEHAVIOUR

Arthur Kleinman

Department of Anthropology
Harvard University

## Introduction

Most research writings on sickness have proceeded at a pace without much attention to the categorization, valuation, personal and cultural significance of illness experience. This failure must seem bizarre to any laymen with personal experience of serious and chronic illness, and to clinicians who treat such problems, since it is a routine experience of the sick and those who care for them (be they family or professionals) that illness both brings particular meanings to a sick person's life world (e.g., the threat of death, the loss of valued body image, a new way of seeing and living in one's world heretofore taken-for-granted) and also crystallizes those special meanings in his/her world that constitute and express a particular form of life (e.g., cancer in the context of a desperately unhappy middle-age marriage, heart disease in the throes of a mid-life crisis that has left a businessman demoralized in his failed quest for lost youth, severe disability in an economically marginal retired couple that threatens bitter catastrophe in what cultural rhetoric has promised should be the "golden years").

Social and biomedical scientists have disregarded this obdurately human aspect of sickness - namely, that we experience symptoms not just with sensations of pain and deliberate choices in help seeking, but with unsettling questions of bafflement and suffering that are freighted with feelings, beliefs and relationships that cannot be divorced from sickness because they are integral to psychophysiological processes constraining both the course of disorder and the response to treatment. Researchers have taken the classical Cartesian tact of reducing sickness to something divorced from meaning in order to avoid the hard and still unanswered technical questions concerning how to actually go about measuring meaning and objectivizing and quantitating its effect on health status and illness behaviour. While such scientific fastidiousness and strict disavowal have their place in the development of a professional field, they must also be viewed as detrimental to the understanding of illness as human experience, since they redefine the problem to subtract that which is most innately human - beliefs, feelings, symbolic communication - and replace it with a fabricated strawman, more straw than man or woman. In contrast, as Plessner (1970) brilliantly shows, the essential feature of being human is the mediated nature of physical experience in which bodily processes are mediated by our understanding of them as meaningful relations in our lives, and that understanding (in a non-Cartesian, recursive, interactionist manner) becomes part of the bodily process itself.

The meaning and experience of illness must be part of any investigation of illness behaviour that conceives of that subject in any way commensurate with real life. Rather than surreptitiously slip meaning back into clinical and social science studies through such slight of hand euphemisms as symptom definition, the cognitive dimension of illness behaviour, algorithms of help seeking and clinical judgement, the appraisal process in stress, the perception of support, the transmission of information between patient and health professional - all interesting lines of research, to be sure, we must study illness meanings per se (head on, so to speak). What are the meanings of an illness episode? How do we construe them in order to measure them? How do we assess their sources and consequences? Given the "interpretive turn" in the social sciences (Geertz, 1983) this may be an especially appropriate time to address these questions.

A clinical vignette may help project the points raised and illumine the major issues in the study of illness meanings:

Consider a middle-aged American, white Protestant minister's wife with chronic neck pain of five years duration. She attributes her pain to an auto accident five years before. Her orthopedic surgeon, who has operated on her cervical spine four times in pursuit of pain control, holds the same view. But whereas he sees the problem wholly and solely as local pathology to the posterior cervical spine, which after the four surgeries is only now becoming detectable on X-ray, the patient sees her problem as a punishment from a severe, uncompromising God for her adultery and separation from her husband to follow a life-long aspiration to be a creative writer.

Examination of the medical records in different physician's offices show, surprisingly, that the patient began to complain of pain in her neck almost a full year before the accident. Her retrospective narratization of her disorder is no more a purposeful lie than is that of her surgeon, but rather represents a common problem in illness interpretations. We build stories to make sense of our lives that are selective fictions, taking up what we regard as the most important landmarks and most distressing circumstances in our life experience as we see it at particular moments in the continuing trajectory of our life course. But not just patients do this. This is the very stuff of clinical work and even of research. Nelson Goodman, (1984), the American philosopher, referring to physical science writes, "... but where truth is too finicky, too uneven, or does not fit comfortably with other principles, we may choose the nearest amenable and illuminating lie. Most scientific laws are of this sort: not assiduous reports of detailed data but sweeping Procrustean simplifications."

The orthopedist's account began when there was no demonstrable pathology in the cervical spine, again not as a lie, but as a particular kind of clinical construction of reality that will lead inexorably toward the solution - a framework within which orthopedists have been socialized and by which they make a living, and therfore, the one holding most relevance for them: whether or not to operate.

The psychoanalytic psychotherapist whom the patient had been seeing twice weekly for several years built her analysis around a history of cold and aloof parents, a lonely childhood, repressive character and unfulfilled dependency needs. Since the patient had been part of a psychological research study of the life course, however, we were able to read the very thorough research records, which disclosed little evidence of unfeeling and unresponsive parents, loneliness or unfulfilled dependency needs in childhood. Quite the opposite, these descriptions from the patient's childhood show her to have had an engaging and supportive family and to have been an indulged and much loved child with little evidence at the time of loneliness or unhappiness. But how do we treat this conflict between later interpretation and a contemporary research record from childhood? Where is the distortion: in the analyst's account or in the records? [Raffel (1979) writes, "It is not that records record things but that the very idea of recording determines in advance how things will have to appear."]

The pain clinic's behavioural scientists had related the patient's persistent pain, against which all treatment proved unavailing, to current life stress, especially an active disability suit. But, opposite to what they predicted, after resolving her marital conflict to her satisfaction and winning the disability suit the pain persisted.

This case makes a shambles of easy and superficial assessments of meaning. It throws in the face of its interpreters grave questions of what meaning is and how it can be established. But most problematic of all it makes unavoidable confrontation with a conclusion that Goodman (1984) again has aptly put:

> "For there is, I maintain, no such thing as the real world, no unique, ready-made, absolute reality apart from and independent of all versions and visions. Rather there are many right world-versions, some of them irreconcilable with others; and thus there are many worlds if any. A version is not so much made right by a world as a world is made by a right version. Obviously rightness has therefore to be determined otherwise than by matching a version with a world."

Goodman's argument would not deny the psychobiological processes constraining illness experience, but it would declare that our knowledge of those processses as well as of the illness experience is constructed in keeping with culturally and historically derived lay and professional understandings.

In response to the vexing problems that emerge from the clinical vignette and from Goodman's statement, an outline of how the study of illness meanings might be fostered as part of clinical and social studies of the phenomenology and epidemiology of illness behaviour (normal and anomalous) will be outlined in this chapter. First, some technical definitions of illness and disease will be introduced, and then an analysis will be presented, relying on materials obtained largely in empirical research on chronic somatization in Chinese and American societies.

## Illness and Disease

By illness, one means the human experience of suffering: the way the sick person and the members of her or his social network come to perceive, live with and respond to symptoms (Kleinman, 1982). Illness is first engaged in lay society, where the sick person and family draw from paradigms of every day practical knowledge and culturally approved management strategies that they learned locally as part of being socialized into shared competencies as members of a local cultural system. These particular paradigms and strategies have been deployed in others' illnesses and in earlier illness experiences of their own. Such practical activities are always a remaking or reworking of existing local beliefs and values as a response to the concrete contexts of personal experiences and actual social situations within which illness is embedded. These paradigms and strategies orient the sick person to his/her bodily complaints, as well as to therapeutic options, including various institutional settings of care. In this perspective, illness behaviour is merely the way social scientists have operationalized illness in the analytic terms of a relatively recently legitimized language of social behaviour.

By disease, in technical contrast to illness, one refers to the process of interpretation which occurs where patients suffering illness visit practitioners of one kind of another. Practitioners, as it were, reconstruct illness by refracting it through the theoretical lenses of their therapeutic professions. Hence, biomedical practitioners construct disease by reinterpreting the patient's meaningful phenomenological experience of illness in the sanctioned biomedical meaning system of dysfunction or structural abnormality in biological processes. This is the orthodox biomedical vision (cf. Foucault, 1973). Within biomedicine itself, physicians who apply the narrow medical model and those who apply the wider biopsychosocial model construct distinctive diseases. Most importantly, biomedical definitions of disease are the basis for the bureaucratic definitions of disability in society (Starr, 1984).

In this perspective then, both illness and disease embody meanings: the former from person (the patient) and local culture; the latter from person (the practitioner) and professional culture. While disease meanings are of increasing interest to medical social scientists who study the culture and institutions of biomedicine, and who have demonstrated that local cultural norms significantly influence professional culture (Townsend, 1978; Gaines, 1979, 1982), this paper focuses on the particular significance that illness experiences hold for patients.

## Types of Illness Meanings

Illness meanings are perceived from a variety of distinctive frameworks:

First, there is the ostensible, overt meaning of the symptom (e.g., rash, chest pain, headache, shortness of breath) as pain, deformity, disfigurement, disability. These shared meanings, which are open to group communication and commentary, are more or less standardized in a local culture. As a result, when we speak of pain and disability we are understood. Those understandings may be fairly subtle - in each social group there are a number of different ways to talk about, for example, headaches and these differences may make a difference in the way the sick person's circle responds to her or him.

A second sense of illness meanings, one developed by phenomenologists (Buytendijk, 1974; Plessner, 1970), has to do with the deeper, usually hidden personal and cultural significances of particular symptoms as suffering. Here religious and moral idioms of distress available in local cultural settings colour the experience. Suffering in Buddhism and in more traditional Christian theology is not a wholly disvalued experience, but the basis for transcendence. These meanings are quite at odds with those held by professionals attending illness in modern secular, medical, bureaucratic settings.

Much of the work of psychiatrists and psychologists studying medical disorders throughout this century has centered on the peculiar personal meanings of illness. Freud's writings are filled with examples of this genre, which still preoccupies many consultation psychiatrists. Here amplification of symptoms is interpreted in the terms of the patient's character structure; the special meanings of illness as threat, loss, gain, punishment, etc., are drawn on to explain how personality and its psychodynamic consequences lead to the damping of symptoms. The search for personal illness metaphors in the biography of a life has become commonplace in our time (Balint, 1958), but its provenience is ancient in the West, and there are cross-cultural counterparts in not a few non-Western societies (Kleinman, 1980; Crapanzano, 1981; Reid, 1983).

Third, illness meanings refer to the culturally marked salience of particular symptoms in particular societies. Symptoms of cancer in contemporary Western society are especially fearful and threatening (Sontag, 1976). In the technological society where rationalization and control diffuse to affect all aspects of life, and where the lowest level of risk is seemingly unacceptable, the pressure of a poorly explained, often uncontrollable, highly malignant disease is a societal-wide threat. Consider the specially stigmatized signs and symptoms of smallpox and leprosy in late medieval Europe (Gottfried, 1983), venereal disease in the Victorian age in Euro-American society and AIDS in the United States today (Brandt, 1984), mental illness in China over the millenia and neurasthenia in China today (Kleinman and Lin, 1982), the "vapors" and neurasthenic sensibility in the Guilded Age in America (Feinstein, 1983). Each of these disorders holds unique significance and salience in the particular societies mentioned. These disorders bring particular meaning to involved persons which constitutes the illness experience.

A fourth meaning of illness is almost the opposite of the cultural meaning that illnesses confer. Each illness, especially chronic illness, as it becomes embodied in a particular life trajectory, absorbs personal and social significances from the sick person's local context in Western society. For example, heart disease for a failed businessman can become embedded in: a disintegrating marriage; alcohol abuse; a demoralizing relationship with a boss; a mid-life crisis in which change in body image and coming to terms with one's mortality assault a fragily constructed ego. Or in Chinese society, think of a 30-year-old, deeply disaffiliated worker, a former Red Guard and rusticated youth, whose bitterness, cynicism and mourning over the multiple losses in the Cultural Revolution are absorbed into the symptoms of a chronic illness. Therefore, the assessment and treatment of physical complaints must take into consideration the psychological and social distress that are likely sources of symptom amplification.

Fifth, another meaning of illness is how the clinician and researcher interpret the illness behaviour of a particular person in a particular situation at a particular time. Here the emphasis is on how clinicians and researchers come to see the social uses and functions of illness (owing to their own subtle and not so subtle emphases on the particular person, setting, or the particular aspect of illness behaviour - coping processes, support system, help-seeking choices and resources). As every clinician knows, chronic illness is overdetermined and conveys several and often many meanings: not just this or that, but this and that ... and that. For example, a chronic illness like asthma may serve to authorize and sanction failure (in work, school, marriage), may mobilize social support otherwise unavailable (e.g., love and aid from an estranged spouse), may sanction the expression of anger, may provide time out and away from difficult circumstances that one feels she or he can no longer tolerate (Kleinman, 1982; Kleinman and Kleinman, 1985). Illness may empower the relatively powerless, such as the wife of a physical abusive husband whose symptoms authorize her otherwise unattended demands that her husband share in the burdensome round of daily household labour. A number of studies have documented the use of symptoms in the workplace to express worker alienation and, through the disability process, provide workers with some, otherwise unavailable, leverage over the work setting. But how do clinician and researcher decide in any given case which meanings are primary and which secondary? That process of selective interpretation reflects the interests of the observer-professional. Here the interests of the interpreter constrain the interpretation as much as do the interests of the actors.

A sixth meaning of illness might be called retrospective narrative: that is, the creating of stories whose function is to make sense of sickness bafflement (Amarisingham, 1982). Here the narrative may function as much to relate illness to life history as to relate life history to illness. One sees retrospective narratization particularly after the trajectory of an illness has been completed or when a chronic illness has settled down into an established pattern. It is especially common among the elderly, who frequently weave illness episodes into the fabric of the plot of their life stories whose denouement they are constantly revising. Retrospective narratization is also common in situations where an illness has ended in a catastrophic outcome, or when such an outcome has been barely avoided. Here the narrative at times holds a moral purpose, acting something like a secular ritual. It may reaffirm threatened core cultural values, point up and bring to conclusion structural tensions, and give shape to a loss (Turner, 1967) and may even function as a political commentary (Taussig, 1980). For these reasons, retrospective narratization can be easily shown to distort the actual happenings of the illness experience, since its raison d'etre is not fidelity to the historical reality of the illness and its treatment, but rather validity for a life history and life circumstances. Retrospective narratives of a more ominous kind occur in the recasting of illness and treatment experience to suit the purposes of disability suits, medical-legal suits and other legal actions. There is a reciprocal process in physician explanation and recording, where cases are at certain times reconstructed with an eye to offical examination of a record so as to protect the practitioner from bureaucratic criticism. In an era of medical-legal and peer review pressures, we can expect this aspect of illness meanings to take on increasing significance.

Finally, illness holds particular meanings for clinicians and researchers based on their special interests (therapeutic, scientific, professional, financial). Therefore, the very ways illness accounts are audited influence the account themselves. This influence affects the telling as much as the hearing. Patients are quite aware of the "demand characteristics" of different settings - their homes, a neighbour's room, public clinic, private office, hospital room, factory clinic, courtroom - and these help cast the story in a certain form. Similarly, health professionals also respond to the "demand characteristics" of different settings (e.g., a busy urban emergency ward, a surgeon's office, an industrial hygiene clinic, or a psychiatrist's consulting room). These demands lead to selective attention to the patient's account such that some aspects are carefully listened for and heard (sometimes when they are not even spoken), whereas other things said are literally not heard. One way of understanding this phenomenon is to view clinical reality - the definition of the problem at hand and the response to it - as constructed differently by different health professionals interacting with different patients (Kleinman, Eisenberg, and Good, 1978; Kleinman, 1980). A saddening dimension of care in America is that increasingly financial issues loom much larger than they should. These issues have become influential in clinical encounters and distort clinical communication and therefore practice. Clinicians and researchers need to unpack their own interpretive schemas, the versions of the clinical world they create, to be certain where therapeutic interests are being altered by concerns of theory validation, research publication, making a living, or professional advancement. These human interests, like the more widely talked about counter-transference responses of clinicians as individuals to patients as individuals, need to be the subject of on-going self-reflexive scrutiny by the interpreters of patient accounts to ensure that the interpretations of those accounts are not biased. This is a large problem in clinical research and practice that has never been adequately addressed.

## RESEARCH ON ILLNESS MEANINGS

Most of the above will seem old hat to seasoned clinicians, albeit illness meanings per se have not been written about much. After all, this is the very stuff of clinical practice which a competent physician develops an intuitive skill in handling. But to the researcher this must appear like a nightmare, something that needs to be eliminated if measures of validity and reliability are to provide some control over clinical data. This soft, messy "subjective" aspect of illness needs to be transformed into a "harder", neater set of behavioural variables before it can undergo statistical manipulation and take on at least the superficial appearance of respectable data. What is routinely done is simply to discount meanings, to define them outside the problem framework and, therefore, to keep them from contaminating the solution framework. For some highly technical purposes, concerned with disease determination, this research strategy may be quite acceptable, but if the purpose is the study of illness, then, to leave the meanings out of the paradigm greatly impoverishes the subject and the findings.

To illustrate how clinical research can take illness meanings into account several studies will be reviewed. In his authoritative and subtle evocation of Tahitian personality and culture, Robert Levy (1973), a physician-anthropologist, draws from psychoanalytic interviews with a small number of informants over a decade to write a description of certain illness meanings and their role in shaping illness experience that reads much like the best qualitative ethnographic and clinical accounts. As noted elsewhere (Kleinman, 1983), this format for the presentation of research data is acceptable in certain quarters (anthropology and psychoanalysis) but not in others (most biomedical research settings and certain social science ones). The increasing number of medical ethnographies (Fabrega and Silver, 1973; Lewis, 1975; Janzen, 1976; Kleinman, 1980: Lindenbaum, 1980; Estroff, 1981; Reid, 1983: among many others) indicates the usefulness of such a format for reporting research findings, but clearly this is still a minor stream even in the study of illness experience. Moreover, ethnographic descriptions of illness frequently employ quantitiative as well as qualitative measures in order to enhance their reliability and replicability. Nonetheless, like detailed single case descriptions and historical accounts, there is a role for qualitative description and hermeneutic interpretation per se in medicine, even though this role heretofore has been only marginal (Kleinman, 1980; Good and Good, 1981; Fabrega, 1974). Quantitative and statistical techniques per se do not a science make.

If the ethnography of meaning is not legitimated in medicine, then meaning will not receive a scientifically appropriate assessment in medicine. Ethnography, the core methodology of anthropology and widely used in other social sciences, is the systematic description of both qualitative and quantitative types. Quantitative ethnography includes mathematical scaling techniques, ethnoscientific eliciting frames and their statistical analysis, sociolinguistic assessment techniques, and formal measurement procedures of time, space, change and other co-ordinates of behavoiur and communications. Qualitative description, taken together with various quantitative measures, can be a standardized research method for evaluating validity. It is especially valuable in studying social and cultural significance of medically relevant events, e.g., illness beliefs, interaction norms, social gain, ethnic help-seeking, and treatment responses. It is the appropriate method to describe the work of doctoring. Attribution research in psychology, survey research in sociology, and ethnoscientific studies in anthropology are quantitative approaches to meaning to which statistical evaluation can be applied. But these techniques are less appropriate to the study of the symbolic meaning of chronic illness experience and its treatment consequences than ethnography and psychodynamic exploration, or interpretive sociological and historical inquiry. Moreover, there are established ways of assuring competent qualitative ethnographic accounts. These include: linguistic facility; accurate and detailed field notes available for scholarly review; the response of research subjects to research reports; follow-up studies by other ethnographers; audio and video taping; utilization of structured interview; and so forth.

To illustrate the use of qualitative means to study meaning, consider studies of somatization (Kleinman and Kleinman, 1985). Somatization is the presentation in a somatic idiom of bodily complaints and medical help seeking by the patient and the family of personal and social distress (e.g., serious problems in family, social network, school, work, or medical relationships). Chronic somatization is chronic illness behaviour that either occurs in absence of demonstrable disease or more commonly as amplification either of the pathophysiology of chronic disease or the psychopathology of chronic stress. Here somatization has become a sickness career. Even though it may be possible to diagnose a psychiatric disease (depression, anxiety, personality disorder) as a contributing problem, the treatment for this disease component frequently will not end the chronic illness behaviour.

In chronic somatization - chronic pain syndrome in the United States, neurasthenia in China, or "functional complaints", worldwide - interpersonal and institutional uses of the sick role, along wih its personal and cultural significance, create persistent disability. In China (Kleinman and Kleinman, 1985), through clinical interviews and ethnography in clinic and workplace, it has been learned that chronic somatization in three-fourths of patients studied, functioned to give workers some limited leverage over an extremely tightly contolled work-disability system (insofar as chronic illness behaviour enables workers to take sick leave with pay, change difficult and demoralizing jobs, or retire early). It also functions to change untenable family situations, to express political disaffiliation covertly in a society where it cannot be expressed overtly, to emblematize suffering and remorse over the tragedies of the Cultural Revolution, and it has other culture wide significances as well. These meanings are known to astute clinicians intuitively. They are not described by questionnaires. Patients often remain unaware of these covert social dimensions of sickness. Financial gain, for example, (even if it is in the awareness of the patient) cannot be openly announced because it directly contravenes the requirements of the sick role that the sick person must want to get better. For the same reason, structured interviews with patients may be unavailing. The uncovering of psychodynamic significance may require the building of trust over a long period. The ethnographic uncovering of social significance may mean interviewing family, friends, co-workers, observing the patient in his/her daily life, and studying patients in community as well as clinic and in relation to broader social themes in the society. Using each of these techniques (Kleinman and Kleinman, 1985), were able to determine the characteristic significances of illness behaviour among neurasthenic patients in Hunan (People's Republic of China). A similar combined approach in research with chronic pain patients in Boston included: quantitative measurements of psychological, psychiatric and physical status; survey measures of stress, social support, work and family functioning; and qualitative in-depth interview assessment and observation in the clinic, family and even in the work setting. Here ethnography provides crucial information on the institutionalization of somatization and on the immense social significance of somatization as chronic illness behaviour that alters our research understanding of the problem under study. Ethnography is also the heuristic basis for hypothesis generation and changes the analytic framework and even the instruments used to conduct a study.

Applying ethnography has had the additional advantage of broadening the analytic framework beyond a narrow biomedical understanding of neurasthenia with its inherant distortions. It forces one to grapple with basic questions ranging from what constitutes validity and reliability of psychiatric assessment to the critical examination of social and psychological hypotheses concerning social behaviour and its determinants. These concerns have fostered a more rigorous, systematic, psychosocially sophisticated analysis of clinical issues and, therefore, a more "scientific" understanding of a clinical problem. Medical anthropology and sociology have already developed critical discourses on stress, behavioural deviance, social supports, family structure and function, help-seeking, illness behaviour, and on many other social dimensions of health and sickness that offer medicine more than just additional researchable variables. These social science discourses are also frameworks for interpreting research data, integrating them with major bodies of findings and analytic concepts for making sense of findings, generalizing data-based ideas within wider academic contexts, and providing established standards of academic criticism. That is to say, learning social science approaches to the study of illness meanings is much more than learning how to use certain research instruments. It is learning a way of handling concepts about illness experience, systematically thinking about illness problems, and creating a context of criticism that links illness to core concerns in social theory regarding the meaning of social behaviour.

In a recent study by Manson and colleagues (1985) anthropologists and psychiatrists investigated the significance of depression among several American Indian groups by first translating standard psychiatric inventories into Hopi and other tribes' conceptual and value frameworks. The purpose was to create a culturally valid psychiatric epidemiologic assessment instrument. Then they conducted ethnopsychological and ethnomedical studies of how these local cultures labeled and coped with problems like depression. From this they derived a culture specific survey instrument to assess prevalence and types of culture specific categories. Finally they conducted an anthropological epidemiology using both sets of instruments in order to compare the findings from indigenous and professional psychiatric assessments of depression. The result is a much more refined, valid and reliable assessment of depression in these societies. Good and Good (1985) have used ethnography, clinical assessments and survey instruments to triangulate affective disorder among Iranian immigrants to the U.S. They detected both core universal types and significances of depression, along with culture-specific patterns of behaviour and meaning. Both of these studies as well as that by Kleinman and Kleinman (1985) gather information on the relationship of illness to disease, on the one side, and illness to society, on the other.

## ILLNESS MEANINGS: CLINICAL ISSUES

In comparative cross-cultural and historical perspective, it can be seen that somatization is organized into distinctive styles (Barsky and Klerman, 1983; Kleinman, 1984). These styles seem to result from the intersection of psychobiological processes with personal and cultural illness meaning. The neurasthenic pattern still popular in China is a weakness-exhaustion style that was popular in the West earlier this century, but that has slowly given way to other styles: chronic pain, bowel preoccupation, and cosmetic preoccupation styles, among many others. Historians have shown how the weakness-exhaustion style fit in well with the cultural orientations of the Victorian period (Sicherman, 1977; Feinstein, 1983). Anthropologists have described culturally dependent forms of somatization such as heart distress in Iran (Good, 1977) and shinkeishitsu in Japan (Reynolds, 1976); while cross-cultural psychiatrists have described somatization as the commonest presentation of mental illness (especially depressive and anxiety disorders) in the non-Western world (Kleinman, 1982). Numerous studies have documented the high prevalence of somatization in primary care settings in the West (Katon et al, 1982,1984; Kirmayer, 1984).

Hence, it is essential that clinicians be able to diagnose somatization and to interpret its sources (psychopathology, coping style, cultural values and beliefs, social gain, etc.). Heretofore, it has been assumed that physicians intuitively learned how to interpret chronic illness behaviour. Recognizing that somatization makes up half of a primary care practitioner's practice, the following recommendations are advanced to systematize the clinical assessment of illness meanings in any illness experience. Clinicians will want to expand or contract this approach based on the chief issues in the care of particular patients, but the framework has been found to be a useful one generally in patient care, and especially in the care of patients with chronic somatization.

The first step is for the physician to elicit the patient's and the family's explanatory model of the illness. In a supportive and open-ended manner, the clinician solicits patients' and families' views about the causes, names, pathology, course and desired treatment of their disorder, including what they most fear about the illness and its treatment and how the illness has most seriously affected their family, work, school, recreational, and personal life. In turn the clinician will want to examine how local cultural systems have differentially placed patients at risk or buffered them against societal wide forces controlling distribution and access to resources. Where such forces can be altered to the benefit of patients, physicians will include social intervention in clinical work.

Second, the clinician can then relate this understanding of the illness to the patient biography and the family history, as well as to the current situation. This is a somewhat slow process that requires knowledge of patient and family acquired over time. Past experiences of illness and other "troubles" that disclose styles of coping, interpreting, and somatizing are especially valuable sources of information.

Third, the clinician who has assembled this information can then review it in terms of the seven kinds of meaning outlined earlier. This includes self-conscious evaluation of what the illness has meant to clinicians: others and him/herself.

Fourth, in the case of a patient with chronic illness, the practitioner sorts out over time which meanings are most salient, seem to best account for exacerbations and remissions, can lend themselves to intervention of clinical, educational or social kind, and provide a framework with which she or he can engage the patient and family. The measure of "truth" of illness meanings should not be thought of simplistically as correspondence between meaning and "real" word, but in terms of their pragmatic utility, their coherence, their aesthetic representation. The physician's task is: (1) to interpret (and help patient and family interpret) illness meanings in such a way as to assist remoralization and to enhance the healing process; (2) to provide them with understanding of the sources of symptom amplification and damping, so that where feasible they can gain mastery over these; and (3) to control and explain disease and treatment in terms patients and families can assimilate and act on. The clinician's work also involves the witnessing of suffering and the sources of distress in those cases where effective intervention is not available. He or she may be able to assist patients and families to make sense of the illness experience and even undertake certain sociopolitical and economic actions as required.

The clinician becomes privileged to understandings of both the obdurately human sources of misery, and the changing sociopolitical and economic sources that characterize a local cultural system. At times he or she may want to engage in social action to address these sources of illness experience. At other times, a physician may be faced with problems involving malingering or suicidal threats which need to be addressed in a bureaucratic framework.

Attention to illness and disease meanings should help assure that the cultural, professional and institutional values implicit in these activities are systematically analyzed. There is no "technological fix" solution to illness meanings as there may be for disease. Rather physicians are forced to confront the ambiguities, ambivalences, uncertainties, ironies and paradoxes that are central to sickness and healing as human experiences. The clinician's mandate to heal must be interpreted in a broader sense here. In chronic illness, after remedial disease and illness problems are addressed, the physician's task includes listening intensely, struggling to empathetically understand, helping to sort out alternatives, sharing the burden of suffering. The physician will always tinker with an illness experience in the hope of improving the patient's situation. Validating and interpreting illness meanings may or may not lead to practical therapeutic options. Even where they do not, simply engaging in these ancient and cross-cultural aspects of healing is an essential part of care and of the work of doctoring. In that health professionals also have preventive, health planning, program development and other wider social responsibilities, the knowledge gained from the confrontation with illness meanings may be applied to social activities within and without medical systems. Finally, through the knowledge gained about self, social system, and profession, the physician's engagement in the web of illness meanings holds out the possibility of self-knowledge and through it liberation from the internal and external sources of our own oppression.

## REFERENCES


Amarisingham, L. R. (1982). Movement among healers in Sri Lanka. Culture, Medicine and Psychiatry, 4, 71-92.

Balint, M. (1958). The doctor, his patient and the illness. New York: International Universities Press.

Barsky, A., and Klerman, G. (1983). Overview: Hypochondriasis, bodily complaints and somatic styles. American Journal of Psychiatry, 140, 273-283.

Brandt, A. (1984). Venereal disease in American society. New York: Oxford University Press.

Buvtendijk, F. J. J. (1974). Prologomena to an anthropological physiology. Pittsburg: Duquesne University Press.

Crapanzano, V. (1981). Tuhami. Chicago: University of Chicago Press.

Estroff, S. (1981). Making it crazy. An ethnography of psychiatric clients in an American Community. Berkeley: University of California Press.

Fabrega, H. (1974). Disease and social behavior. Cambridge: MIT Press.

Fabrega, H., & Silver, D. (1973). Illness and shamanistic curing in Zinacantan. Stanford: Stanford University Press.

Feinstein, H. (1983). Becoming William James. Ithica, New York: Cornell University Press.

Foucault, M. (1973). The Birth of the clinic: An archaeology of medical perception. New York: Random House.

Gaines, A. (1979). Definitions and diagnoses. Culture, Medicine and Psychiatry, 3, 381-418.

Gaines, A. (1982). Cultural definitions, behavior and the person in American psychiatry. In A. Marsella & G. White (Ed.), Cultural conceptions of mental health and therapy. Dordrecht: D. Reidel.

Geertz, C. (1983). Local knowledge. New York: Basic Books.

Good, B. (1977). The heart of what's the matter. Culture, Medicine and Psychiatry, 1, 25-58.

Good, B., & Good, M. J. (1981). The meaning of symptoms. In L. Eisenberg & A. Kleinman (Eds.), The relevance of social science for medicine. Dordrecht, Holland: D. Reidel.

Good, B., & Good, M. J. (1985). The interpretation of Iranian depressive illness and dysphoric affect. In A. Kleinman, & B. Good (Eds.), Culture and depression. Berkeley: University of California Press.

Goodman, N. (1984). Notes on the well-made world. Partisan Review, 2, 276-288.

Gottfried, R. (1983). The black death. New York: Free Press.

Janzen, J. (1976). The Quest for therapy in the lower Zaire. Berkeley: University of California Press.

Katon, W., et al. (1982). Depression and somatization. American Journal of Medicine, 72(1), 127-135, 72, 241-247.

Katon, W., et al. (1984). The prevalence of somatization in primary care. Comprehensive Psychiatry, 25(2), 208-215.

Kirmayer, L. (1984). Culture, affect and somatization. Transcultural Psychiatry Research Review, 21(3,4), 159-188, 237-262.

Kleinman, A. (1980). Patients and healers in the context of culture. Berkeley: University of California Press.

Kleinman, A. (1982). Neurasthenia and depression. Culture, Medicine and Psychiatry, 6, 117-189.

Kleinman, A. (1983). The cultural meanings and social uses of illness. Journal of Family Practice, 16, 539-545.

Kleinman, A. (1984). Somatization. Referential Journal of Psychiatry. (in Chinese).

Kleinman, A., Eisenberg, L., & Good, B. (1978). Culture, illness and care. Annals of Internal Medicine, 88, 251-258.
Kleinman, A., & Kleinman, J. (1985). Somatization. Interconnections between Chinese culture, depressive meanings and the experience of pain. In A. Kleinman, & B. Good (Eds.), Culture and depression. Berkeley: University of California Press.
Kleinman, A., & Lin, T. Y. (Ed.). (1982). Normal and abnormal behavior in Chinese culture. Dordrecht, Holland: D. Reidel.
Levy, R. (1973). Tahitians: Mind and experience in the society islands. Chicago: University of Chicago Press.
Lewis, G. (1975). Knowledge of illness in a Sepik society. London: Athlone.
Lindenbaum, S. (1979). Kuru sorcery; Disease and danger in the New Guinea highlands. Palo Alto: Mayfield
Manson, S. et al. (1985). The depressive experience in American Indian communities. In Kleinman & Good (Eds.), Culture and depression.
Plessner, H. (1970). Laughing and crying: A Study of the limits of human behavior. Evanston: Northwestern University Press.
Raffel, S. (1979). Matters of fact: A sociological inquiry. London: Routledge & Kegan Paul.
Reid, J. (1983). Sorcerers and healing spirits. Canberra: Australian National University Press.
Reynolds, D. (1976). Morita psychotherapy. Berkeley: University of California Press.
Sicherman, B. (1977). The uses of a diagnosis: Doctors, patients and Neurasthenia. The Journal of the History of Medicine, p. 33-54.
Sontag, S. (1976). Illness as metaphor. New York: Farras, Strauss and Giroux.
Starr, P. (1984). The social transformation of American medicine. New York: Basic Books.
Taussig, M. (1980). Reification and the consciousness of the patient. Social Science & Medicine, 14B, 3-13.
Townsend, J. M. (1978). Cultural conceptions of mental illness. Chicago: University of Chicago Press.

# EXPLANATORY MODELS AND CARE-SEEKING: A CRITICAL ACCOUNT

Byron Good

Department of Social Medicine and Health Policy
Harvard Medical School

This chapter is based on research not primarily devoted to utilization or care-seeking. For the past ten years, the author has been interested in the relation between meaning and illness. Carrying out field research in a small Turkish town in Iran (Good, 1977; Good and Good, 1982), consulting with psychiatrists and primary care practitioners in the management of depressed Iranian immigrants, discussing the relation of health care to their lives with members of a small community on the north coast of California, and talking with medical students and research physicians about the work of doctoring, he has been interested in how people face the "reality shock" of illness, how they make sense of the experience and revise their understanding of the world in light of that experience. From the perspective of symbolic anthropology, the primary focus of cross-cultural research is considered to be the study of the relation of human action to its sense, rather than behaviour to its determinants. "Many social scientists," Geertz wrote in 1983 (p. 19), "have turned away from a laws and instances ideal of explanation toward a cases and interpretations one, looking less for the sort of thing that connects planets and pendulums and more for the sort that connects chrysanthemums and swords." Medical anthropology, from this perspective, is a meaning-centered or interpretive program. Medical anthropologists attempt to understand how members of a society bring to meaning those disorders that appear as fundamental and unwelcome realities, how they construe the relationship of those realities to previous and concurrent difficulties in their lives, how illness idioms articulate the experience of disorder, and how individuals seek and engage in therapies in an effort to transform those illness realities.

This may appear to be an odd attitude to bring to the study of illness behaviour. In few domains of the social sciences have social physics advanced further. Stress researchers have shown that individuals are bombarded by demands, which they appraise and respond to with particular coping resources and levels of health-care utilization. Health belief researchers have shown that perceptions of threat of illness, of benefits of particular behaviours, and of barriers to performing those behaviours significantly predict preventive health activities, compliance, and rates of clinic utilization. Here the anthropologist seems to be in the presence of real science, more akin to planets and pendulums than chrysanthemums and swords. Cross-cultural studies can help identify local instances of universal stressors, supports, and beliefs about threats and benefits, but the field seems to have passed beyond interpretation and hermeneutics to real science.

Rather than focusing primarily on data and research findings, this chapter addresses at a rather deeper level some assumptions about the nature of health-care beliefs and explanatory models, on the one hand, and the nature of care-seeking decisions on the other. First, it provides a brief discussion of the paradigm shift involved in moving from the social psychological research on the Health Belief Model and utilization to an interpretive or meaning-centered approach for analyzing explanatory models and care-seeking. Second, it reviews a debate that has developed in the anthropological literature over the nature of care-seeking decisions in cross-cultural contexts. Finally, the chapter outlines new approaches that have been developed in the author's work and that of other anthropologists and cross-cultural psychiatrists working in this field. In particular, it addresses the issue of how we might use an interpretive approach to study illness behaviour cross-culturally, what hazards are posed for research by failure to adequately conceptualize meaning and beliefs, and whether there is method to a disciplined craft of interpretation that can be replicated and integrated with other forms of research.

Anthroplogists, of course, are not alone in their interest in cultural meanings associated with symptoms and illness behaviour. However, there are important differences in the field on the conceptions of "meaning". In part, these differences grow out of the settings that frame the research; while most of the sociologists or psychologists who study cognitions and behaviours related to pain, cancer, or smoking can treat a whole series of cultural variables as constants and leave them unexamined, this is not the case for the anthropologist who works in a non-Western society. It is the source of both great methodological challenge and of insight that the anthropologist can assume almost nothing to be a constant or an obvious equivalent. Anthropologists often find themselves in the world of Alice in Wonderland where croquet games turn out to be played with hedgehogs.

## HEALTH BELIEF MODEL RESEARCH

In a volume of the Health Education Quarterly of 1984, Becker and Janz reviewed the Health Belief Model (HBM) research of the past decade (Janz and Becker, 1984). Because of the apparent similarity of the notions "health belief model" and "explanatory model of illness", it will be useful to contrast the two. The HBM approach was developed in the 1950's by a group of social psychologists influenced by Kurt Lewin, in response to efforts by members of the Public Health Service to increase utilization of widely available preventive measures for diseases such as tuberculosis - and later, rheumatic fever, polio, and influenza (Rosenstock, 1974). In close accordance with various behaviourist theories of motivation and decision-making the model predicted that behaviour depends largely upon the value placed by an individual on a particular goal, and upon the individual's estimate of the likelihood of an action resulting in the goal (Maiman and Becker, 1974). More specifically, the model hypothesized that perceived susceptibility to a disease and perceived severity of that disease, combined with perceived benefits of preventive actions minus perceived barriers to taking those actions, explained the likelihood of an individual taking preventive health measures, complying with prescribed regimens, or utilizing medical services.

It is particularly instructive to note that at a time when anthropologists, historians, and literary scholars are devoting renewed attention to the role of cultural meanings in the experience of and response to illness - from the social history of venereal disease (Brandt, 1985), to the symbolic import of obesity (Ritenbaugh, 1982), to the metaphors associated with cancer (Sontag, 1977), HBM research seems to have run its course. As Janz and Becker, the leading figures of this field, conclude in their recent review (1984, p. 45): "Given the numerous survey-research findings on the HBM now available, it is unlikely that additional work of this type will yield important new information."

Why is this the case? Why has the HBM research failed to cast light on the profound cultural values that influence American beliefs about AIDS, or the pattern of care-seeking that has made weight reduction a multi-million dollar industry, or dramatic social class and racial differences in utilization of prenatal care responsible for dramatic differences in infant mortality? What is the theory of culture and meaning in which the health belief model is embedded, and how has this theory inhibited researchers studying cultural beliefs from pursuing such issues?

The theory of culture assumed by health belief model researchers has two characteristics. First, HBM theories are quite explicit versions of "subjective utilitarianism". Its actor is a universal Economic Man, proceeding rationally toward the goal of positive health, a preference only slightly modified by health beliefs. The actor weighs the costs and benefits of particular behaviours, engaging in a kind of "threat-benefit analysis", then acts freely on his perceptions to maximize his capital. As Sahlins (1976, p. 102) has noted, in such utilitarian theories culture is "taken as an environment or means at the disposition of the 'manipulating indiviual,' and also a sedimented result of his self-interested actions." Although purportedly Lewinian in its focus on the perceptions of individuals, the theory analyzes the structure of health beliefs and thus health culture only to the extent that they contribute to the rational calculus of the care-seeker who is ultimately free to make voluntary choices and whose beliefs are subjective qualities influencing the evaluation of goals and the perception of efficacy.

Second, HBM theories have assumed biomedical knowledge as the norm. Developed specifically to help public health specialists convince people to act more rationally - to use preventive services, to obey the doctors' orders, or to utilize medical care "appropriately" - such theories evaluate health beliefs for their proximity to empirically correct knowledge concerning the seriousness of particular disorders and the efficacy of particular behaviours or therapies.

Thus, in the HBM research, the analysis of cultural beliefs is made doubly subservient, relativized to the privileged perspective of current medical knowledge, and placed in the service of a utilitarian theory of illness behaviour.

## BELIEFS AND CARE-SEEKING: THE ANTHROPOLOGICAL DEBATE

While anthropological theories on health beliefs and care-seeking vary dramatically from those of the HBM theorists, their origins are closely related. As public health specialists of the 1950's enlisted social psychologists in campaigns to increase acceptance of immunizations and other preventive measures, so they invited anthropologists to work along side them in international public health programs (Paul, 1955; Foster, 1982). Also as the social psychologists argued that health beliefs shape the terms of rational decision-making, so anthropologists argued that a society's local, culturally-grounded illness theories shape its members' illness behaviour and choices they make among traditional therapies, folk healers and biomedical practitioners. For example, refusal to boil water in a Peruvian village indicated not irrationality but behaviour grounded in an alternative form of rationality, one which included theories of balances between hot and cold essences, passed along from Galen to the Muslim universities in Spain and carried by Spanish priests to the New World (Wellin, 1955). Choices among traditional curers, nativist Christian healing rites, and European medicine in the Admiralty Islands follow a "hierarchy of resort," as patients and their families evaluate the likely cause of an illness, then seek appropriate treatments, following a culturally prescribed sequence until a cure results or the treatment of last resort has been exhausted (Romanucci-Ross, 1969). The logic of care-seeking in American ethnic communities varies from the standard Anglo pattern because of the presence of beliefs in folk illnesses - such as susto or fallen fontanel in the Mexican American community (Rubel, 1964) or ataques de nervios in the Puerto Rican community (Harwood, 1977; Garrison, 1977) - which provoke resort to traditional cures (cf. Harwood, 1981). Unlike the work of the social psychologists, anthropological reports focused on placing health beliefs in the context of a culturally constituted local health-care system and on elaborating the full range of potential therapeutics and the logic of decisions among the options.

From these early studies, two paradigms of care-seeking have emerged in the anthropological literature. The first has elaborated the early interest in strategies of resort among the variety of popular, folk and professional therapies available in most societies, using various forms of decision analysis. Such studies have provided increasingly elegant models of choice points in complex traditional societies (Kunstadter, 1975), of the cognitive or conceptual schema used for categorizing types of illness by cause and severity (Fabrega and Zucker, 1979; J. Young, 1978, 1981), of the role of the lay referral network or the therapy management group in the care-seeking process (Chrisman, 1977; Janzen, 1978), of perceived qualities of the treatments offered (Nichter, 1980), and ultimately of formal characteristics of resulting treatment choices (Young and Garro, 1982).

The second position, grounded in political economic theories, criticizes these decision-modelling theories, arguing that characteristics of the objective social order, not subjective factors, play the decisive role in determining care-seeking patterns, and that the voluntarism assumed by such decision theories is more characteristic of our tacit social constructs than of the actual conditions of most persons seeking health care. For example, Morsy (1978, 1980), an Egyptian-American anthropologist, found that the position of the Egyptian village within the power structure of the household predicted possession by spirits and resort to curers. Individuals who were either wives of the sons of the household head, or the brother of the household head - that is, those with the least power in the household - were by far the most likely to suffer possession. Here, structural conditions were analyzed not as stressors impacting on de-socialized individuals, but as an ordered aspect of local power relations. She goes on to argue that other aspects of care-seeking are predominantly constrained by power relations in Egyptian society and open onto global power relations.

Both parties to this debate - the decision theorists and the political economists - share an anthropological perspective. They begin with a holistic, non-normative view of health culture. They consider the full range of available care-seeking options, not simply the professional sector. And they begin by exploring the internal organization of cultural meanings, rather than prematurely searching for local instances of universal variables such as perceived severity, threat, or benefits.

While making significant contributions, however, both the decision model and the political economy model of health culture and care-seeking have important limitations. The political economy critics of decision theories are correct: decision theories often make empirically false assumptions about the freedom of individuals to make voluntary decisions, thus reducing attention to the overwhelming social constraints. As a result, decision model research may reproduce our conventional, ideologically-grounded understandings of individuals as rational and voluntaristic actors (cf. A. Young, 1980). On the other hand, political economists often treat culture as epiphenomenal or as a quality of subjective experience and seldom provide empirical studies of individual care-seeking.

The remainder of this paper outlines new directions for research that follow from recent work of interpretive anthropologists, beginning first with research on explanatory models, and secondly examining their relation to care-seeking.

## EXPLANATORY MODEL RESEARCH

During the mid-1970's, Kleinman and his colleagues developed the notion "explanatory model" as a clinical application of an anthropological concept and as a research tool for clinically applied research (Kleinman, Eisenberg and Good, 1978; Kleinman, 1980; Good and Good, 1981a, 1981b). Explanatory models provided a means of exploring patients' understandings of their conditions, for explicitly comparing and contrasting the perspectives of clinicians and patients, for investigating how cognitive orientations open or close avenues of care-seeking, for research into the micro-level changes in patients' understandings, and for comparisons across cultures and across ethnic groups. While some have argued that explanatory model researchers make assumptions about the rationality of behaviour similar to those that have been criticized in this paper (A. Young, 1981), a careful examination of the work of Kleinman and his colleagues shows little similarity with that of health belief model research or even earlier anthropological research designed to represent whole cultures or ethnic groups in terms of characteristic "beliefs". Rather, the focus has been on the use of explanatory models to interpret troubling social conditions or body experience, the construction or negotiation of "illness realities" through discourse employing explanatory models, and their embeddedness in "semantic illness networks" and socially organized power relations.

Current explanatory model research is leading in three directions: toward studies of explanations or illness representations as emerging in situated discourse; as interpretive operators, rather than simply motives for acts; and as embedded in semantic networks. Each of these areas of research indicate important aspects of paradigm differences between rationalist theories and current work in explanatory models and medical discourse. Examples from work in each of these areas will be briefly described.

First, a number of contemporary medical anthropologists are focusing their research on illness behaviour and explanatory models as forms of situated discourse. That is, the telling of illness narratives is itself a special form of illness behaviour, governed by cultural rules and social context. For example, Early (1982) sat with women in a poor neighbourhood of Cairo and recorded their naturally occurring discussions of present and past illnesses and their encounters with professional or folk medical specialists. She began to find that these accounts had a particular narrative structure. "Therapeutic narratives," as she called them, were organized to provide biographical context and experiential reference for the perception and diagnosis of illness. These narratives made sense of symptoms or illnesses by relating them to the life histories of the women, connecting troubling life circumstances with shared cultural knowledge about illness. Some narratives, she found, were used to make sense of a current ambiguous situation and negotiate an approach to therapy; others, she found, "form a codified, elaborated version (of past events) affirming cultural truths" about such central concerns as envy and sibling rivalry. Early's research focused on both the particular narrative structures of these naturally occurring discourses and on the principles that generated the narrative.

Other researchers interested in the relation of explanatory models to situated illness discourse have focused on differences in illness narratives across social and communicative contexts. These interests are generated by findings that differing contexts within culture may be as important as differences between cultures in determining the nature of symptom presentation of idioms of complaint. For example, investigating the issue of somatization in Chinese culture, Cheung has shown that illness narratives in physicians' offices are quite different from those in other settings (Cheung, Lau, and Wong, 1984). It is not that individuals in Hong Kong fail to experience psychological symptoms, she argues, but that social norms and linguistic conventions play a critical role in determining what idiom will be used in particular communicative contexts. Research such as this indicates important issues for empirical research in areas such as the study of somatization, a classic focus of illness behaviour research. Naturalistic accounts of illness narratives in culturally-marked communicative contexts may help us understand whether propensity to "somatize" is a cultural characteristic, a psychological trait of some individuals, or a characteristic of particular communication contexts within a culture. Studies of language rules that determine in what contexts members of a particular society are to be introspective and in which contexts somatic expressions are deemed appropriate may provide surprising benefits to our understanding of the relation of somatization and psychologization to care-seeking.

Furthermore, studies such as these provide new questions for explanatory model research. How are the explanatory models that are elicited embedded in narrative form; how do these narratives vary - over time, as people struggle to control their illness; and in different relationships, as people try to accomplish different rhetorical and practical ends with their narratives; and across cultures? To what extent do these really provide motives for care-seeking behaviour rather than efforts to rationalize or make meaningful past experiences and previous attempts to receive effective treatment?

These questions lead to the second characteristic of explanatory models that is currently under investigation. Explanatory models are not simply static beliefs, but are "interpretive operators" or cultural models used to interpret some aspect of reality. For example, they are used to interpret bodily sensations or feelings, linking potential causes with predicted consequences, thus defining the nature of the symptom and determining appropriate action. They are also used for retrospective interpretations, enabling an individual or therapy management group to construct and revise "etiological interpretations" of a condition at various points in its treatment (Good and Good, 1982). For example, "stress" is one of the most popular current explanatory models in American culture - both professional and popular. "Stress" serves as a classic etiological operator, used to link troubling events in individuals' lives to painful symptoms or illnesses.

This analysis suggests a complex relationship between belief and motivation. Schutz (1971:I, pp. 70-72) distinguished "in-order-to" motives - that is, those means of framing a situation in terms of the end to which an action is to be directed - from "because" motives, those retrospective elaborations on why particular actions were undertaken. The distinction between the two, he notes, is often disregarded in ordinary language. Certainly in many anthroplogical analyses, retrospective accounts are treated as equivalents of motives for action, disregarding the many changes that have occurred in interpretation before an authoritative narrative account becomes fixed. Elicitation of an individual's beliefs or explanations of the cause of a condition is often believed to provide the data necessary to understand why an individual selected a particular form of treatment. If an interpretation of cause is correlated with treatment choice, as in the work of Young and Garro (1982), it is argued that perceived cause motivated action. This may well be the case; however, since data is collected retrospectively rather than prospectively, "because motives" - the retrospective accounts - cannot be distinguished from the "in-order-to motives" of the patient at the time of the decision to seek care. In addition, the role of narrative type (the kind of account the patient chooses to give of the condition) and means of relating the illness or symptom to deep cultural meanings in producing the explanation are seldom considered seriously in typical rationalist studies of the relation of patient beliefs to care-seeking.

Explanatory models are thus not simply beliefs that one has - like pieces of furniture - nor are they dispositions or enduring characteristics of individuals. Rather, they are frames provided by culture that we do things with. This is true of even the classic anthropological examples of folk illnesses. Elsewhere, Good and Good (1981a) have provided an analysis of a clinical case of a Mexican-American woman in California who believed her baby had caída de la mollera or fallen fontanel illness. This "folk illness" is based in a popular cultural belief that there is in infants a small floating bone that can be dislodged and drop down against the upper palate and block the oral passage. Unless treated by a folk healer to return it to its place, it can kill an infant. In the case observed, a mother brought her infant for emergency care, demanding immediate treatment because she feared the baby was about to die. An older woman who specialized in treating fallen fontanel had seen the infant, made the diagnosis, and treated the baby. The mother continued, however, to be anxious for the baby's safety. When he learned of the folk belief involved, the physician caring for the baby and mother believed he had learned the motive for care-seeking and sought to reassure the mother. When she would not be reassured, the physician was very frustrated. In the following weeks, a more complex story of the meanings of the baby's condition emerged. From birth, the infant had had a "skull asymmetry" (a dent in her forehead, probably caused by positioning of the fetus in the womb). The mother had been told recently by a specialist that the abnormality would probably right itself, and that it was probably not dangerous, though he noted in passing that the condition should be watched because should the suture line of the skull happen to close early it might not allow for normal brain growth. Not surprisingly, the mother was not reassured by this. The infant had been hospitalized for a hernia operation some weeks earlier, adding to the mother's concern. It was also learned that the mother had not had an infant for seven years and was generally concerned about her mothering abilities, and that her insecurity was heightened by lack of support from her husband. It gradually became clear that the mother's conviction that the infant suffered fallen fontanel was not simply a popular explanation of a set of symptoms (upset stomach, depression of the fontanel). It was rather an attempt to make meaning of a broader set of medical and social difficulties, all of which were interpreted as the underlying cause of the present perceived crisis. The problem for the practitioner was thus not simply negotiating between discrepant beliefs. The cultural frame "fallen fontanel" was being used to interpret very real medical concerns and social problems in the life of the mother. No amount of "education" to change beliefs would make these go away.

We are thus interested in how explanatory models are used interpretively, and in how they construct the definition of a situation both retrospectively and as an orientation to action.

Thirdly, current researchers are investigating the relationship between explanatory models and semantic networks - those ordered networks of meaning that provide the deep structure of culture (Good, 1977). One example will illustrate. There are a wide variety of explanatory models of obesity in our popular culture and in our clinics. Popular theories of "set points", of the importance of the number of fat cells created through infant feeding patterns, of the need to balance calorie intake and calories expended, and many others motivate dieting and exercise for losing weight. In clinical settings, explanatory models include theories of illness behaviour, models of the role of self-perception and body image, behaviourist models of eating activities, psychoanalytic theories of the origins of orality and self-loathing, and many others. What is intriguing to the anthropologist is the extent to which a few fundamental symbols appear in both the popular culture and in clinical discourse. Control, self-control, responsibility, and self-worth all appear as central issues in the explanation and treatment of fatness. Cutting across all these diverse explanatory models is a deeper level symbolic order - a semantic network - that links body size and beauty to central concerns of Western culture about self-control. Large body size has become a symbol for unwillingness to control the self, its passions, and its appetites. The intensity of feelings about being fat - the fear and loathing it generates, and the incredible care-seeking frenzy it produces - are thus accidents of our hidden symbolic associations. Individual explanatory models of body size are constructed to tie together aspects of personal biography - personal meanings - with central concerns of American society.

These current explanatory model studies take us far from the old HBM studies, as well as from many traditional anthropological studies of health beliefs, and raise complex theoretical and methodological issues. They suggest a need for studies of illness discourse in natural settings, for studies of the relation of explanatory models to semantic networks, and for on-going microanalyses of individuals over time and across social contexts, not unlike the approach to stress research currently employed by Lazarus and his colleagues (e.g., Lazarus, 1984). Such studies as these will provide a richer understanding of the explanatory model side of the explanatory model/care-seeking relationship.

## CURRENT DIRECTIONS IN CARE-SEEKING RESEARCH

A few words are in order about the care-seeking side of that relationship. Throughout this paper "decision model" approaches to the study of care-seeking have been criticized for their assumptions about the importance of individual care-seekers as decision-makers, about their freedom to make voluntary choices, and about the role of rationality and cognitive beliefs as motivating and constraining behaviour. The criticism of this perspective is not simply that such studies fail to consider, for example, medical costs or distance to the doctor - variables accounted for in the old health belief model studies as barriers - though these are systematic constraints on choices and are often neglected in studies of the influence of beliefs on care-seeking. The criticism also is meant to point to other systematic constraints on individual care-seeking decisions.

First, it is remarkable how seldom studies examine the extent to which our medical institutions are impervious to patients' decision-making efforts. Patient-dumping - the sending of patients who are unable to pay for care to poorer quality public institutions - is a major reality in the current American scene and is likely to grow as the market place increasingly dominates care provision. Patients in such situations are hardly free to make voluntary choices. The same is often true about the patient's ability to discuss psychological or psychosocial problems with their physicians. A wide range of formal and informal tactics are often used to discourage "brief psychotherapy" (i.e., long discussions with the doctor) or other treatments which cannot be reimbursed. For example, the diagnosis "depression" is not reimbursable for family physicians by many California third-party payers, despite the fact that it may well be the most common diagnostic problem seen in primary care. While physicians are experts in writing diagnoses that are most likely to produce revenue ("weakness and tiredness" is accepted as a diagnosis by many of the same insurance companies in California that refuse to reimburse for treatment of depression by primary care practitioners), the systematic economic rewarding of a physician's undertaking medical procedures and similar discouraging of "talk therapy" not only places constraints on practitioner's behaviour; but also systematically constrain the patient's autonomy and ability to choose the clinical agenda.

In addition to medical institutions constraining the autonomy of the care-seeker, there are major social, cultural and subcultural differences in who makes health-care decisions and how they are made. This of course comes as no surprise to students of illness behaviour. In fact, the illness behaviour model of care-seeking was developed primarily to examine precisely such influences on health-care decisions. This model holds, essentially, that the individual experiences bodily sensations, appraises these (or makes illness attributions) using available illness representations (or explanatory models), then makes treatment choices in consultation with members of a lay referral network. Mechanic (1982) outlines this approach:

> "Illness behaviour ... describes the manner in which persons monitor their bodies, define and interpret their symptoms, take remedial action, and utilize the health care system. People differentially perceive, evaluate, and respond to illness, and such behaviours have enormous influence on the extent to which illness interferes with usual life routines, the chronicity of the condition, the attainment of appropriate care, and the co-operation of the patient in the treatment of the situation."

It would seem that this model could accommodate and highlight differences among cultures. But is this the case?

In a study by Lin and his colleagues (Lin, Tardiff, Donetz, and Goresky, 1978), which examined care-seeking pathways followed to mental health services, only one of the three ethnic groups studied fit easily in this model. The study examined the help-seeking patterns typical of severely disabled psychiatric patients from Anglo, Chinese, and American Indian groups in Seattle. The Anglo-Saxon and middle European ethnic group individuals experienced symptoms, consulted their family members, reviewed available resources, and chose mental health or social service resources, following a pattern very close to that outlined by the illness behaviour model. They often re-evaluated and changed care-providers if they were unhappy.

The two other groups studied, however, do not easily fit the pattern outlined by the model. For the ethnic Chinese, there were early and prolonged efforts by the family to manage problems in each episode without encouraging the sufferer to seek professional care. Many were isolated in the home and allowed few contacts. Remarkably advanced psychiatric symptoms were often present before any outside care was sought. Later, medical intervention occurred, although intervention by legal or social agencies were rare. In the Chinese case, the family unit seems to be far more than a "lay referral group" consulted by the individual making health-care choices. Indeed, the family unit is the decision-making entity rather than the individual who has problems; family members seem to evaluate symptoms, determine their meaning, and organize the active suppression of mental health care-seeking.

The American Indian patients followed quite a different pattern. These patients were most commonly among Seattle's street people, with neither a family to organize care-seeking choices, nor the ability to actively organize their own care. They were often transferred between social service agencies and police, who became the major groups responsible for "care-seeking decisions" rather than the patients themselves.

This study raises significant questions about what seems to be our most culture-free models. At very least, the "therapy management group" - those responsible for making decisions - varies across social and cultural groups, and the ability of the individual to appraise symptoms, review available resources, then make voluntary choices is simply a myth for many in our society and in other societies. The model of the rational, autonomous care-seeker organizing treatment choices to maximize perceived benefits to the self is thus hardly a value-free model. It is rather a model of how members of our society are believed to act - an ideological model - which serves best when used to study middle-class Anglo Americans. When the sampling domain is limited, the illness behaviour model accounts for important aspects of the care-seeking behaviour. Furthermore, it clearly points toward important variables that will be of value in cross-cultural research. However, studies such as those reviewed in this paper suggest the need for new theoretical models and research strategies that can incorporate major social structural conditions as well as culture-specific patterns of organizing treatment as central to the paradigm, rather than maintaining these as aspects of social context or as external factors that impact on the autonomous individual decision-maker.

## REFERENCES

In this paper it is argued that we need to turn away from research that simply reproduces conventional knowledge of individuals, free to make health-care choices, influenced by beliefs, and to move beyond constructing highly restricted research contexts that simply highlight those variations that fit into the conventional utilitarian model. The chapter outlines alternative directions research into explanatory models and care-seeking should pursue. Illness narratives need to be examined in natural settings. Such research would reframe the study of explanatory models, attributions, and health beliefs as analysis of meaning construction - the process by which individuals and social groups link personal biography to cultural meanings in their reflections on their illness and treatment experiences. It would also focus critical attention on the narratives through which we have access to this process. Careful comparison of illness discourse across social contexts is needed if we are to make progress in understanding whether such phenomena as somatization are characteristics of individuals, are particular idioms salient in some cultures, or are characteristic of particular discourse settings or relationships which define communicative context. Finally, much more focused and finely detailed cross-cultural studies are needed of illness meanings and the organization of the care-seeking process. Such research can help to move beyond the ethnocentrism which often characterizes it now and open richer perspectives on illness behaviour.

## CONCLUSION


Brandt, A. M. (1985). *No magic bullet: A social history of venereal disease in the United States since 1980*. Oxford: Oxford University Press.

Cheung, F. M., Lau, B. K. W., & Wong, S. (1984). Paths to psychiatric care in Hong Kong. *Culture, Medicine and Psychiatry*, *8*, 207-228.

Chrisman, N. J. (1977). The health seeking process: An approach to the natural history of illness. *Culture, Medicine and Psychiatry*, *1*, 351-377.

Early, E. A. (1982). The logic of well being. Therapeutic narratives in Cairo, Egypt. *Social Science and Medicine*, *16*, 1498-1499.

Fabrega, H., & Zucker, M. (1979). Components of illness and type of medical practitioner: A comparative study. *Social Science and Medicine*,*13A*, 13-24.

Foster, G. (1982). Applied anthroplogy and international health: Retrospect and prospect. *Human Organization*, *41*, 189-197.

Garrison, V. (1977). The "Puerto Rican syndrome" in psychiatry and *espiritismo*. In V. Crapanzano and V. Garrison (Eds.), *Case studies in spirit possession* (pp. 383-449). New York: John Wiley.

Geertz, C. (1983). *Local knowledge*. New York: Basic Books.

Good, B. (1977). The heart of what's the matter. The semantics of illness in Iran. *Culture, Medicine, and Psychiatry*, *1*, 25-58.

Good, B., & Good, M. (1981a). The meaning of symptoms: A cultural hermeneutic model for clinical practice. In L. Eisenberg & A. Kleinman

(Eds.), The relevance of social science for medicine (pp. 165-196). Boston: Reidel.
Good, B., & Good, M. (1981b). The semantics of medical discourse. In E. Mendelsohn & Y. Elkana (Eds.), Anthropological and historical studies of the sciences (pp. 171-212). Boston: Reidel.
Good, B., & Good, M. (1982). Toward a meaning-centered analysis of popular illness categories: "Fright illness" and "heart distress" in Iran. In A. J. Marsella & G. M. White (Eds.), Cultural conceptions of mental health and therapy (pp. 141-166). Boston: Reidel.
Harwood, A. (1977). Rx: Spiritist as needed. A study of a Puerto Rican community mental health resource. New York: Wiley.
Harwood, A. (Ed.). (1981). Ethnicity and medical care. Cambridge: Harvard University Press.
Janz, N. K, & Becker, M. H. (1984). The health belief model: A decade later. Health Education Quarterly, 11, 1-47.
Janzen, J. (1978). The quest for therapy. Medical pluralism in Lower Zaire. Berkeley: University of California Press.
Kleinman, A. (1980). Patients and healers in the context of culture. Berkeley: University of California Press.
Kleinman, A., Eisenberg, L., & Good, B. (1978). Culture, illness and care. Clinical lessons from anthropologic and cross-cultural research. Annals of Internal Medicine, 88, 251-258.
Kunstadter, P. (1975). Do cultural differences make any difference? Choice points in medical systems available in northwestern Thailand. In A. Kleinman, P. Kunstadter, E. Alexander, & J. Gale (Eds.), Medicine in Chinese cultures. Comparative studies of health care in Chinese and other societies. DHEW Publication No. (NIH) 75-653.
Lazarus, R. S. (1984). Puzzles in the study of daily hassles. Journal of Behavioral Medicine, 7, 375-389.
Lin, T., Tardiff, K., Donetz, G., & Goresky, W. (1978). Ethnicity and patterns of help-seeking. Culture, Medicine, and Psychiatry, 2, 3-14.
Maiman, L. A., & Becker, M. H. (1974). The health belief model: Origins and correlates in psychological theory. In M. H. Becker (Ed.), The health belief model and personal health behavior (pp. 9-26). Thorofare, NJ: Slack.
Mechanic, D. (1982). Symptoms, illness behavior, and help-seeking. Trenton, NJ: Rutgers University Press.
Morsy, S. (1978). Sex roles, power, and illness in an Egyptian village. American Ethnologist, 4, 137-150.
Morsy, S. (1980). Body concepts and health care: Illustrations from an Egyptian village. Human Organization, 39, 92-96.
Nichter, M. (1980). The layperson's perception of medicine as perspective into the utilization of multiple therapy systems in the Indian context. Social Science and Medicine, 14B, 225-233.
Paul, B. D. (Ed.). (1955). Health, culture, and community. New York: Russell Sage Foundation.
Ritenbaugh, C. (1982). Obesity as a culture-bound syndrome. Culture, Medicine, and Psychiatry, 6, 347-362.
Romanucci-Ross, L. (1969). The hierarchy of resort in curative practices: The Admiralty Islands, Melanesia. Journal of Health and Social Behavior, 10, 201-209.
Rosenstock, I. M. (1974). Historical origins of the health belief model. In M. H. Becker, (Ed.), The health belief model and personal health behavior (pp. 1-8). Thorofare, NJ: Slack.
Rubel, A. (1964). The epidemiolgy of a folk illness: Susto in hispanic America. Ethnology, 3, 268-283.
Sahlins, M. (1976). Culture and practical reason. Chicago: University of Chicago Press.
Schutz, A. (1971). Collected papers. In M. Natanson (Ed.), Volume I: The problem of social reality. The Hague: Martinus Nijhoff.
Sontag, S. (1977). Illness as metaphor. New York: Farras, Strauss and Giroux.

Wellin, E. (1955). Water boiling in a Peruvian town. In B. D. Paul (Ed.), Health, culture, and community (pp. 71-106). New York: Russell Sage Foundation.
Young, A. (1980). The discourse of stress and the reproduction of convention knowledge. Social Science and Medicine, 14B, 133-146.
Young, A. (1981). When rational men fall sick: An inquiry into some assumptions made by medical anthropologists. Culture, Medicine, and Psychiatry, 5, 317-335.
Young, J. (1978). Illness categories and action strategies in a Tarascan town. American Ethnologist, 5, 81-97.
Young, J. (1981). Medical choice in a Mexican village. New Brunswick, NJ: Rutgers University Press.
Young, J., & Garro, L. Y. (1982). Variation in the choice of treatment in two Mexican communities. Social Science and Medicine, 16, 1453-1466.

# DECISION-MAKING MODELS OF TREATMENT CHOICE

Linda Garro

Department of Social and Preventive Medicine
University of Manitoba

When people perceive themselves as ill, they may do a number of things. They may do nothing. They may try to treat the illness by themselves or within the family. They may consult with friends and relatives about what they should do. They may seek care from a number of different sources, including but not limited to physicians. Indeed, studies carried out in North America and Great Britain indicate that roughly 70 to 90 percent of all illness episodes are never seen by a physician (Hulka, Kupper, and Cassel, 1972; White, Williams, and Greenberg, 1961; Zola 1972, 1973). Many of these illness episodes are treated within the family, yet little attention has been given to this dimension of health care by researchers (Dean, 1981; Kleinman, 1980). Another alternative to the physician is traditional or folk healers. Anthropologists working in a variety of cultural settings have detailed how folk healers relate, interact and contrast with people seeking help and other providers of health care (e.g. Garro, in press; Janzen, 1978; Kleinman, 1980; Lock, 1980; J. Young, 1981a). Additional alternatives that vary across cultural settings include pharmacists, osteopaths, chiropractors, faith healers, health food and vitamin vendors, and quacks.

Anthropologists have used a number of different methodological and theoretical approaches to study how the decision to seek help is made and how treatment choices are made from available alternatives. A variety of different approaches to this issue will be described in this paper. Comparing different approaches will facilitate an understanding of how different data are used and how approaches differ on what constitutes an explanation of illness behaviour. One of these approaches, the decision-making approach, focuses on the considerations individual actors bring to illness situations and attempts to discover the shared standards of choice underlying treatment decisions. Once elicited, these standards can be used to build a model that can be tested through measuring the correspondence between the model and observed behaviour. There has been some confusion in the anthropological literature on what is a decision modeling approach and how it is distinct from other approaches (Stoner, 1985). This paper is intended to clarify some of this confusion. In addition to comparing different approaches, a detailed example of a decision-making study of illness behaviour is provided. Finally, suggestions for future directions of decision modeling approaches will be made.

## APPROACHES TO THE STUDY OF TREATMENT CHOICE

Anthropologists interested in what leads an individual to a given treatment source have generally adopted one of three perspectives. These three approaches - the correlational approach, the explanatory models approach, and the decision-making approach - are not the only perspectives in anthropology that center on explaining help-seeking behaviour. However, associated with each of these approaches are theories, methods and supporting evidence that are well integrated. Examples of other perspectives include descriptive studies of the stages of help-seeking behaviour (e.g. Chrisman, 1977; Fabrega 1973, 1974; Igun, 1979) and work stressing the importance of the larger political and economic context in accounting for illness behaviour (Frankenberg, 1980; A. Young, 1982). Although authors writing from these two latter perspectives have been able to marshal related research to support their positions, neither has developed into a full-fledged explanation of treatment choice. The stage accounts, as they center on the process of illness episodes, have not attempted to explain how treatment choices are made in a manner distinguishable from other approaches (e.g., correlational, decision-making). As well, although the importance of political and economic circumstances constraining the availability of treatment alternatives and an individual's ability to make treatment choices should not be under-estimated, theorists adopting a political economy perspective have yet to propose explanations of why the same individual will use different treatment sources at different times. Therefore, although these two latter perspectives have much to contribute in understanding treatment choices, they will not be reviewed in the present paper.

### The Correlational Approach

Investigators adopting the correlational approach focus on the "determinants of use of care" (Kroeger, 1983). The term "correlational" is used in a general sense, since not all studies, especially those in anthropology, have employed explicit statistical procedures. Their common feature is the discovery and/or assertion of some characteristic(s) of either the illness, the people seeking, or the treatment alternative itself, that tends to co-vary with the use of treatment alternatives, and on the basis of this association, to attribute to such characteristics causal significance in people's decision making. The majority of this work has been done in medically pluralistic settings where both Western medicine and traditional or folk health care are practiced. Kroeger (1983) provides a recent summary of this literature (also see Stoner 1985) in which he categorizes existing anthropological data using a modified version of Andersen's (1968) generic behavioural model. The generic behavioural model is considered the most widely adopted and empirically assessed model of health care utilization in medical sociology (Wolinsky, 1980, p. 142). The explanatory variables used by Kroeger are of three types. Predisposing factors, or characteristics of the health-care seeker, may be measured by such things as age, sex, socioeconomic level, education, ethnicity, and occupation. Characteristics of the disorder and their perception include the chronicity and severity of the disease, its etiology, and the expected benefits for a given type of treatment. Enabling factors relate to factors which facilitate or discourage the use of particular health services such as geographical accessibility and costs associated with given alternatives.

One example of a correlational explanation can be found in work done by a number of researchers linking treatment choice to the acculturative status of the choice makers (e.g. DeWalt, 1977; McClain, 1977; Woods and Graves, 1973). Characteristics of individuals such as age, wealth, and education are used as measures of acculturation and are correlated with observed patterns of treatment choice. On the basis of observed regularities in usage, these researchers argue that people who are more acculturated (and therefore younger, wealthier and better educated) will use Western treatment facilities to a greater extent than those who are less acculturated.

Aside from problems inherent in defining a concept such as acculturation using measurable characteristics, the correlational approach is not a full account of treatment choice. Typically such studies account for a proportion and usually only relatively small proportion, of all treatment choices (Mechanic, 1979, 1982; J. Young, 1981b). In part, this is because the explanation is necessarily couched in terms of the specific variables the investigator chooses to examine. If data is collected on demographic and economic characteristics only, then the explanation of treatment choice will of course be made in these terms. While it is conceivable that one might collect data on 'all' factors potentially relevant to treatment choice, in practice only a few are examined in any one study.

However, a more important drawback to the correlational approach is that the link between what people think and what people do is ignored. Attention is focused on the phenomenal order (Goodenough, 1964); that is, on the observable, statistically describable pattern of events and the regularities apparent in them. Conversely, the ideational order, which consists of the standards and principles of action that the people observed have in mind in producing these events, is neglected. Since the same outcome may be chosen for different reasons, investigations which are limited to the phenomenal order are imprecise, and often incorrect about the ideational basis of observed behaviour.

## The Explanatory Model Approach

Explanatory models are the ideational in nature, since they are the sets of beliefs and knowledge about illness that provide explanations of sickness and guide behaviour. A. Young (1982) has pointed out that in spite of similar concerns, different investigators often have different interpretations of what an explanatory model is and how it is to be studied. Here, the approach will be defined in a broad sense, including studies coming out of Geertz's (1973) "thick descriptive" hermeneutical approach (e.g. B. Good, 1977; B. Good and M. Good, 1981; Janzen, 1978) and those more directly concerned with clinical applications of the approach (e.g. Blumhagen, 1980; Kleinman, 1978, 1980).

The clearest definition of explanatory models is provided by Kleinman (1980). According to him, explanatory models are not generalized notions about illness, although they often draw upon more general culturally patterned knowledge systems. Rather, they are tied to individuals involved in a particular illness situation at a particular time and reflect significant aspects of cultural context and social relations. Explanatory models are held by all involved in a given illness situation, including individuals treating the illness. However, in explaining treatment choice, it is the study of patient and family which explanatory models hold the most promise. Here these tell us "how they make sense of given episodes of illness, and how they choose and evaluate particular treatments" (Kleinman, 1980, p. 105). Explanatory models can be elicited in interviews that center on five issues "etiology; onset of symptoms; pathophysiology; course of sickness (severity and type of sick role); and treatment" (Kleinman, 1978, p. 87-88). Explanatory models are what generate statements about illness and informant's statements about illness are used by the researcher to discover the explanatory model.

An explanatory model thus provides an interpretive framework for understanding treatment decisions that are developed through an in-depth investigation of people's understandings concerning specific illness episodes and events leading up to them. With the emphasis on illness as an individualized process, this approach has direct clinical implications and has been proposed as a means to alert physicians to the social context of illness and the network of meanings brought by the patient and family to a clinical interaction (B. Good and M.Good, 1981; Kleinman, 1981). It has been most extensively applied to chronic illnesses, "difficult" cases, or to other particularly complex and prolonged illnesses.

Explanatory models can also be used to investigate social network influences and cues or "triggers" (Zola, 1973) to action in illness episodes. A good example is Janzen's (1978) study of therapeutic decision-making among the BaKongo of Lower Zaire. Although predating the widespread use of the explanatory model label, Janzen's work belongs to this tradition. He presents only a small number of illness cases in great detail, as he felt that this approach was best suited to understanding the complex influences and processes behind treatment decisions. Janzen follows his cases through time and interprets the choices made using informants' "explanatory models" and information about the social position and personal history of the patient. The cases Janzen chooses are unusually complex and problematic, and his descriptions richly portray the social context and native logic involved in treatment choices.

The explanatory model perspective has been criticized by those concerned with how political and economic determinants shape the experience of ill health and its treatment (Frankenberg, 1980; A. Young, 1982). According to this critique, since explanatory model writers are primarily concerned with the beliefs and knowledge individuals bring to illness situation, they pay relatively little attention to the objective social order as a critical determinant of medical behaviour. Thus, with the emphasis on how individuals interpret treatment choices, on the ideational basis of behaviour, the explanatory model approach is of limited usefulness in understanding treatment choices.

In addition, the fairly complicated types of illnesses used by writers to illustrate the explanatory model perspective do not form a representative sample on which to build a generally applicable model of treatment choice. Such a model must also account for the more routine, but also significant, illness episodes that people deal with in daily life.

Both of these difficulties arise because the explanatory model approach, like the correlational approach, does not attend to the link between the phenomenal and ideational orders. Unlike the correlational approach, the bias is towards the knowledge behind individual treatment decisions, but this by itself fails to account for observable regularities in treatment decisions within a cultural setting. An explanation of treatment choice should demonstrate the interdependence of the ideational and phenomenal orders.

Decision-Making Approaches

Attention to everyday health-care problems and their resolution characterizes decision-making approaches. Decision-making explanations of treatment choice come out of work done primarily in economics and psychology with the aim of constructing decision theories that will account for all types of choice-making behaviour. Two general types of theories have been proposed - normative and descriptive.

Normative decision theory views choice-makers as rational beings who evaluate alternatives in a systematic fashion and ultimately select the best or optimal alternative for a given choice situation. Normative decision theorists often construct complex mathematical models of choice and use these to predict expected behaviour (e.g., C. Gladwin, 1975). One example of a normative approach to illness treatment choice (Fabrega, 1973, 1974) proposes that people are able to subjectively estimate probabilities with some degree of accuracy, that they use these probabilities to compare the benefits and drawbacks of different treatment alternatives and reach the optimal decision, subject to whatever constraints are operative.

Descriptive decision theorists, on the other hand, argue that models of the normative type are not psychologically realistic, as they attribute unrealistic information-processing capabilities to the decision maker (Quinn, 1978; Tversky, 1972; Tversky and Kahneman, 1974). To take the place of probability estimations, descriptive decision theorists claim that people develop strategies or heuristics which simplify the decision-making process. Further, they state that because of these simplifying procedures, the actual choices people make are often quite different than those predicted by normative models (Simon, 1957). Anthropologists, who have adopted this approach to study decision-making in natural settings, have argued that in recurrent choice situations, like that of illness, where people must regularly choose among alternative courses of action, the members of a given group often come to have a common set of cultural standards used in choice situations. These shared standards of choice can be discovered through examining how information is evaluated by individual actors and what considerations are involved in their choices of treatment. Descriptive studies can be differentiated on whether they attempt to formally model the decision process or not. Informal approaches describe types of strategies or heuristics. For illness treatment, some examples of heuristics include fixed strategies associated with particular illnesses, fixed treatment sequences or hierarchies of resort in the case of commonly occurring illnesses, and treatment by analogy to a known illness under novel situations (see Mathews 1982 for a full discussion of different kinds of heuristics). Work on the nature of cognitive scripts, a concept coming out of artificial intelligence work directed at simulating human thought processes (Schank and Abelson, 1977), may provide insight into the knowledge structures and processes that underlie decisions (Abelson, 1976).

The formal modeling approach, henceforth referred to as the decision modeling approach, grew out of cognitive anthropology's interest in the relationship between the phenomenal and ideational orders. The majority of studies employing this perspective are not concerned with treatment choice, but cover a wide variety of decision situations (e.g. Geoghegan, 1973; C. Gladwin, 1976, 1984; H. Gladwin, 1975; Quinn, 1975, 1978; Randall, 1977). Decision models are built out of informants' statements about considerations involved in treatment choices. The model itself is a formal representation of these considerations and represents an attempt to describe the standards of choice in an explicit and testable manner. Once constructed, the model can be compared against independently collected data on actual choices made by members of the community. This data provides a measure of the model's validity. The decision modeling approach will be illustrated by a study of illness treatment choice in a Mexican village done by the late James Clay Young and the author (for more details of this work see Garro and Young, 1983; Young 1980, 1981a, 1981b; Young and Garro, 1982).

## A MODEL OF TREATMENT CHOICE

Pichátaro is a rural community of approximately 3,000 people of Tarascan Indian background located in the west-central Mexican state of Michoacan. As in many rural Third World communities, people in Pichátaro use sources of health care representative of both modern Western medicine and traditional or "folk" medicine. This does not mean that only two treatment alternatives are available to the Pichátaro. At the time of the fieldwork, the principle alternatives available to them included self-treatment, local herbal curers, local unlicensed practitioners of Western medicine called <u>practicantes</u>, and physicians practicing in a town some twenty miles distant. As physician services are not available in Pichátaro, the choice to consult one involves a bus trip or taxi ride to another town. In addition to transportation costs, fees must be paid for physician services which may be considerable relative to household resources. Prescription-type drugs, however, are available for purchase without a prescription from the practicantes and pharmacies. Although the folk curers and the practicantes also charge for treatment, in contrast with the physician, fees are minimal and these individuals are often willing to wait for payment. Both folk curers and practicantes are easily accessible, as several practice in Pichátaro.

In order to build the model, a series of interviews were carried out with a core group of approximately fifteen informants. The initial interview was designed to elicit the criteria used in selecting one treatment option over another. This was done by systematically contrasting each pair of treatment alternatives using the following question:

> If you or another person in your household were ill, when - for what reasons - would you (consult) (use) _________ instead of (consulting) (using) _________?

Four criteria were consistently cited as important considerations in the choice of treatment: 1) the gravity or the seriousness of the illness; 2) the knowledge and experience possessed concerning the given type of illness and its appropriate remedy; 3) the _fe_ ('faith', 'confidence') one has in the effectiveness of folk treatment remedies as opposed to Western medical treatment in treating a particular illness; and 4) the expenses associated with some alternatives and the availability of resources to meet them.

The nature of two of the criteria listed above were explored in further interviews. In order to understand how informants judge and classify the seriousness of symptoms and illnesses, a card sorting task was developed. Two sets of cards were used, one with the symptoms people in Pichátaro recognize as indicative of illness, and the other with illness labels. Informants were asked to sort one of the decks into groups on the basis of seriousness. Although no instructions were given on how many groups were to be formed, in general, a three level division of seriousness was used by informants. These three levels can be referred to as nonserious, moderately serious, and grave, even though the actual terms used by Pichatareños are somewhat different. Overall, symptoms were more easily and consistently assigned to the same group across informants, indicating that they are more important in assessing seriousness than the illness label.

In order to investigate the nature of faith judgments, a special interviewing procedure was created. Informants ranked cards with the names of treatment alternatives written on them, according to how likely successful treatment would be for each of 13 illness types. These rankings are analogous to less formal statements people make when they say one alternative is _más cierto_ ('more certain' or 'more sure') than another. Across all rankings, treatment by physician received the highest average rank (1.5) meaning that it was the alternative thought most often to offer the highest relative probability of cure. Treatment by _practicante_ and curer received similar average rankings (2.6 and 2.7 respectively), and self-treatment was ranked lowest (3.2). With the exception of a few folk illnesses such as _mollera caída_ ("fallen fontanel") and _mal de ojo_ ("evil eye"), physicians are seen by Pichatareños as representing the greatest likelihood of cure for most illnesses.

Another interview involved a series of hypothetical situations. These were constructed in order to obtain information on the order of use of treatment alternatives. Three of the four considerations mentioned previously - seriousness, available resources, and knowledge of appropriate remedy - were used to create an illness scenario and informants were asked what the probable sequence of actions would be. The "faith" consideration was not included as we wanted to see for what choices it would be cited as relevant.

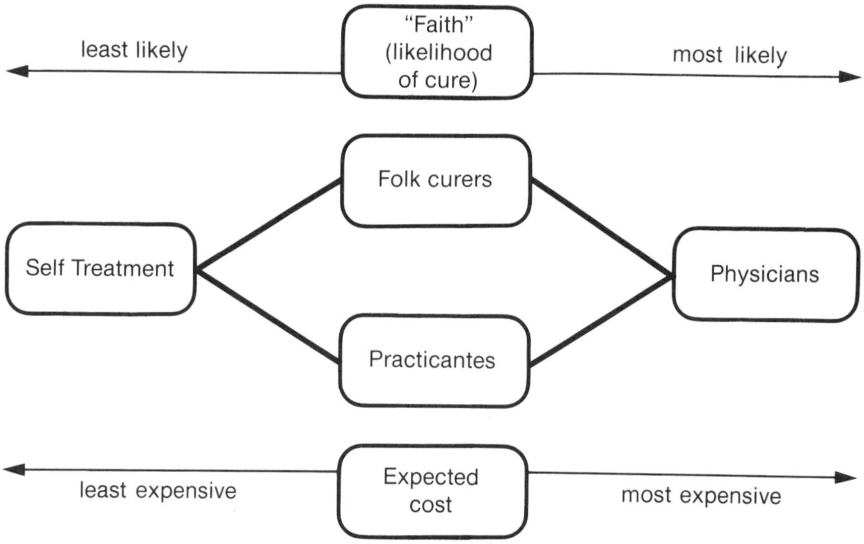


FIGURE 1

In these hypothetical situations, each consideration assumed one of two values: seriousness was either grave or minor; available resources were either abundant or scarce; and the illness had either been successfully treated before within the household or else it was unknown. Since there were three considerations, each with two values, a total of six hypothetical situations were presented. After each reply, informants were asked what they would do if the action just taken had been ineffective. This question was repeated until they finally said nothing more could be done.

The answers people gave to the hypothetical situations yielded the two orderings of treatment alternatives portrayed in Figure 1. These orderings apply for most, but not all illness types. One is based on faith or probability-of-cure and the other on cost. The two orderings are inverses of each other. Self-treatment is judged the least costly, but also as the least likely to bring about a cure. Treatment by a physician is generally considered to be the most certain source of successful treatment, but also as the most expensive. The curer and the practicante options are intermediate on both characteristics. Since they are approximately equal in cost, whether one of these is used in a given situation depends upon the faith one has in folk or Western medical treatment for the specific illness at hand. When the illness is not serious, the general pattern is to use the treatment alternatives in the order of their cost, from least expensive first to most expensive only as a last resort. When the illness is judged to be serious, the preferred pattern is to use the alternative most likely to result in a cure, with cost a much less important consideration. The principal exceptions to these two rank orderings are a few illnesses thought to be

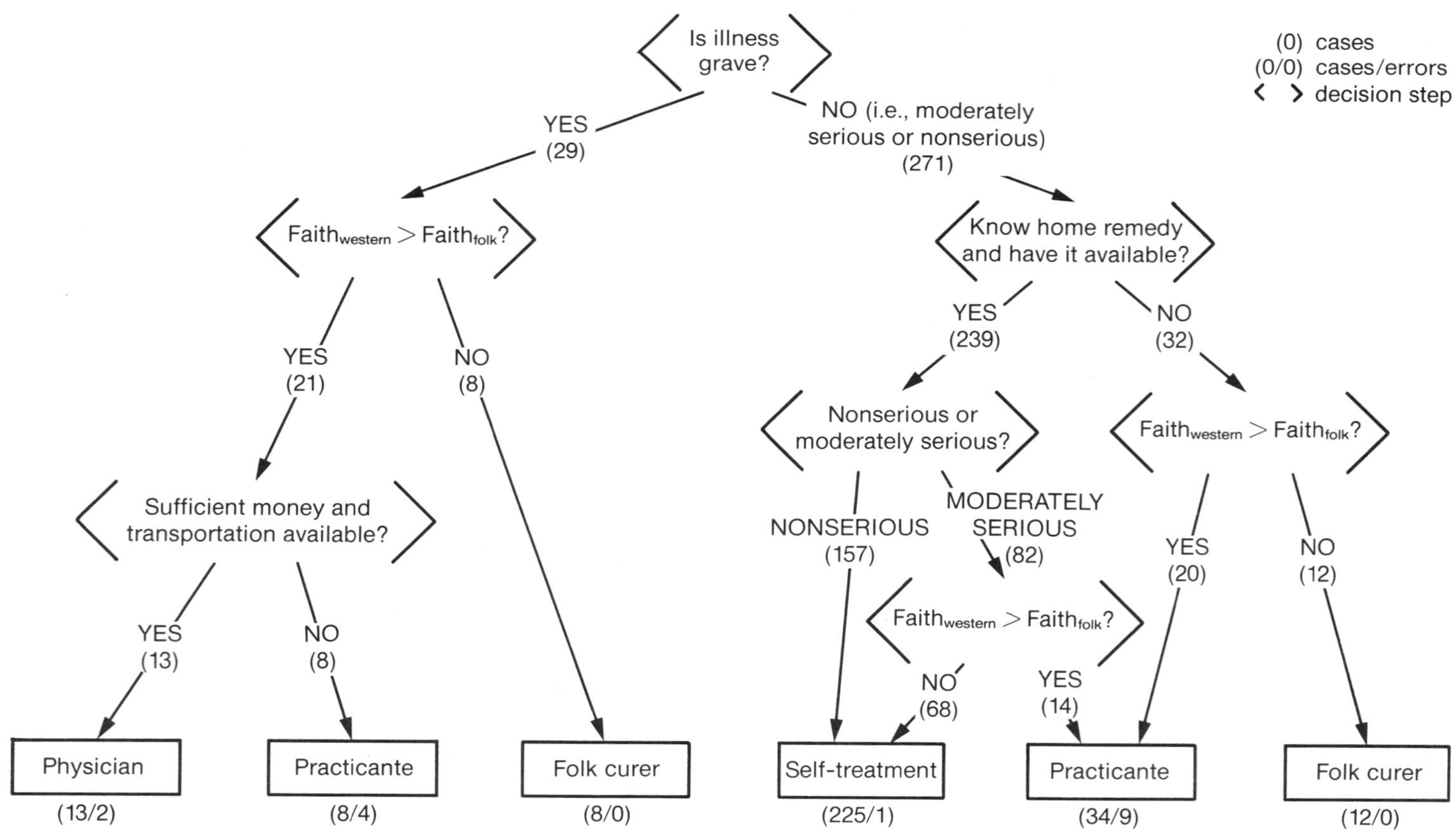


**FIGURE 2.** Decision model for the initial choice of treatment

incurable with Western medicine (mal de ojo or 'evil eye', mollera caída or fallen fontanel and witchcraft related illnesses). However, as these are diagnosed infrequently, and rarely the first diagnosis assigned to an illness case, they do not greatly detract from the explanatory value of the two orderings.

These rank orderings represent ideal patterns and of course there are exceptions to them, especially when the means are not available to realize a particular choice. For example, when a serious illness occurs in a household with scarce economic resources, even though the preferred choice would be the alternative with the highest likelihood of cure, economic limitations constrain choices towards lower costs, thereby approximating a cost-ordered sequence. The formal model incorporates these basic patterns of preferred sources of treatment in different illness situations, and details the variety of constraints that at times lead to the choice of less preferred alternatives. It might be helpful to think of the two basic orderings as representing the objectives or goals people have in mind when making treatment decisions. Embedded in the cost-ordering strategy is the goal of becoming well, but with the least expense. For the probability-of-cure strategy, the goal is to become well but as quickly as possible, leading one to select the alternative with the highest likelihood of achieving a cure. These two goals are implicit in informants' statements about treatment choice.

Decision models can be displayed in a number of formats; here, a hierarchical decision tree is used. Figure 2 presents the model for initial choices of treatment and Figure 3 that of subsequent choices. In these figures, the four decision criteria appear in brackets. With the exception of illness gravity which has three values (reflecting informants' judgments of seriousness in the card sorting task), criteria are represented as binary variables. The decision path on the left side depicts a probability of cure based ordering since the illness is assessed as being grave at the highest node. The next step on this path represents a judgement favouring either folk or medical treatment for the specific illness at hand. A determination that folk remedies are more likely to result in a cure lead to the decision to consult a curer. Alternatively, if the decision maker has greater faith in Western remedies, the next consideration is whether money and transportation are available for physician consultation. If they are, a physician is consulted; if not, a practicante is the predicted choice.

On the right side of the tree, the model depicts the cost-based preference ordering since the illness is not judged as grave. In the situation where a home remedy is known and the illness is considered non-serious, self-treatment is given; if the illness is moderately serious, either self-treatment or a practicante will be chosen depending on an intervening faith judgment for folk or Western remedies. If no home remedy is known or available, and dependent again upon a faith judgment, the expected choice is one of the next least costly alternatives, either a curer or a practicante.

The decision tree for subsequent illness choices, Figure 3, can be read in much the same way. An additional consideration in this tree is the preceding unsuccessful choice, which may lead to shifts in the faith judgment toward the previously unselected mode of treatment.

To sum up the model, it is the gravity of the illness which determines whether a probability-of-cure based sequence or a cost-order sequence is preferred. One's faith establishes the relative ordering of Western versus folk remedies for the particular illness case. Not knowing an appropriate remedy constrains self-treatment. Economic and transportation factors relating to accessibility determine whether a physician's help will be sought.

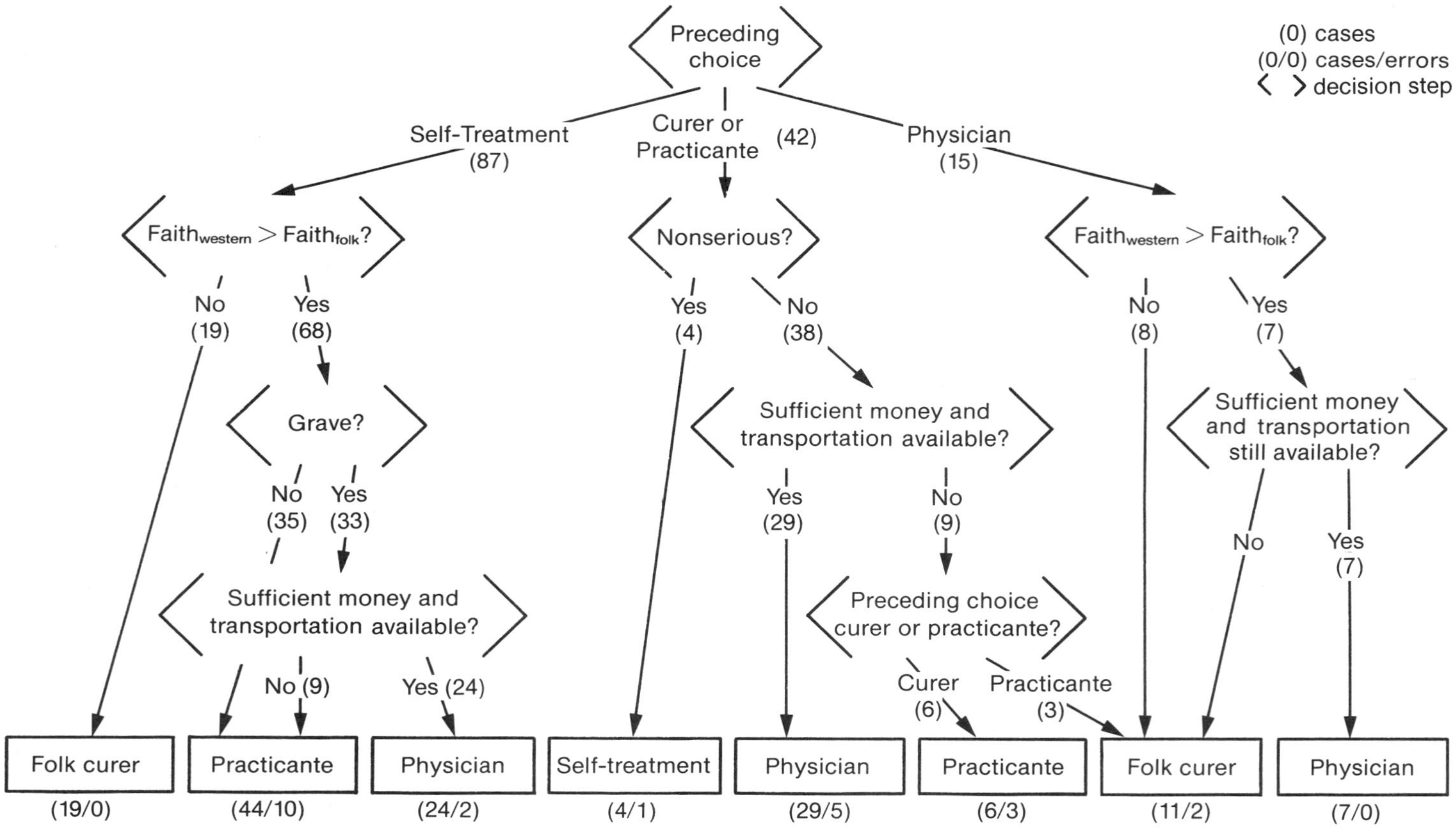


**FIGURE 3.** Decision model for subsequent choice of treatment

In order to evaluate the decision model case histories were collected from a random sample of households that were independent of those used in building the model. Sixty-two households were visited on a bi-weekly basis over a six-month period, and records were made of all illness occurrences for each household during this time. These cases were used to test the model by comparing the actual treatment used with what the model would predict. The scoring was a fairly complex procedure in which information about past illnesses in the household, detailed descriptions provided by household members for each illness episode, and independent wealth rankings of the households, were all taken into account. The numbers appearing in the two decision trees represent the outcomes of these scoring procedures and the number of cases at the bottom of each tree summarize the number of cases scored through that path and the number of errors in predictions. Overall about 90 percent of the choices made in the test cases were consistent with the model. Even if the choices involving initial self-treatment are eliminated from consideration, as this is a quite routine and hence easily predicted action, over 80 percent of the choices conform to what the model would predict. This predictive ability of the model links the explanatory accounts to behavioural outcomes. The high percentage of predicted illness decisions would seem good evidence for the basic validity of the model, and for the contention that the considerations embodied in it indeed represent important aspects of how these choices are actually made.

## EVALUATING THE DECISION MODELING APPROACH

It has been argued that the cognitive decision-making approach provides a view, from the perspective of the decision maker, of the logic involved in choices, and not just data on which to infer that logic. It makes explicit the shared considerations and real-world constraints that interact in producing treatment choices. In contrast to many anthropological methods where there are no external criteria for evaluating theories, a major strength of the decision-making approach lies in a testing procedure that is both quantifiable and potentially replicable. This evaluation process links together the ideational and the observable in a way difficult to accomplish through any other means. Decision models are applicable to a wide range of illness cases and can be used to explain treatment choices in a high proportion of these.

Through the verification procedure, aspects of the decision-making process in need of further refinement may be highlighted. For example, the model of treatment choice developed in Pichátaro was less successful in predicting which of the two middle ranked options - the curer or practicante - would be selected in a given situation. Because these two options are fairly equivalent on the cost ranking, decisions between these two options occur on the basis of faith judgements. Future research on the nature of the faith judgements could help to clarify how these are made and improve both the explanatory and predictive ability of the decision model.

An additional benefit of the decision-making approach is that it provides data with which to evaluate the relative influence of cultural beliefs and external constraints on treatment choices. The literature on illness behaviour among rural Third World peoples has provided two interpretations for the low rates of physician utilization and continued resort to traditional healers. The first points to the importance of cultural factors, such as traditional practices and beliefs about illness, which act as barriers to the use of Western medicine. The second regards low physician utilization rates as a consequence of restricted access to Western medicine, because of socioeconomic marginality and local inavailability of services. There are a number of implications resulting from the application of either of these views. The most important is that the cultural barriers position places the primary responsibility for low utilization rates on the people themselves; the marginality position places the responsibility on the providers of health care.

The study in Pichataro provides several lines of evidence supportive of the marginality position. The first involves the faith rankings discussed previously which showed that for most illnesses physicians were seen by informants as the alternative with the greatest likelihood of producing a cure. The second type of evidence concerns the frequency of folk-specific illnesses. In discussions of the medical beliefs and practices of rural Mexicans, frequent mention is made of illness like 'evil eye', 'fallen fontanel', and witchcraft related ailments. Since these illnesses are thought curable only through folk methods or by traditional healers, and this result was obtained in the faith rankings, such diagnoses preclude the possibility of treatment by physician. However, to then conclude that adherence to beliefs of this type represents a pervasive barrier to the use of Western health care is to overlook the possibility that the incidence of folk-specific illnesses may be quite infrequent. In the case histories collected in Pichataro, it turns out that in less than 10 percent of all cases recorded was the illness considered to be of a type curable only through folk methods. The remaining 90 percent were considered potentially curable through either folk or modern treatment. Whether a given illness in fact received modern treatment was largely a matter of whether it was considered serious enough to justify the expenditures such treatment would entail.

It is also possible to trace individual illness cases through the decision tree and isolate the considerations involved in a person's decision not to seek a physician's treatment when a physician is a plausible choice - given an understanding of the standards by which such choices are made in Pichátaro. For the 38 cases of this type, the distribution of each of three critical considerations is as follows: in 8 (21 percent) of the cases, greater faith in folk medicine was the basis for the decision. In 22 (58 percent) instances, non-use was due to inaccessibility, either the person did not have enough money, and/or transportation out of the village was not available. In the remaining 8 (21 percent) cases, doctor's treatment had just been given without success, leading to a choice to explore other means of treatment.

As these results show, the most common constraint on physician utilization was the <u>perceived inaccessibility</u> of such treatment. A greater faith in folk medicine was the crucial factor in only one out of five cases. Thus, in Pichátaro, it is not cultural beliefs which can be seen as the primary cause of low use rates of Western medical treatment, but rather restricted access to these alternatives.

These results led to comparative work in Uricho (Young and Garro, 1982), a village neighboring Pichátaro and likewise of Tarascan Indian background, but having much better access to primary health services, including a free physician-staffed clinic nearby. Illness case histories for the preceding two months were collected from randomly selected households in both communities. After determining that the distribution of informants' judgements concerning illness gravity were quite similar across the two communities, it was found that people in Uricho sought a physician's treatment in twice as many illnesses, and had an average number of physician visits per household nearly three times as great, as for the comparison household sample in Pichátaro. Illness beliefs in the two towns were investigated using two formal interviewing methods (triads similarity judgements and a term-frame substitution interview) and responses represented using a computer modeling technique, multidimensional scaling. There were no significant, systematic differences in the illness beliefs of the two samples. The illness beliefs of people in Uricho, which were just as "folk" and no more oriented to Western medical theory than was true of Pichátaro, clearly presented no barrier to the use of Western medicine when it was made physically and economically more available. A study with a similar design done in Pichátaro after a government run health clinic was built in the community reached the same conclusion (Garro, 1985).

Nonetheless, as in any research framework, a decision-making approach emphasizes certain aspects of help seeking behaviour while minimizing others. For example, because the focus is on explaining treatment decisions, less attention is given to the processes leading up to a decision to seek help. Missing is specific information on how lay referral systems affect treatment decisions (McKinlay, 1981) and on cues to action that lead an individual to move beyond self-care and seek help from other sources. In addition, decision-making models, to some extent, minimize the contribution of past experiences with an illness condition in explaining current actions. This becomes problematic when a significant proportion of choices to be explained are related to illnesses that are chronic in nature, as is the case in the author's current work in an Ojibway Indian community in Manitoba. Although it is possible to incorporate actions taken with respect to these illnesses into a decision model (Garro, 1984), in order to more fully understand current treatment actions for chronic illness conditions, it is also necessary to understand the often rich and complicated histories associated with them and the belief systems generated through previous experience. Attention to these aspects of choice might clarify what leads individuals to seek alternative forms of treatment at the times they do.

For these reasons, the author's current research involves supplementing the decision modeling approach with explanatory model interviews. As both address directly the ideational basis of illness behaviour, they complement each other. Indeed, in cognitive anthropology, there is much recent interest in folk theories, which are similar in many respects to explanatory models (Nardi, 1983; Quinn, 1983; Quinn and Holland, in press). A folk theory can be defined as a cognitive structure, acquired from everyday experience by nonspecialists, used to provide explanations and guide behaviour. It is expected that using both approaches will lead to a greater understanding of help-seeking behaviour than either approach by itself.

As these last remarks indicate, this paper was not intended to argue the methodological or theoretical superiority of one approach or another. Rather, the central point is that explanations of treatment choice must account for both the ideational and phenomenal orders. The decision modeling approach was presented as one example of how this can be accomplished. In addition, the decision modeling approach provides a base for further research into aspects of treatment choice which may be investigated through other means.

## ACKNOWLEDGEMENTS

Work on this paper was supported by the National Health Research and Development Program of Canada through a Postdoctoral Fellowship to the author (6608-1314-48) and in part by an operating grant from the Manitoba Health Research Council (6278). Figure 1 is from an article by James C. Young (1980) and is reproduced by permission of the American Ethnological Society, a division of the American Anthropological Association, from <u>American Ethnologist</u> 7(1): 106-131, 1980. Figures 2 and 3 are also from an article by James Young (1981b) and are adapted with permission from <u>Social Science and Medicine</u>, 15B: 499-507, 1981. Not for further reproduction.

## REFERENCES


Abelson, R. P. (1976). Script processing in attitude formation and decision making. In J. Carroll & J. W. Payne (Ed.), Cognition and Social Behavior. Hillsdale, NJ: Erlbaum.

Andersen, R. (1968). A behavioral model of families' use of health services. Research Series No. 25. Chicago: University of Chicago, Center for Health Administration Studies.

Blumhagen, D. (1980). Hyper-Tension: A folk illness with a medical name. Culture Medicine and Psychiatry, 4, 197-227.

Chrisman, N. (1977). The health seeking process: An approach to the natural history of an illness. Culture, Medicine and Psychiatry, 1, 351-377.

Dean, K. (1981). Self-care responses to illness: A selected review. Social Science and Medicine, 15A, 673-687.

Dewalt, K. M. (1977). The illnesses no longer understand: Changing concepts of health and curing in a rural Mexican community. Medical Anthropology Newsletter, 8, 5-11.

Fabrega, H. F. (1973). Toward a model of illness behavior. Medical Care, 11, 470-474.

Fabrega, H. F. (1974). Disease and social behavior: An interdisciplinary perspective. Cambridge: MIT Press.

Frankenberg, R. (1980). Medical anthropology and development: A theoretical perspective. Social Science and Medicine, 14B, 197-207.

Garro, L. (1984, November). Issues in modeling treatment choice: Examples from Canada and Mexico. Paper presented at the annual meetings of the American Anthropological Association, Denver, Colorado.

Garro, L. (1985). Decision Models and Variation in Treatment Choice Over Time. Unpublished manuscript.

Garro, L. (in press). Intracultural variation in folk medical knowledge: A comparison between curers and non-curers. American Anthropologist.

Garro, L. & Young, J. C. (1983). Atencion de Salud en Minorias Etnicas Rurales: Algunas Observaciones Antropologicas. Boletin de la Oficina Sanitaria Panamericana, 95, 333-344.

Geertz, C. (1973). Thick description: toward an interpretive theory of culture. In Geertz, C. (Ed.), The interpretation of cultures (pp. 3-30). New York: Basic Books.

Geoghegan, W. (1973). Natural Information Processing Rules: Formal Theory and Applications to Ethnography. Monographs of the Language - Behavior Research Laboratory, No. 3. Berkeley, CA: University of California Language - Behavior Research Laboratory.

Gladwin, C. (1975). A model of the supply of smoke fish from Cape Coast to Kumasi. In S. Plattner (Ed.), Formal methods in economic anthropology. Special publication of the American Anthropological Association, No. 4. Washington, D.C.: American Anthropological Association.

Gladwin, C. (1976). A model of plan Puebla: An application of hierarchical decision models. American Journal of Agricultural Economics, 58, 881-887.

Gladwin, C., (Ed.). (1984). Frontiers in hierarchical decision making. Human Organization, 43, 198-276.

Gladwin, H. (1975). Looking for an aggregate additive model in data from a hierarchical decision process. In S. Plattner (Ed.), Formal methods in economic anthropology. Special publication of the American Anthropological Association, No. 4. Washington, D.C.: American Anthropological Association.

Good, B. (1977). The heart of what's the matter: The semantics of illness in Iran. Culture, Medicine and Psychiatry, 1, 25-28.

Good, B. & Good, M. J. Delvecchio. (1981). The meaning of symptoms: A cultural hermeneutic model for clinical practice. In L. Eisenberg &

A. Kleinman (Eds.), The Relevance of Social Science for Medicine. Dordrecht, Holland: Reidel.
Goodenough, W. H. (1964). Introduction. In W. H. Goodenough (Ed.). Explorations in cultural anthropology. New York: McGraw-Hill.
Hulka, B. S., Kupper, L. L., & Cassel, J. C. (1972). Determinants of physician utilization. Medical Care, 10, 300-309.
Igun, U. A. (1979). Stages in health-seeking: A descriptive model. Social Science and Medicine, 13A, 445-456.
Janzen, J. (1978). The quest for therapy in Lower Zaire. Berkeley and Los Angeles: University of California Press.
Kleinman, A. (1978). Concepts and a model for the comparison of medical systems as cultural systems. Social Science and Medicine, 12B, 85-93.
Kleinman, A. (1980). Patients and healers in the context of culture. Berkeley: University of California Press.
Kleinman, A. (1981). On illness meanings and clinical interpretation: Not 'rational man', but a rational approach to man the sufferer/man the healer. Culture, Medicine and Psychiatry, 5, 373-377.
Kroeger, A. (1983). Anthropological and socio-medical health care research in developing countries. Social Science and Medicine, 17, 147-161.
Lock, M. M. (1980). East Asian medicine in urban Japan. Berkeley and Los Angeles: University of California Press.
Mathews, H. (1982). Illness classification and treatment choice: Decision making in the medical domain. Reviews in Anthropology, 9, 170-180.
McClain, C. (1977). Adaption in health behavior: Modern and traditional medicine in a West Mexican community. Social Science and Medicine, 11, 341-347.
McKinlay, J. B. (1981). Social network influences on morbid episodes and the career of help-seeking. In L. Eisenberg and A. Kleinman, (Eds.), The Relevance of Social Science for Medicine. (pp. 77-107). Dordrecht: Reidel.
Mechanic, D. (1979). Correlates of physician utilization: Why do major multivariate studies of physician utilization find trivial psychosocial and organizational effects. Journal of Health and Social Behavior, 20, 387-396.
Mechanic, D. (1982). The epidemiology of illness behavior and its relationship to physical and psychological distress. In D. Mechanic (Ed.), Symptoms, Illness Behavior, and Help-Seeking. New York: Prodist.
Nardi, B. (1983, November). The use of extended natural discourse in cognitive studies. Paper presented at the annual meetings of the American Anthropological Association, Chicago, Illinois.
Quinn, N. (1975). Decision models of social structure. American Ethnologist, 2, 19-45
Quinn, N. (1978). Do mfantse fish sellers estimate probabilities in their heads. American Ethnologist, 5, 206-226.
Quinn, N. (1983, November). What discourse can say about culture: Convergent evidence for a cultural model of American marriage. Paper presented at the annual meetings of the American Anthropological Association, Chicago, Illinois.
Quinn, N. & D. Holland. (1986). Cultural models in language and thought. Cambridge, England: Cambridge University Press.
Randall, R. (1977). Change and variation in samal fishing: Making plans to 'make a living' in the southern Philippines. Unpublished doctoral dissertation, University of California, Berkeley.
Schank, R. C. & Abelson, R. P. (1977). Scripts, plans, goals and understanding: An inquiry into human knowledge structures. Hillsdale, NJ: Erlbaum.
Simon, H. A. (1957). Models of man: Social and rational. New York: Wiley.

Stoner, B. P. (1985). Formal modeling of health care decisions: Some applications and limitations. _Medical Anthropology Quarterly_, _16_, 41-46.
Tversky, A. (1972). Elimination by aspects: A theory of choice. _Psychological Review_, _79_, 281-299.
Tversky, A. & Kahneman, D. (1974). Judgment under uncertainty: Heuristics and biases. _Science_, _185_, 1124-1131.
White, K. L., Williams, T. G., & Greenberg, B. G. (1961). The ecology of medical care. _New England Journal of Medicine_, _265_, 885-892.
Wolinsky, F. D. (1980). _The sociology of health_. Boston: Little, Brown & Co.
Woods, C. & Graves, T. D. (1973). _The process of medical change in a highland Guatemalan town_. Latin American Studies Series, Vol. 21. Los Angeles: University of California Latin American Center.
Young, A. (1982). The anthropologies of illness and sickness. In B. J. Siegel, A. R. Beals, & S. A. Tyler (Eds.), _Annual Review of Anthropology_, _11_, 257-285.
Young, J. C. (1980). A model of illness treatment decisions in a Tarascan town. _American Ethnologist_, _7_, 106-131.
Young, J. C. (1981a). _Medical choice in a Mexican village_. New Brunswick, NJ: Rutgers University Press.
Young, J. C. (1981b). Non-use of physicians: Methodological approaches, policy implications, and the utility of decision models. _Social Science and Medicine_, _15B_, 499-507.
Young, J. C. & Garro, L. (1982). Variation in the choice of treatment in two Mexican communities. _Social Science and Medicine_, _16_, 1453-1465.
Zola, I. K. (1972). The concept of trouble and sources of medical assistance. _Social Science and Medicine_, _6_, 673-679.
Zola, I. K. (1973). Pathways to the doctor: From person to patient. _Social Science and Medicine_, _7_, 677-689.

# PART IV    ILLNESS BEHAVIOUR:  SOCIOPOLITICAL ISSUES

# ILLNESS BEHAVIOUR AND DISABILITY

Monroe Berkowitz

Professor of Economics
Rutgers University

The recent crisis in the administration of the Social Security Disability Insurance (DI) program in the United States highlights the failure of social scientists in general and economists in particular to influence the development of public policy in this crucial area. Perhaps the DI experience is only one of many illustrations of how difficult it is to have complex human conditions responded to by welfare decisions which are attuned to individual circumstances yet are explicit, predictable, challengeable and politically palatable (Bolderson, 1985).

In 1980, under the Carter administration, Congress passed legislation (P.L. 96-265) mandating reviews of the status of persons who were receiving DI benefits. The Social Security administration (SSA) under the Reagan administration, responded to the prevailing conception that many persons were on the rolls who did not belong there and began the re-examination of the eligibility of the beneficiaries.

At least two issues presented themselves for decision. Which cases should be selected for review and what standards ought to be applied? SSA chose what seems to have been sound managerial options. They decided to put their money where the action was likely to be and gave the priority for review to those cases most likely to be terminated. In March of 1981, a study by the General Accounting Office showed that 20 percent of the beneficiaries on the rolls were not disabled (General Accounting Office, 1981). SSA chose to look first at cases whose "profiles" indicated that they might not belong on the rolls. As to the standards to be applied, SSA studies revealed that there had been inconsistencies in past decision-making and it was recognized that standards varied among states. SSA chose to apply the standards prevailing at the time of review. People on the rolls were to be judged in exactly the same way as persons who were seeking to get on the rolls.

The results of this eminently logical approach to the reviews mandated by Congress were chaotic. In three years time, nearly one million cases were reviewed and nearly half of these were found to be ineligible and, for the most part, their benefits were terminated (Committee on Finance, 1983). Many of these persons had been on the rolls for years and thought their pensions secure. The media publicized the cases of mentally ill persons left without any means of support and cases of suicide were attributed to the seemingly arbitrary withdrawal of benefits. Shocks were felt throughout the .pl 77 entire administrative system. SSA's decision to terminate benefits was challenged and reversed over 200,000 times in various stages of the appeals process. States which have responsibility for making initial eligibility decisions began to defy SSA and refused, in some instances, to participate in the review process.

The pressures on Congress to do something to alleviate the situation were intense but it was not until 1984 that Congress was able to agree on the Social Security Disability Benefits Reform Act of 1984 (P.L. 98-460). Some of its provisions were to be applauded in that they strengthened administrative procedures, but, on the whole, Congress embraced the "medical model" of disability. Once on the rolls, beneficiaries could not be removed unless there was substantial evidence that the individual had medically improved. Granted that the amendments also provided other grounds such as showing of fraud, or that the individual had been the beneficiary of advances in medical, vocational therapy or technology, Congress seemed singularly unimpressed with the notions of sociologists and economists that disability was a socioeconomic phenomenon which could be understood only by looking at a complex interaction between the individual's medical condition and a host of environmental variables.

From an economist's point of view, one can make sense out of what might be termed the disability system only in terms of a model which allows for the full impact of an individual's differential reaction to identical physical or mental medical conditions. Following Nagi (1969) and Haber (1984) the essential aspects of this model are set out using some accepted distinctions among terms which have been used by researchers and those persons engaged in surveys of disabled persons. Following a brief look at the numbers of disabled persons some of dimensions of disability expenditures in the United States are outlined together with some idea of the growth in these expenditures over the years. It is concluded that the social scientists have emerged from their examination of the system with intellectually satisfying explanations for the phenomena they observe which apparently have proven to be quite useless in the practical policy debates of the 1980's.

## Definitions of Terms

Disability can be defined as the loss in the ability to perform socially accepted or prescribed tasks and roles due to a medically definable condition. The sequence leading to disability begins with this physical, mental or emotional condition which is the state of active pathology. In some (relatively few) cases, the condition leaves a person with some residual impairments, some physiological, anatomical or mental loss or abnormality which persists after the condition has stabilized. In some cases (again, relatively few) these residual impairments cause a person to have functional limitations. The person, because of physical impairments, is unable to lift, carry, walk, or has not the strength or endurance to perform certain tasks. An emotional impairment may leave the person in such a state that he or she is simply unable to relate to his or her fellow-workers. Some persons may be prevented by these functional limitations from performing their expected roles, and hence, are classified as being disabled.

Note that to determine whether a person has a physical condition, an impairment, or a functional limitation, one has only to examine the person himself/herself. To determine whether he or she has a disability may be a more complex task since the inability to perform expected or prescribed roles may be due to functional limitations interacting with a whole host of other factors in that person's environment. While conceptually clear, the complex interaction of factors may be most difficult to translate into the kind of easily understood practical rules and regulations required for the administration of a mass-production type of benefit plan. This point will be returned to later.

It is not enough to talk about this continuum from condition to disability without recognizing that there is a time dimension. A person acutely ill with a cold accompanied by chills, aches and fever has no difficulty in identifying their physical condition or impairment. He or she is probably completely functionally limited and certainly disabled in the sense that they cannot fill any role except that of the supine patient. But, happily, these episodes are self-limiting and usually of short duration. It is when the condition leaves the person with more or less permanent impairments and functional limitations that one becomes involved with disability issues. Attention is confined to permanent or long-term disabilities, usually those which last six months or longer. In the DI program, a person's impairment is expected to last for more than 12 months or to be permanent, and a person must have been out of the labour force for five months before he can collect benefits. Any dividing line must be arbitrary, and it is recognized that long-term disabilities begin with short-term episodes.

There is yet another difficulty with these conceptually clear definition which are difficult to translate into practice. The difficulty has to do with the terminology, the names that are applied to the various stages of the sequence. Different terms are used in various pieces of legislation or by various organizations. Once again, relatively clear-cut concepts fall prey to real world usage. The World Health Organization (1980) chooses to use disabilities to mean what has herein been called functional limitations and the term handicaps to denote what has been called disabilities, but their concepts, if not their terminology is similar to the more traditional terms employed in the United States. Far more serious confusion occurs because of entrenched but nonuniform usages in various programs. The Rehabilitation Act's definition of handicapped pertains not only to a person who has an impairment which limits a person's major life activity, but also a person with a record of such impairment, or a person who is regarded as having such an impairment.

To choose another example, persons with physical and mental impairments which began at birth or developed early in life may benefit from services under the Developmental <u>Disabilities</u> legislation although the concept fits more neatly under the definition of impairments. Under most state workers' compensation laws, a person will be examined after his/her medical condition has stabilized. If he/she is left with some physical impairment or with some functional limitation, he/she may be eligible for a weekly cash benefit. But, whether the amount of that benefit is rated in accordance with the extent of the physical impairment, or according to some measures of functional limitations, it is likely to be called a permanent partial <u>disability</u> benefit. When it is awarded on the basis of one's actual loss of wages due to one's inability to perform all of the duties of his job, then it conforms exactly to the concepts outlined, but the terminology remains the same, regardless of the basis of the benefits.

The definition of disability could conceivably apply to a person's inability to perform any social role, but it fits most comfortably with the inability to work at a job - the concept underlying the DI program and most, but not all, income replacement programs. But work is obviously only one of the many roles a person carries on in their daily living. This is not to say that other aspects of a person's life are not of equal importance. It is difficult, however, to determine if a person is, say, recreation disabled. Most individuals have some physical or mental condition that prevents them from performing some sports role as adeptly as would be liked. As a practical matter, the problem becomes marked as one deals with older age groups which have many persons retired from work. For such people, it is peculiarly necessary to specify the role to which the disability measure will apply. Since it is not easy to find one central role which the retired person performs, it is most difficult to apply disability concepts to such retired persons. Whatever the problems in measuring work disability, it is easier to measure than any of the alternative concepts. Thus, it is no accident that basic information about disability prevalence comes from labour market or social security surveys which are confined to respondents in the labour force age groups, and which define disability as some variant of the inability to work.

## The Numbers of Disabled Persons

It is futile to search for an unambiguous precise count of the number of disabled persons. Even if one confines oneself to the least ambiguous concept, that of work disability, one is confronted by moving targets - changing circumstances which influence the count. The whole economics of disability and for that matter the whole concept of illness behaviour rests on the notion that disability resides as much in external circumstances as it does in the person himself/herself. If that goes too far, then, at least, the social scientist would insist that to ascertain whether a person is disabled or not, one needs to know more than a physician's evaluation of his physical or mental condition. The point can be illustrated in countless ways, but it is quite obvious that the prevalence of a condition, say, Multiple Sclerosis is one thing and the number of persons disabled by MS quite another.

Estimates of the number of disabled persons derive, for the most part from survey information as persons are asked if they are limited in the amount and kind of work they can do, or, if their physical or mental condition prevents them working at all. One could compile a long list of what is wrong with that question and, it should come as no surprise to find that estimates derived from various surveys differ widely.

Attention is focused on the "severely disabled" (defined as those not working or not working regularly). Haber (1984) estimates on the basis of the 1978 Social Security Survey that 5.8 percent of the noninstitutional population, ages 18 to 64 can be classified as disabled. In 1983, the noninstitutionalized population ages 18 to 64 in the United States was approximately 142 million. Using the 5.8 percent prevalence figure, it is estimated that 8,353,000 persons were classified as disabled in this restricted meaning of the term.

The 5.8 percent prevalence rate is higher than was found in the 1980 census where 4.4 percent of the population aged 16 to 64 was found to be disabled. Although the census used similar questions, the 1978 survey had the advantage of better screening questions and more highly specialized interviewers. The 1982 Current Population Survey (CPS) used a broader definition including persons who left a job because of health reasons, persons receiving certain benefits as well as those who reported health problems that limit or affect their work. Under this broader definition, the CPS found 8.9 percent of the population to be work disabled. No matter which of these survey results are used disability emerges as an important problem which affects a not inconsiderable percentage of the working-age population in the United States.

The response to the phenomena of disability has been a welter of rather diverse programs which pay cash benefits, provide medical care and other services. In addition, the United States has adopted some general policies relating to access and opportunities for disabled persons which will be briefly examined. One way to make some sense out of almost confusing array of programs is to examine disability expenditures.

## Disability Expenditures

Disability expenditures are classified into three broad categories - cash transfer payments, medical care payments and other direct service payment. All expenditures which arise because of the long-term disability of persons in the labour force age groups are included. For the cash transfers and the medical care payments, one can inquire into the rationale for these payments. Why is that society in the United States and in most other countries, is willing to transfer funds to disabled persons?

One reason is that persons insure against the contingency of becoming disabled. This insurance may be compulsory as in the DI program or voluntary as in private insurance, or, possibly a little of both under some employer-provided or collectively bargained plans. In any of these situations, a person who is insured becomes entitled to these payments upon a showing of disability status. Obviously, here is part of the problem in the DI controversy. Persons on the rolls, having once qualified for benefits feel that their entitlement ought to continue undisturbed. Having qualified for their tickets out of the labour force, perhaps after long months of interrogation, application and examination, they do not look kindly at any attempts to take them away.

Quite a different rationale for transfers exist in the case of persons who are damaged by the negligence of others. In the United States, where we have developed the arts of litigation to a higher degree than most other nations, this is an important reason to transfer funds and to provide medical care services to persons so disabled. In addition to the traditional negligence cases, personal injury or medical malpractice, the no-fault programs such as workers' compensation are included.

The third reason to transfer funds and provide medical services is simply that of need. Some funds from the public purse go to those persons who can demonstrate they are poor regardless of the reason for that state, but the larger categorical programs are reserved for those whose poverty can be ascribed to a particular cause. Disabled persons qualify as members of the "deserving" poor, and, upon showing of need, qualify for payments from the federal program confined to disabled persons and those 65 years of age and over.

It is estimated that the total U.S. disability expenditures among persons ages 18 to 64 were nearly $122 billion in fiscal 1982, about 4.7 percent of Personal Income in the U.S. (M. Berkowitz, 1985). A little more than half the amount is accounted for by cash transfers. As might be expected, the DI program, accounted for a substantial portion of these cash transfers, about $18.8 billion. However, another $18 billion was paid out in all the private and employer-provided insurance programs including those provided by various levels of government for its employees. One of the problems of measuring disincentive effects of the DI program is that it obviously does not exist in isolation. Many persons receive benefits from more than one program and some people fall between the cracks and may not be eligible for any.

Cash transfers also include the indemnity payments. The concept of these is broad including payments under "no fault" schemes as well as the traditional tort liability payments. Payments to veterans for service-connected injuries are also placed here. Adding all of these indemnity-related transfers together results in a total of $23.3 billion for 1982 - a sum greater than that paid out in DI, although not greater than that of DI and the individual and employment insurances combined.

In the last cash transfer category are the income support programs - veterans' pensions, Supplemental Security Income (SSI) and Aid to Families of Dependent Children (AFDC) - all programs in which recipients must demonstrate need. In these calculations only that portion of the total payments which can be ascribed to disability are included. The total for 1982 is $7.3 billion, about 11 percent of the estimated $67.4 billion of disability transfers for that year. (See Table 1).

TABLE 1

CASH DISABILITY TRANSFERS IN FISCAL 1982

| Source | Amount | Percentage |
|---|---|---|
| Social Insurance | $18.8 billion | 28% |
| Individual and Employer-provided Insurance | 18.0 | 27% |
| Indemnity Payments | 23.3 | 34% |
| Income Support | 7.3 | 11% |
| Total | $67.4 | 100% |

## Medical Care Costs

Unlike transfer payments, medical care costs involve the use of real resources, be they the time of physicians, the use of hospitals, or the purchase of prescription equipment and drugs. The objective is to calculate those sums which would be eliminated if disabilities were somehow magically eradicated. But, even if that state were to come about and disability as is known was gone, the formerly disabled persons would still incur a certain amount of medical expenses.

The matter might be put another way. Disabled persons must meet a certain amount of medical expenses because of their chronic condition or conditions which underlie their disabled status. In addition to these expenses, they probably have to pay medical bills because of conditions that have nothing to do with their medical impairments. E. Roberts, former director of the California rehabilitation program, is impaired. He cannot go far from his iron lung without some breathing apparatus - but he is fond of noting that it has been months since he has seen a doctor. He may be impaired, or even disabled, if one uses that term loosely, but he is not sick.

It is estimated that the total medical care costs for the disabled population for fiscal 1982 were $51.2 billion. As with transfers, that sum represents the total expenditures for the disabled population, ages 18 to 64, as best as these age adjustments can be made. Those programs which deal only with short-term illnesses have been eliminated, but one cannot be confident that all the expenditures for these short-term, self-limiting episodes of illness have been eliminated in programs such as Medicaid and Medicare (where both acute and chronic conditions are covered).

As with transfers, one can divide medical care costs into categories dependent upon the reasons for the payment. In the social insurance category, one includes only the Medicare program, which, since 1973, has covered DI recipients after a two-year waiting period. In 1982, Medicare paid out $9.8 billion in hospital and supplementary medical insurance payments to persons on DI or those qualifying for the special End Stage Renal Disease Program.

As in transfers, medical payments are made when persons insure against the contingency - by taking out a private policy, by subscribing to one of the Blue plans, or by having this type of coverage provided through one's employer. It is relatively easy to estimate the total paid out by private insurers and the Blue plans. It is not as easy to estimate the proportions of the total paid out for medical care usage by disabled persons. The best that one is able to do is to utilize data on health-care utilization by age and by disabled-nondisabled status and to adjust the reported figures accordingly. It is estimated that about $24 billion were paid out in this private and employer provided category. That total includes $60 million, an estimate of the amount spent under the several Department of Defense programs which serve disabled dependents.

The indemnity category includes a host of veterans' programs and the federal and state workers' compensation programs. The amounts paid in tort settlements is not reported separately, since we cannot distinguish them from other amounts paid under the private insurances where the vast bulk of these payments are made. The total in this category is $6.4 billion.

The last category is that of income support where the prominent program is Medicaid and where $11.7 billion was paid in 1982. (See Table 2).

Medical care payments are summarized in Table 2.

TABLE 2

MEDICAL CARE PAYMENTS IN FISCAL YEAR 1982

| Source | Amount | Percentage |
|---|---|---|
| Social Insurance | $ 9.8 billion | 19% |
| Private and Employer-provided Insurance | 24.0 | 46% |
| Indemnity | 6.4 | 12% |
| Income Support | 11.7 | 23% |
| Total | $51.9 billion | 100% |

## Disabled Persons' Proportion of Medical Care Costs

Even though medical care costs for disabled persons are only a small portion of total medical care costs, the disabled population accounts for a disproportionately large share of total medical payments. We have some information about this from the 1980 National Medical Care Utilization Survey (NMCUES).

Out of a total population between the ages of 18 to 64 of 127.6 million, NMCUES found that about 10 percent of 12.5 million persons classified themselves as disabled. But this 10 percent of the population accounted for one-third of the total medical expenditures - some $26.2 billion out of a total of $78 billion. The average yearly medical expense for a disabled person was $2,214.00, nearly four times larger than the medical bills paid by the average nondisabled person. The impact on disabled persons is softened somewhat because a larger share of their medical bills were paid for by third parties. Nondisabled persons paid 27 percent of their medical bills out of their own pocket, whereas disabled persons met 18 percent of their expenses themselves. Nonetheless, the average yearly out-of-pocket expenses for disabled person was $441.00, nearly three times greater than the $155.00 yearly out-of-pocket expenses incurred by nondisabled persons.

## Disincentives and Medical Care Payments

One other aspect of medical care for disabled persons might be mentioned. Receipt of cash transfers constitute a potential disincentive to persons going back to work. In evaluating the seriousness of that problem, it is estimated, with some degree of confidence, the amount of cash transfers a person might receive. (These amounts cannot be estimated with 100 percent accuracy because of the uncertainty as to how many different types of benefits a person might receive). But any forecasts as to future medical care payments is beclouded with greater uncertainty since it is dependent, not only on program eligibility, but also on a person's medical condition which might change over the years. A disabled person might be persuaded to give up a monthly DI check for hourly wages, but be more cautious about relinquishing Medicare eligibility if faced with some unknown future medical liability. It is no accident that Congressional amendments aimed at disincentives assure workers of continuance of Medicare for some limited period and easy return to the rolls should the worker find it impossible to continue at the job.

## Other Direct Services

Medical care costs are one form of direct services separated, in part, because of their magnitude. Also, we are able to categorize medical expenditures according to whether they arise because of social or private insurance, indemnity or income support, but one is unable to classify other direct services quite as easily. Provision of these services rests on a different footing than cash transfers or medical care payments. Certain of these services are designed to restore persons to the labour market. Their obvious rationale is that they are a good investment - that they will return to government an amount greater than their costs. Whether such claims can stand a great deal of scrutiny is another matter, but such has been their historic rationale (Berkowitz and Berkowitz, 1983).

Prominent among such services are vocational rehabilitation. In fiscal 1982, it is estimated that about $1.1 billion was spent for vocational rehabilitation and closely related services out of a total of an estimated $3 billion for all direct services.

Services for veterans are placed in another category and separate veterans' programs are identified. Among these programs are the separate vocational rehabilitation programs for veterans, programs to supply adapted vehicles, housing and prosthetic appliances and various programs at the federal and state level to provide domiciliary care. These veteran's direct service programs are estimated to cost about $406 million.

In a separate category there are a number of miscellaneous programs designed to provide services to persons with specific impairments. Historically, the government has provided services to blind and deaf persons, and in more recent years, has extended the provision of services to the mentally ill and to persons afflicted with developmental disabilities. Possibly there are two reasons for such provision of services. These services are provided in response to political pressures by, or on behalf of particular groups. Deaf persons and blind persons have been successful in persuading government to provide particular education, rehabilitation and other services. Parents of mentally retarded children have organized and been able to persuade legislators to include their children in the mainstream school systems and to provide other services.

The "mainstreaming" aspect to the appeals or demands of the developmental disabilities movement contain a clue to the rationale for these expenditures. Disabled persons are asking government to provide services designed to repair or to compensate for any difficulties they may encounter in competing in education, activities of daily living or the labour market.

Persons in wheel chairs argue that providing attendant services will allow them to work and not be a charge on the community. The expenditures for all these programs cannot be accurately determined, but it is estimated that, in fiscal 1982, approximately $141 million was spent on these programs with the largest amount, some $52 million, allocated for the developmental disabilities programs.

The difficulty in making cost estimates in this field occurs, in part, because certain of these expenditures are paid under general programs which pay benefits to disabled and nondisabled persons. Some attendant care is paid for out of Medicaid or social service block grants. In addition, there are general federal programs, such as the food stamp program, where allocations are made on the basis of need and where a number of persons qualify because of their disability status. The assumption is that these persons are in need, or are receiving the services because of their disabling condition. In 1982, it is estimated that $663 million was spent on food stamps received by disabled families and that about $405 million was spent on social services for a total of about $1.1 billion in this category.

Disabled persons are also served by the several employment assistance programs. Included here are the programs for handicapped persons working for the federal government as well as the various employment or jobs programs such as the Comprehensive Employment and Training Program (CETA) and its successors and predecessors. In some of these programs designed to return people to the labour market, or to encourage their entry for the first time, a specific dollar amount is set aside to serve handicapped persons. In other programs, it is necessary to estimate the amounts spent on disabled persons. It is estimated that in all of these employment assistance programs, approximately $300 million was spent for services to disabled persons (in 1982).

The total of some expenditures incurred are missed because of laws which are designed to provide functionally limited persons access to jobs, housing, public buildings and transportation facilities. Sections 503 and 504 of the 1973 amendments to the Rehabilitation Act require covered employers to make accommodations for disabled persons so as to allow them access to job opportunities. Collingon (1985) has made some estimates of accommodation expenditures and the Bureau of Economic Research at Rutgers in compiling information on housing and transportation modification costs, but reliable data in these areas are not available. These are important outlays, not necessarily because of their amounts, which are undoubtedly small as compared to transfers and medical care costs, but because they signal a significant policy initiative. In a sense, this is a response to the disability rights activists whose plea has been that it is society and not they who are disabled - that with equal access and accommodations, they can function efficiently. They couch their demands in terms of nondiscrimination against the new minority of disabled persons.

The expenditures for which information is available are summarized in Table 3 that follows:

TABLE 3

DISABILITY EXPENDITURES - 1982

| Source | Amount (billions) | Percentage |
|---|---|---|
| Transfer payments | $ 67.4 | 55.5 % |
| Medical services | 51.2 | 42.1 |
| Direct services | 3.0 | 2.4 |
| Total | $121.5 | 100 % |

Granted that the estimates in the area of direct services are most problematical, direct service expenditures are a rather paltry portion of the total. For the most part, any preventative and remedial services would fall into this category. It is quite clear that the U.S. government preference is to pay cash benefits and provide medical services but not to spend a great deal on rehabilitation or other corrective type services.

## Trends in Expenditures

Looking at one year's expenditures is limiting. Public policy is influenced by trends in expenditures and the perception has been that these expenditures have been growing at a rapid rate. It was these perceptions which influenced the 1980 legislation providing for the Social Security Disability Insurance reviews. The reality is that expenditures in 1982 were 400 percent greater that in 1970. The years of explosive growth were in the 1970's and the rate of growth has slackened off in recent years. This is not the place to explore the several reasons for these trends except to note that disability expenditures increased faster than inflation rates, gross national product or other welfare expenditures.

## The Economic Model of Disability

The essence of the concept is that behaviour of the person affected is not mandated by that person's medical condition as diagnosed and described by a physician. The model requires that a distinction be made among the condition, the impairment, the functional limitations and finally, the disability, as these terms are defined above. The economist would stress the choices the functionally limited person have to become disabled or not become disabled. A sociologist would place less emphasis on "choice" and more on familial and societal influences on the person. But these are details , the question is whether the model is useful? Does it help us understand the world a little better?

The model does help explain some commonly observed disability-related phenomena. For example, the March 1982 Current Population Survey presented information on the ages and educational levels of persons who reported themselves as disabled. As would be expected, the reported prevalence of a work disability increases with age. About 5.4 percent of men, ages 25 to 34, reported the presence of a work disability but men in the older age group, ages 55 to 64, were five times as likely to report such a disability (26.2 percent). That is not surprising since it is known that the prevalence of impairments, such as visual and hearing impairments, and circulatory and respiratory conditions increase with age.

But the CPS data also show a strong negative relationship between levels of schooling and the prevalence of a work disability. For example, among men ages 35 to 44, 17.8 percent with fewer than nine years of schooling report a work disability as against 4.7 percent of those who have completed at least one year of college. Approximately the same relationship between education and disability holds true for women as well. The CPS has data on race, and, with few exceptions, it was more likely for a black man or woman of a given age and level of schooling to report a disability than their white counterpart.

In some cases, the person's physical condition may have forced him or her to abandon his/her schooling at an early age, and such persons may find themselves in low level jobs with a high degree of occupational risk, but there is probably more going on. A given physical or mental impairment, or a given level of limited functioning will knock the blue collar worker out of the labour market. The identical condition may have no effect on the lawyer or physician who can continue his practice. To labour the point, in order to understand the disability, one must know more than the person's physical or mental condition. One must know his/her demographic characteristics and human capital attributes.

The economists's model of disability looks for additional intervening variables which mediate between the level of functioning and the disabled state. With a model which has each person seeking his/her highest level of utility or satisfaction, the person is not indifferent among the several choices he may have among work and not working and collecting benefits. Some, but not all, of the many cash benefit programs alluded to previously require that the recipient withdraw from the labour market. A person, dependent upon the circumstance in which he/she incurred his/her impairment, may be eligible for benefits from more than one of these programs.

The economists' model would predict that if benefits increase, all other things equal, more persons will apply for the program. Leonard (1979) estimated that a ten percent increase in expected DI benefits will increase the number of Social Security DI benefits by 3.5 percent. A relationship between labour force participation rates and benefit levels has also been observed although competent investigators differ over the exact elasticities (Leonard, 1979; Parsons, 1980; Haveman and Wolfe, 1984). It would be difficult to explain why more persons should drop out of the labour market or why more people should apply for benefits as cash benefit levels increase except with some model which recognized factors which are external to the affected person. These examples could be multiplied with observations of the strong positive relationship between unemployment and the disability rate, or the increases in workers' compensation benefit levels and the rate of applications (Worrall and Butler, 1985), but the conclusion would be the same - the model is useful in explaining, at least to the economist, a piece of the real world he/she sees about him/her. Why then has it failed to influence the Social Security DI administrative process, or if it has had some influence there, why has it not been accepted by the appeals system.

## The Economic Model of Disability and the Determinations Process

In order to be eligible to collect DI benefits, a person must demonstrate attachment to the labour force by having a certain number of years of employment in covered industry. After a waiting period of five months, a person must show that he is unable to engage in substantial gainful employment (defined as work which yields a certain wage) because of his physical or mental condition which is expected to last at least 12 months. By quirk of historical accident, the determinations as to disability status are made at the state level (E. Berkowitz, 1979), theoretically, to allow the state vocational rehabilitation agencies to try their hand in restoring the person to the work force. (The differences in allowances among the states which seem to be related to differences in economic conditions can be explained only in terms of the type of an economic model).

Applications are judged on the basis of material in the file and consist largely of reports of medical examinations. The question to be decided initially is whether the applicant meets the so-called "medical listings" a list of medical impairments and symptoms which prior to the 1984 amendments were not public in the sense that government was not required to publish them in the Federal Register. If it is decided that the applicant's medical condition as reflected in reports in the file meets these medical listings, benefits are allowed. If the decision is that the applicant does not meet the listings, benefits might still be allowed and it is at this stage that inquiries are made as to the client's residual functional capacity and factors such as age, skill and education are taken into consideration. As far as can be ascertained, the bulk of the determinations are made by use of the medical listings alone.

The determination process, at least in part, recognizes nonmedical factors, but Congress in the 1984 amendments seems to have dealt the thinking of the social scientists a grievous blow. Why should not a person's beneficiary status change if there is some substantial change in the nonmedical factors which may have a powerful influence on a person's disability status? One is left with the impression that, in trying to extricate the system from the horrible and chaotic condition it found itself in after the review process got underway, Congress had no stomach for trying to understand all of the complexities of the relationship between medical condition and disability.

This was not the first time that Congress expressed some skepticism as to these matters. At one time, Congress embraced the notion that persons, once on the disability rolls, could benefit from vocational rehabilitation services designed to get them into the job market and hence off the disability rolls. In the 1965 Social Security amendments, Congress provided that the state vocational rehabilitation agencies could be reimbursed from the DI trust fund for 100 percent of the funds they spent in rehabilitating DI beneficiaries who met certain elgigibility requirements. The performance of the state agencies in removing persons (Treitel, 1979), or at least their failure to document their successes, led Congress in 1981 to cut off this source of funding for the vocational rehabilitation program. Retraining or the provision of counselling, guidance and placement services was not thought to be worth what they cost.

Such decisions would unlikely be very different if the social science view of the world were more widely accepted. Political decisions are not made under conditions where fine intellectual arguments are persuasive. Yet, the social scientist's model of disability seems to explain so much of what is observed about disability in the real world and this could be more useful in the political and legal decision-making process.

## Some Needed Work on the Economics of Disability Model

At first glance, it might seem that the difficulty with the model is that it embraces too many variables in too complex a fashion. Much of the economists' work has been in the development of multivariate econometric models where the dependent variables are labour force participation, wages, benefit levels, etc. In the professional journals, scholars argue about the appropriate specification of the model, about selection bias, identification problems and other such stimulating issues. Only the initiated who have paid their dues are entitled to take part in these discussions. But before one concludes that this is the problem, one has to account for the fact that the courts seem to be able to handle evidence based on equally complex multivariate models in the equal employment opportunity cases. The courts are accustomed to listening to experts who discourse in learned fashion about matters which adjudicators themselves are not expert in.

Of course, the equal employment cases tend to be class action suits where broad tendencies rather than individual situations come to the fore. Some of the protest against the review process were also class action suits but the determination process is peculiarly an individual one, albeit one which is handled in accordance with rules and regulations appropriate to a mass production benefits program. Granted that the disability models yield results cast in terms of the probability of their occurrence and the individual case demands an answer appropriate to that particular individual, it would still seem that the models should prove of some use to the decision maker.

The difficulty may lie not in the complexity of any model but in the quality of the information in the model itself. The model in some general sense does explain such phenomena as the relationship between levels of education and reported work disability. But that is not enough if the notion is to be widely disseminated and understood. The relationships must be quantified and the separate effects of each of the several factors, age, race, education, training, potential benefit levels, state of the labour market as well as the person's health must be measured. And it is the last item, the state of the person's health where measurement is most questionable.

Estimates of the effects of a rise in benefit levels on some factor such as labour force participation differ in part, in good part, because of the different methods used to standardize for what might be called, for lack of a better term, health. Condition classifications, mortality estimates, activities of daily living scales, self-reported disability, and functional assessment measures have all been used. Condition classifications tell us very little about severity and work limitations; mortality estimates depend upon panel data and may have little relationship to morbidity and work limitations; activities of daily living scales may do well in measuring a persons's skills in performing basic functions but many quadraplegics unable to dress themselves unaided do well in the job market; and self-reported disability defined in terms of the ability to work is hardly the measure to use in determining who can work. The best measure is one of functional limitations, but information in this area is sparse. Scales can be constructed from self-reported information from survey data, but the last comprehensive survey in the United States was in 1978 and that left much to be desired.

In an ongoing project the author and colleagues are employing a scale called the Functional Assessment Inventory (FAI) (Crewe and Athelstan, 1979). While it may do a good job in assessing a person's health in the sense of physical and mental limitations, it must be administered by some person who is familiar with the client or applicant. Unfortunately, most research on this and similar measures of functional limitation has been conducted using the measures in case diagnosis and prognosis and not as a measure of the current state of health (Halpern and Fuhrer, 1984).

Much more needs to be done in the testing and development of measures which can depict a person's mental and physical limitations or in a more positive sense, their residual functional capacities, to use the DI term. Research is needed on both the conceptual and measurement spheres. It is obvious that our attempt to construct the mental disability analogs to the functional limitations in the physical disability area need the most work.

Although the limitations are well recognized, it may be that one has to be content with scales developed from self-reported data. The last full-scale Social Security Administration survey was in 1978 and no new survey seems to be in the offing.

More needs to be done. The whole theory underlying the economics of disability would seem to have a prominent place for rehabilitation efforts. Counselling, guidance, retraining and placement as well as removal of job barriers, physical and psychological, fits in well with the notion that nonmedical factors can cause disability. But here agin, the evidence is quite sparse that rehabilitation is cost effective in restoring persons to the labour market. There have been no large-scale rigorously controlled evaluations of the program. Or, at least, there have been none that are able to convince those who are skeptical about the efficacy of the vocational rehabilitation process.

## CONCLUSION

Public opinion is notoriously fickle. The media, which in the 1970's delighted in portraying the scandal of able-bodied persons receiving DI program benefits, filled its pages in the 1980's with horror stories of the plight of persons arbitrarily removed from the rolls. After much hesitation and floundering, Congress responded in a manner which seemed to reinforce the medical model of disability. If the 1984 amendments are to be given credence, it will be more difficult to remove beneficiaries from the rolls unless an improvement in their medical condition can be shown. That seemed to fly in the face of all that has been learned from the development of the economics of disability over the last decades. A large and complex disability system has evolved providing for cash payments, medical care and direct services and the economic model takes into account their disincentive effects and the influence of a host of nonmedical factors on disability status.

Why have the contributions of the social scientists in general and the economist in particular not been more influential? One recognizes the difficulty of applying findings from probabilistic models to individual cases, but the real problem probably lies in the quality of the models and the basic data on which they are built.

Differences in empirical results when these economic models are tested can be traced to differences in measures of health and the paucity of recent information on such matters as the total receipts from benefit programs. New surveys on these matters would help remedy some of these deficiencies but none are in the offing. Rehabilitation models which promise changes in the disability status of persons with physical and mental impairments desperately need rigorous testing if these ideas are to receive wide acceptance.

The true scholar is probably indifferent as to whether his ideas and theories can or cannot be applied in the real world. However, scientists with a more applied bent await the time where the scholarly inquiries of the social scientist can have more of an impact on public policy than is evident in the 1984 amendments to the Social Security Disability Insurance amendments.

## REFERENCES


Berkowitz, E. D. et al. (1979). The American disability system in historical perspective. In E. D. Berkowitz et al. (Eds.), Disability policies and government programs. New York: Praeger Publishers.

Berkowitz, E. D., & Berkowitz, M. (1983, January). Benefit cost analysis. National Rehabilitation Information Center.

Berkowitz, M. (1985, January). Disability expenditures 1970-1982. New Brunswick, NJ: University Bureau of Economic Research.

Bolderson, H. (1985, March). Disability benefits and administrative law judges in the United States of America. Journal of Social Welfare Law. Sweet and Maxwell.

Committee on Finance. (1983, September). U.S. Senate, staff data and materials related to the Social Security Act disability programs (Senate Print No. 98-93). 98th Congress, 1st Session.

Crewe, N. M., & Turner, R. R. (1984). A functional assessment system for vocational rehabilitation. Functional assessment in rehabilitation. Baltimore, MD: Brookes Publishing.

General Accounting Office. (1981, March 3). More diligent followup needed to weed out ineligible SSA disability beneficiaries. (Report No. HRD81-48). Report to the Congress by the Comptroller General.

Haber, L. (1984, November 29-30). Trends in demographic studies on programs and disabled persons. Switzer Memorial Seminar, New York, NY.

Haveman, R. H., & Wolfe, B. L. (1984). The decline in male labor force participation: Comment. Journal of Political Economy, 92, No. 3.

Hahn, H. (1984). The issues of equality: European perceptions of employment for disabled persons. New York: World Rehabilitation Fund.

Halpern, A. S., & Fuhrer, M. J. (1984). Functional assessment in rehabilitation. Baltimore, MD: Brookes Publishing.

Leonard, J. (1979). The social security and disability program and labor force participation. (Working Paper No. 392). National Bureau of Economic Research.

Nagi, S. (1969). Disability and rehabilitation. Columbus, OH: Ohio University Press.

Parsons, D. O. (1980, February). The decline in male labor force participation. Journal of Political Economy (pp.117-134.)

Treitel, R. (1979). Recovery of disabled beneficiaries: A 1975 followup study of 1972 allowances. Social Security Bulletin, 42, 3-23.

Weaver, C. (1986). Thinking about social security disability policy in the 1980's and beyond. In M. Berkowitz & M. A. Hill (Eds.), Disability and the labor market: Ecomonic problems, policies and programs. Ithaca, NY: ILR Press.

World Health Organization. (1980). International classification of impairments, disabilities, and handicaps. Geneva: World Health Organization.

Worrall, J. D., & Butler, R. J. (1986). Some lessons of workers' compensation. In M. Berkowitz & M. A. Hill (Eds.), Disability and the labor market: Economic problems, policies and programs. Ithaca, NY: ILR Press.

# LONG-TERM CARE: AN ALTERNATIVE MODEL

Stanley Wallack

Center for Health Policy Analysis and Research
Brandeis University

## Introduction

If all individuals acted or behaved in a similar, stable manner, policy development would be a rather simple matter. However, that is not the case. Sociologists, social psychologists, and scientists have pointed out the difficulties of moving between the "micro" and the "macro", or from individual behaviour to national policy and programs. Economists have had an equally difficult time; microeconomics and macroeconomics are derived from different theoretical constructs, and no theorist has been able to build a bridge between the two theories.

The credibility and longevity of the prevailing macroeconomic theory has suffered due to the lack of a clear connection between micro and macroeconomic theory. Keynes built his general theory of the economy upon individual behaviour under uncertainty. Changes in investment behaviour drove the economy, and yet Keynes offered little knowledge about what determined the level of investment by individuals. He viewed investment as so unpredictable that he used the recent past as the best predictor of the future. Keynesian economics fell into disrepute when fiscal policies did not lead to their intended results. The explanation for poor performance was the inability of Keynesian theory to incorporate the expectations of individuals. Keynesian economics has now been replaced by the monetary theory. While no one, including Milton Friedman, understands how the money supply impacts on the performance of the economy, Friedman has noted the limited relationship between changes in the money supply and the performance of the economy. The policy solution offered was to keep the growth in money supply constant, since it was not known how changes in the money supply would affect the economy.

Because monetary theory has not come to grips with the interaction between macro and micro behaviour, the role of government is minimized in solving major social problems. And, the "black box" theory predominates today because economists do not understand how to bridge the macro and micro issues. The need to relate the behaviour of individuals and institutions with national policy is great; for without this change, public policies will be judged inadequate.

Trying to Build the Bridge: Long-Term Care

One of the far-reaching problems facing policymakers today is that of long-term care for the elderly. Finding more appropriate ways to finance and pay for long-term care for the chronically ill and disabled elderly has become one of the most important health policy issues of the 1980's. Currently, long-term care activists have found little support in either government programs or private insurance. Due to the changing perspective of what constitutes long-term care and the problem of adverse selection, few insurance companies have been willing to expand into the long-term care market. Due to the burgeoning elderly population, and the old-old generation, which will grow from about two million to six million by 2040, a re-evaluation at the federal and state level is needed, as well as expansion of the private insurance model.

The population needing long-term care is expected to double in the next thirty years and no one source, whether public programs, private insurance, or individuals will be able to pay for the costs. As the need for long-term care continues to grow, the government's ability to pay for care through future tax dollars will be constrained by budget cuts, changes in Medicare-Medicaid, and low federal initiative. Long-term care needs have not been adequately addressed in the past because of a lack of knowledge about financing and delivery of these services, the lack of a data base for information, and even a lack of understanding of the definition of long-term care.

Public expenditures for long-term care are primarily for nursing home care. Of the approximately 13.45 billion the government spent on long-term care in fiscal 1980, 10.56 billion, or 79 percent, was for nursing home care, whether for a skilled nursing facility or an intermediate care facility (Health Care Financing Administration, 1981). Currently, many patients are in skilled nursing facilities which they not only do not need, but which cost more than an intermediate care facility (Fox, 1983). And, although the figure has dropped in the past few years, over-utilization of nursing homes is still a significant issue. Over 45 percent of nursing home residents whose costs were paid by Medicaid were not initially poor but had their resources depleted as a result of chronic illness. Thus, much of Medicaid's budget goes toward paying for the care of people who become poor because of a lack of insurance. Currently, private insurance is minimal, and public programs for at-home services amount to less than 10 percent of expenditures for long-term care (Meiners and Trapnell, 1984).

For the elderly, long-term care is the leading cause of catastrophic expenditures, forcing many to go on welfare and break-up their homes and families. Financing for long-term care in the United States is so minimal that families either have to pay out-of-pocket, or spend down to go on welfare. Due to the growth of the elderly population and the need for institutional and community care, the demand for long-term care services will continue to increase.

The costs to the federal government and to the states via Medicaid have alerted policymakers to the problem of financing long-term care in the future. By limiting the construction of nursing homes and making stringent certificate-of-need standards, states are tightly regulating nursing home services in an effort to control Medicaid budgets. Sixteen states imposed some form of moratorium on the construction of nursing homes in 1984 (Feder and Scanlon, 1980; Meiners, 1983). Currently, 80 percent of long-term care costs, even in a well-managed system, go to nursing homes, and Medicaid, the major public funding source for long-term care, covers 48 percent of these expenditures (Lave, 1985).

By recognizing the limited growth in public financing, the relevant issue becomes how to foster and encourage private sources of financing, and how to efficiently use existing public dollars. Because of the growing population over 65, the elderly will comprise 22 percent of the population by 2030 (Congressional Budget Office, 1977). Thus, the federal and state governments are faced with the problem of how to meet the health care needs of the elderly in the future and the problem of how to stimulate insurance models which will help finance this care. Private insurance carriers have not been interested in long-term care issues because of the difficulty in predicting the need for care and estimating the costs.

One of the benefits of expanding and developing a model for long-term care insurance is the ability to relieve the burden on Medicaid and the pressure on public budgets by encouraging private insurance models to provide a variety of comprehensive services. If costs could be pooled over an entire population, huge expenditures for an individual would be minimized, and fewer people would have to spend down to Medicaid. Even if risk pooling was limited to only those over 65, affordable protection would be feasible.

## Continuing Care Retirement Communities

One model based on the idea of prepaid health care is the continuing care retirement communities (CCRC's), or life care communities. Approximately 400 to 600 continuing care communities across the United States care for over 100,000 elderly (Raper, 1984). The life care community is an organization established to provide housing, services, and health care, (Winklevoss and Powell, 1984). The community contains independent living units, congregate dining, nursing home facilities, and is based on the idea of continuing health care. Residents pay an endowment fee, plus a monthly fee for maintenance costs. The monthly fees may be higher initially than the cost of services received, but this higher cost, paid by all residents, helps defray nursing home costs at a later date. This policy of prepayment helps to stabilize monthly payments for all residents (Pastalan, 1985). Rather than pooling Medicare and Medicaid dollars, the entry fees are used to cover a broad set of services. In some communities, individuals pay the same monthly rate whether they are in an apartment or the nursing facility. The end result is that no resident spends down to Medicaid. Thus, continuing care retirement communities prove that insurance risk spreading can work.

Some CCRC's guarantee long-term health care, financed through a pooled risk arrangement to a segment of the population who needs protection against the catastrophic costs of long-term care. These communities often have higher levels of nursing home care than those found outside the community. The reasons are many and intertwined; insurance reduces the cost for the individual, the geographic proximity of the nursing home reduces the anxiety of moving from the apartment, and the more attractive living arrangements provide an easier transformation for the resident.

Studies have been conducted at Brandeis University on continuing care retirement communities, as well as on the general community, to understand utilization patterns, and therefore, costs. Through its work with different organizations, Brandeis has been able to gather data on the elderly over a long period of time. By looking at transitions into hospitals and nursing homes, we have been able to analyze how many elderly will enter a nursing home over a lifetime, how much time they will spend there, and how much it will cost to finance the care.

## Utilization of Nursing Homes

At age 65, the lifetime risk of entering a nursing home for a non-CCRC resident is 43 percent (Cohen, Tell, Wallack, in press). This risk increases with age until the age of 80; at the age of 85, the risk begins to decline. This decline occurs because fewer people survive at this age to enter a nursing home. These data, based on the 1977 survey of 4,100 Medicare beneficiaries, included people living in the community, as well as those living in various long-term care facilities.

TABLE 1

LIFETIME RISK OF NURSING HOME ENTRY AT DIFFERENT AGE LEVELS AND CHANGE IN RISK

| | Remaining Risk of Entering an Institution | | | | | |
|---|---|---|---|---|---|---|
| Age | Total Population (%) | | Males (%) | | Females (%) | |
| 65-69 | 43.1 | | 30.5 | | 51.9 | |
| 70-74 | 44.7 | (+1.6) | 30.6 | (+0.1) | 53.4 | (+1.5) |
| 75-79 | 47.7 | (+3.0) | 29.7 | (-0.9) | 57.4 | (+4.0) |
| 80-84 | 47.6 | (-0.1) | 27.6 | (-2.1) | 57.3 | (-0.1) |
| 85-+ | 43.0 | (-4.6) | 22.9 | (-4.7) | 52.0 | (-5.3) |

Table 1 shows the risk of entering a nursing home for males and females at different age intervals, and shows the change in the risk between the intervals. For males, between the ages of 65 and 74, there is only a small increase in the risk rate. The group facing the highest risk of entering a nursing home is aged 70-74, with a leveling off after that period.

For women, the risk of entering a nursing home increases with age until the age of 80. After age 80 the risk declines. Since females tend to live longer than males, their use of nursing homes should be greater, as seen in this table. Characteristics of the population which increase the risk of institutionalization are functional status, age, health status, and marital status. Studies by the National Center for Health Statistics show that the presence or absence of a spouse is a major factor affecting nursing home utilization. In the Center study, only 12 percent of residents of nursing homes had a spouse.

Table 2 shows the rates of CCRC residents in six communities for which there is detailed individual data. The probability of entering a nursing home at least once at a CCRC is much higher than for those residing in the general community, with a range of 67-76 percent. The higher utilization of the nursing home is probably due to easier access at CCRC's, and the insurance built into the system. Not only is there a higher probability of entering a nursing home when one lives in one of these communities, but the average length of time spent in a nursing home is greater as well.

## The Cost of Nursing Home Care

From the nursing home utilization rates and the number of days over a lifetime, we have estimated the expected cost per individual. In calculating the likely cost, we compared the different utilization rates of those living in the general community with those in life care communities. The per capita lifetime nursing home cost in current dollars for a 75-year-old, unmarried female appears to be between $16,000 for non-life care residents and $25,000 for life care residents. While this is not a trivial sum, it would be an affordable premium for many of the elderly, considering their current assets, particularly their homes. If all 75-year-old, unmarried females were to prepay this amount, all those needing care would receive it free of charge, even those needing nursing home care who could contribute in excess of $100,000.

TABLE 2

DISTRIBUTION OF NURSING HOME ENTRANTS BY AGE AT CCRC ENTRY (DEATH ONLY)

| Age at CCRC Entry | No Entry | | At Least One Entry | |
|---|---|---|---|---|
| 65-69 | 19 | (32.8%) | 39 | (67.2%) |
| 70-74 | 56 | (32.0%) | 119 | (68.0%) |
| 75-79 | 90 | (26.5%) | 249 | (73.5%) |
| 80-84 | 85 | (23.8%) | 272 | (76.2%) |
| 85-89 | 41 | (24.1%) | 129 | (75.9%) |
| 90 and over | 20 | (32.8%) | 41 | (67.2%) |

This above example suggests that insuring for long-term care is quite possible. In fact, this type of risk-sharing is exactly what happens in many life care communities. Over the past few years, we have studied a number of mature life care communities. A mature community has an average age of 85, and often about 20 percent of the residents are in the nursing facility. The additional cost of entering a nursing home rather than staying in one's apartment is about $10,000 per year. This cost is spread or shared by all the residents, so that the average per capita cost for nursing home care is about $2,000 (0.2 x 10,000). With each individual paying $200 per month for nursing home care, the community is able to self-insure. The outcome of this type of risk-sharing is that no single individual bears catastrophic long-term care costs. This, in turn, means that no member of the community has to go on welfare.

The total costs of long-term care are not overwhelming, and it is important to make this point clear to policymakers in the public and private sector. However, having such data on the total costs does not allow one to determine the proper strategies in terms of delivery and financing. To do this, one needs to have some idea of the distribution of costs and the predictability on an individual basis. Knowledge of the distribution of expenses provides policymakers with information as to whether an income or benefit program would be more desirable.

Policymakers also want to be able to predict the future use for those living in the community so as to determine future financial liability and delivery system needs. To do this we need a model that goes from individual characteristics to onset of illness, illness to disability, and disability to nursing home use. This chain of events means there are a number of predictive variables that are significant such as age, marital status, and functional status. What is probably more important to policymakers is that our model, as well as that of other researchers, does not predict which individuals will enter a nursing home. No doubt this is related to random variation, thus, a national program would ameliorate this problem. However, part of the problem is related to systemic factors, e.g., delivery system configurations. Finally, a voluntary program, such as private long-term care insurance, would have to build-in significant premiums for possible adverse selection (or unexpected high utilization).

Thus, while the total costs of long-term care are manageable, the variation will stymie public policymakers and the private sector. To move policymakers forward, we need to provide them with a higher degree of certainty. Policymakers will feel more comfortable providing fixed dollar, categorical grants, but this will not be helpful in view of the variation in use. An insurance or benefit program is needed, one that can be predicted to be within a prescribed budget.

## Learning How to Better Predict the Costs

We have learned how to bring about better predictability in health care costs. Cost sharing by consumers, case management and risk-taking by providers all work to create a more efficient system and one that is more predictable in terms of cost and utilization outcomes. However, given the uncertainty of how to best provide and manage long-term care, providers placed at financial risk will probably want to go beyond the usual control mechanisms, preferring to have control over resources as well. The CCRC, with its controls on beds and staff provides a starting point for developing a system, but one capable of serving many more individuals.

Researchers at Brandeis are now working to develop financing and delivery models for long-term care. It is the responsibility of research groups not only to analyze and dissect problems, but also to suggest solutions, and test for validity and effectiveness.

This is how the Social/HMO was conceived at Brandeis. The Social/HMO was developed as a more appropriate health-care program for the elderly, one that meets the needs of the chronically ill. The Social/HMO was built off the medical system (the HMO), adding social and long-term care services to the benefit package and delivery system. Over the past five years, since conceiving the concept, four sites have been developed co-operatively with significant involvement of Brandeis researchers. There are now four Social HMO's operating, and Brandeis is currently evaluating their performance. We expect this critical review will lead to modifications of the sites, and, therefore, alter the future variants of the model.

Over the next two years, it is expected that each site will enroll four to six thousand elderly persons. This opportunity will permit the observation of the care and outcome of about 20,000 elderly. This will lead to new information on how to target the necessary care, and how to best provide this care in light of the health outcomes of these elderly individuals. Other social scientists will have the opportunity to evaluate and critically analyze the Social/HMO.

However, the Social/HMO is only one of many programs that should be evaluated to deal with the chronic health care needs of the elderly. University researchers must be intimately involved in these programs if the results are to be readily translated, and then used in developing the next generation of solutions.

## CONCLUSIONS

Finding more appropriate ways to finance and pay for long-term care for the elderly is becoming one of the most important health policy issues of the decade. There are two major problems with the current financing of long-term care; inadequate financial protection for individuals, which results in catastrophic expenditures for the elderly, and a fragmented financing system which produces significant inefficiency in the delivery of care. Total long-term care costs for our society are not overwhelming. What is overwhelming is the distributional character. Ten to fifteen percent of the elderly account for ninety percent of long-term care expenditures, but we are not able to predict which individuals will need and seek this care. The distributional problem is less troublesome in a compulsory or public program. However, the current fiscal problems of the federal and state governments make it unlikely that adequate public financing will be provided for long-term care for the elderly.

With the level of uncertainty in predicting costs, and the need to foster private financing endeavours, researchers need to develop efficient delivery systems that are able to control utilization. With today's limited knowledge, only life care communities which have control over all the necessary resources, offer the needed risk-sharing and services. By analyzing their performance as well as other long-term care efforts, researchers should be able to develop models that private and public sector policymakers will find attractive enough to encourage large scale experimentation.

## REFERENCES


Cohen, M. A., Tell, E. J., Wallack, S. S. (in press). The lifetime risk and costs of nursing home use among the elderly. Medical Care.

Congressional Budget Office. (1977). Catastrophic health insurance. (#052-070-03882-9). Washington, D. C.: U. S. Government Printing Office.

Feder, J., & Scanlon, W. (1980). Regulating bed supply in nursing homes. Milbank Memorial Fund Quarterly, 58, 54-88.

Fox, P. D. (1983). Long-term care: A bird's eye view. Pride Institute Journal, 2, 23-30.

Health Care Financing Administration. (1981). Long-term care: Background and future directions. (DHHS Publication-HCFA 81-20047). Washington, D. C.: U. S. Government Printing Office.

Lave, J. R. (1985). Cost containment policies in long-term care. Inquiry, 22, 7-23.

Meiners, M. (1983). The case for long-term insurance. Health Affairs, 2, 55-79.

Meiners, M. R., & Trapnell, G. R. (1984). Long-term insurance. Medical Care, 22, 901-911.

Pastalan, L. A. (1985). Retirement communities. Generations, 9(4), 26-30.

Raper, A. T. (1984). National Continuing Care Directory. Washington, D. C.: American Association of Retired Persons.

Winklevoss, H. E., & Powell, A. V. (1984). Continuing care retirement communities: An empirical, financial, and legal analysis. Homewood, IL: Richard D. Irwin.

# ILLNESS BEHAVIOUR - A POLITICAL ANALYSIS

Irving Zola

Department of Sociology
Brandeis University

This chapter examines the nature of medicine and the political context of the terms "health" and "illness". More specifically, issues of power will be addressed. Power will be illustrated on the macro level by the phenomenon of medicalization and on the micro by the encounter between health-care provider and patient.

The term "medicalization" has been defined as the growing power of medicine in the twentieth century (Conrad and Schneider, 1980; Zola, 1972a). Medicine has become an institution of social control and has led to increasing application of the labels "health" and "illness" to social problems, as well as to widening areas of everyday life. At least some of the concern with this problem is political (Crawford, 1977, 1979, 1980; Zola, 1975). For the "medical model", whatever else, has a very individualistic focus. Thus, as medical diagnoses are used to describe social problems and troublesome people, whole series of actions and connotations come with them. Illness is almost universally perceived to be bad, not good, and as such not something to be treasured or even pondered over, but something to be treated and gotten rid of. So, too, with medicalized social problems and "sick" troublesome people (Zola, 1975). Moreover, if a problem gets defined on the medical/individual level then it becomes less likely that treatment/ intervention will occur on any other (e.g., political, social) level.

The medical position of power is due to a number of forces. Many other institutions, such as law and religion, (which were major arbiters of moral values), have no longer the influence they once had (Rieff, 1968). Medicine has also become more meaningful in the everyday life of the population. As Henderson (1935) has claimed, up until the early part of the twentieth century, if a random doctor met a random patient with a random disease, the patient had about a 50-50 chance of benefiting from the encounter. That this situation is no longer true is due to many factors - some medical, some societal (Dubos, 1961, 1965). In any case, with a gain in perceived efficacy, medicine sought to consolidate its position (Brown, 1979; Starr, 1982) by more exclusively controlling who was a physician and what he/she could do (Freidson, 1970a, 1970b, 1976; Stevens, 1971) and thus, by definition what others cannot do. There are, for instance, relatively few other areas of work where one can be arrested for practicing without a license.

This power differential is continued in the actual practice of medicine. First, you can certainly tell the players by the uniforms they wear, with varying insignia (some subtle, like in certain institutions the not wearing of a uniform) distinguishing the ranks. Patients on the other hand are, in all senses of the word, often stripped of their identity (Goffman, 1961) thus losing any symbols which might designate or elevate their status. The distancing is perpetuated in the forms of address. The providers of care are most often referred to by title whereas patients are most often referred to with inappropriate terms of endearment, belittlement and familiarity. Consider the following example. A colleague of the author once had the following encounter when she had to undergo an emergency hospitalization. The examining physician upon entering introduced himself, "I am Dr. Robinson. How are you, Marcia?" She looked up at him. She said, "I am fine, Richard. How are you? My name is Dr. Millman." He then said to her, "I was only trying to make you more comfortable by calling you ... ", to which she replied, "I was only trying to make you more comfortable". The women's movement (Boston Women's Health Book Collective, 1984) has pointed out the further distancing, if not humiliation, that too often comes in the manner of questioning or the position one is in, when being questioned.

Anthropologists have long emphasized the importance of turf and territory in delineating control and power. Thus, the shift in location (Gibson and Kramer, 1965) of the medical encounter from the home to the office, and medical center is a shift of great import. No claim is made that power was all in the hands of the patient when the visit was in the home but it certainly "looked" differently. The author personally recalls his mother dealing with her anxiety, as any person might, by getting up and walking around or even leaving the room for a minute to compose herself. She reasserted control as well as hospitality by offering the physician a cup of coffee and a cookie. Not only are these features absent in a typical encounter but they have not been replaced by anything which might restore the loss and thus some balance.

It should be no surprise that aspects of this imbalance are perpetuated in the kind of research and concepts that are generally used. In fact, it would be quite a surprise if that did not take place. It is a sociological truism that people in power tend to perpetuate themselves in word and in deed. (1)

The perpetuation of this distancing is more subtle where the nature of research and research concepts is concerned, but it is still there. This argument is not that there is imperiousness and conspiracy, but rather that ideas and models, once in place and if left unexamined, often take on a life of their own. Mechanic (1986, this volume) defines illness behaviour as involving "the manner in which persons monitor their bodies, define and interpret their symptoms, take remedial action and utilize various sources of help as well as the more formal health-care system." And yet, if one reviews bibliographies on illness behaviour these deal almost entirely with the formal health-care system. Thus, the tendency has been to look at how people utilize medical facilities, and the nature of the encounters considered are encounters with physicians. Little attention is paid to the encounters with

---

1. An example is the 2nd International Conference on Illness Behaviour. The presenters were predominantly white, male, either M.D.'s or Ph.D.'s speaking to an audience which was a little less white, clearly less made up of M.D.'s and Ph.D.'s and males. Moreover, they are speaking about people who are even less likely to be male, and more likely to be female of lower socioeconomic classes, and of very different ethnic groups.

any other health professionals such as nurses or occupational therapists. Maybe there is an assumption that the nature of that encounter would be the same. It is, however, an assumption not supported by much data.

Other "illness behaviour" research suffers from the same questionable focus. Decision-making invariably refers to the decision to seek medical aid. Though not excluded by Mechanic's definition, there is little study of alternative healers - except to discredit them or their utilizers. (See Garro, this volume for an exception). Few papers on illness behaviour address the issue of self-care specifically (Levin and Idler, 1983). When recognition is given to such behaviours it is often perceived as a stage in getting to a provider of care (and occasionally as a barrier to it). The questions follow suit with the emphasis on when self-care activities occurred and what or where they led. Garro (this volume) documented that the vast majority of all actions in response to a bodily "disturbance" was self-care, and not done on the way to somewhere else but as an end in itself. Dunell and Cartwright (1972) reported interesting findings from a systematic study of self-care. They noted that people using self-care often felt that it was quite efficacious. Many of them even perceived it as more efficacious than a medical visit. At least part of this lack of investigation of self-care must be explained in terms of who controls the research monies and what kinds of research are regarded as important. Zola (1966, 1973) has noted enormous data on self-care, but without a framework (Zola, 1983) there were enormous difficulties in interpreting this data.

Power issues translate implicitly into who are studied. Consider the three-volume study, New Directions in Helping by DePaulo, Nadler, and Fisher (1983). In the second volume titled Help-Seeking, one thing that was taken as sine qua non was that help-seeking involved at least two parties and one of the parties was the helpee and the other party the helper. Much of this research was related to characteristics of the helper; personally, sociodemographically, and attitudinally. All of these qualities were regarded by the authors as having an effect on how help is received and whether or not people even go for help.

As Kessler (this volume) noted, one's cognitive framework often determines not only what variables are considered but how they are examined. When reviewing the data on utilization of health facilities by gender, Kessler found that many investigators did not design their studies with gender differences in mind, and if they had done so, might have analyzed their data differently. There is little doubt that there are significant differences in the way men and women use and are used by the health-care system, even though general rates of utilization may not differ. As a start, researchers might ask women what they think are the most important aspects of the health-care system as it impacts upon them. The writings of the Boston Women's Health Book Collective (1985) might prove a useful source. DePaulo et al. (1983) reported gender differences, such as in the kind of information that would be transmitted and how this might be influenced by the gender of the provider of care.

In order to study the effects of certain variables (gender, race, ethnicity, socioeconomic class) it is not sufficient to use them as demographic variables in one's ongoing analyses. One must first think through, from the person or group's perspective, how the system may impact upon them. Their questions may not be the researcher's questions and may be considered unimportant and even rejected. If researchers adopt this position they should be prepared to defend it.

Some of the ways that research as well as conceptualization of illness behaviour might be re-oriented needs to be addressed. A priority issue in this regard is language. It can obfuscate as well as elucidate. There is a form of address and reference used in "illness behvaiour" research of which one should be wary, namely, the term "patient". There are times, indeed, when the people studied are "patients", and that label and its connotations are central to the theme under discussion (for example, an individual in a medical setting is functioning in a "patient role"). But when the sample is derived merely because someone has a specific condition then it is important, as both the women's movement and the disability rights movement have pointed out, that he/she is not the condition. References to these samples as patients convey associations of dependency or victimization. They may inadvertently colour one's perceptions and ultimately one's assumptions and what is studied (Crawford, 1977).

Much is made in current research literature about the "experience of illness" and the need to capture that experience vividly from the person's perspective (Conrad, in press). Many of the standard instruments are quite detrimental to this aim. Symptom check lists are a good example. They are often used to determine the presence or absence of certain conditions, and thus the experience. Such check lists, no matter how sophisticated, are derived from "medically relevant" concerns, usually derivative of or correlative with some important diagnostic category. If one is attempting to understand the categories of experience "out there", then one must proceed from a very different perspective. The vocabulary of trouble (Emerson and Messinger, 1977; Kahne and Schwartz, 1978; Zola, 1972b) may be a much more appropriate starting point. Specifically, be aware that the researcher's objective is to map a universe that describes the individuals's reality (anthropologists avoid this pitfall) rather than trying to determine whether the individual's reality fits with the researcher's conceptualization (questionnaire studies are particularly susceptible to this bias).

As for the professional education of health-care workers, it is essential for anyone in the business of caring/healing to deal with the issue of vulnerability. That is, consider what it feels like to be a patient, to feel impotent and helpless and to realize what one can and cannot do. (2) There are "sensitivity" training groups and simulation exercises that can assist in promoting this awareness.

Finally, consider the implications of the actual visitation to health-care providers. This encounter places the potential patient in a position of considerable vulnerability, generates anxiety, exacerbates feelings of ignorance and even worthlessness (Zola, 1973, 1981). There are at least several things that can be done to redress the balance and regain control. First, as in any learning situation there are tools appropriate to the situation. Given the anxiety of the situation it would be helpful to encourage the writing down of questions. Similarly, the provision of written explanations or instructions by health-care providers would be advantageous. Second, there should be more time for patients to consider information about their diagnosis, their prognosis, and care. Patients should have an active choice in how their treatment proceeds. (3) Third, the view that a medical encounter requires advocacy should be encouraged. Given all the power imbalances, anxiety, and information transmitted, one could argue that one should never go for a medical visit alone. This is especially true where

---

2. See DePaulo et al., 1983. This reference includes separate chapters on topics such as embarrassment and feelings of inadequacies in help-seeking.

3. As the women's movement has taught us - e.g., re the relationship in time between a biopsy and a "necessary" mastectomy (Kushner, 1980; National Cancer Institute, 1979, New England Journal of Medicine, 1979).

certain medical conditions as well as treatment regimens involve a person's family and significant others. This must be taken into consideration when the implications of a particular diagnosis and its treatment are explained. Without taking responsibility away from the individual one can encourage and allow the presence of others during all phases of the medical encounter. There has been a tendency to overprivatize the medical interview to the detriment of all concerned.

Many years ago, Tom Lehrer wrote a song with the following lyrics, "I don't care where they go up, only where they come down. That's not my department said Werner von Braun." The issue of "where it comes down", (how the concepts of illness behaviour are used), is however everyone's concern. Unless we make it our business, we will someday find ourselves facing the dilemma of Walt Kellys' Pogo, who upon realizing what had gone on, said, "We have met the enemy and he is us."

## REFERENCES


Boston Women's Health Book Collective. (1984). The new our bodies, ourselves. New York: Simon & Schuster.

Brown, R. (1979). Rockefeller medicine men: Medicine and capitalism in America. Berkeley: University of California Press.

Conrad, P. (in press). The experience of illness: Recent and new directions. In J. A. Roth & P. Conrad (Eds.), Research in the sociology of health care Vol. 6. The experience and management of chronic illness. Greenwich, CT: JAI Press.

Conrad, P. & Schneider, J. W. (1980). Deviance and medicalization: From badness to sickness. St. Louis, MO: C. V. Mosby.

Crawford, R. (1977). You are dangerous to your health: The ideology of victim blaming. International Journal of Health Services, 7, 663-680.

Crawford, R. (1979). Individual responsibility and health politics. In S. Reverby & D. Rosner (Eds.), Health care in America: Essays in social history. Philadelphia: Temple University Press.

Crawford, R. (1980). Healthism and the medicalization of everyday life. International Journal of Health Services, 10, 365-388.

DePaulo, B. M., Nadler, A., & Fisher, J. (Eds.). (1983). Help-Seeking, Vol. 2 of New Directions in Helping. New York: Academic Press.

Dubos, R. (1961). The mirage of health. Garden City, NY: Anchor.

Dubos, R. (1965). Man adapting. New Haven, CT: Yale University Press.

Dunnell, K., & Cartwright, A. (1972). Medicine takers, prescribers and hoarders. London: Routledge and Kegan Paul.

Emerson, R. M., & Messinger, S. L. (1977). The micro-politics of trouble. Social Problems, 25, 121-134.

Freidson, E. (1970a). Profession of medicine. New York: Dodd-Mead.

Freidson, E. (1970b). Professional dominance: The social structure of medical care. New York: Atherton.

Freidson, E. (1976). Doctoring together: A study of professional social control. New York: Elsevier.

Gibson, C. D., & Kramer, B. M. (1985). Site of care in medical practice. Medical Care, 3, 14-17.

Goffman, E. (1961). Asylums. New York: Anchor.

Henderson, L. J. (1985). Physician and patient as a social system. New England Journal of Medicine, 212, 819-823.

Kahne, M. J., & Schwartz, C. G. (1978). Negotiating trouble: The social construction and management of trouble in a college psychiatric context. Social Problems, 25, 461-475.

Kushner, R. (1980). The treatment of primary breast cancer: A patient's viewpoint. Connecticut Medicine, 4, 437-440.

Levin, L., & Idler, E. (1983). Self-care in health. Annual Review of Public Health, 4, 181-201.

National Cancer Institute. (1979). The treatment of primary breast cancer: Management of local disease. National Institute of Health Consensus Development Conference Summary (Vol. 2, No. 5).
Rieff, P. (1968). Triumph of the therapeutic: Uses of faith after Freud. New York: Torchbook, Harper-Row.
Starr, P. (1982). The social transformation of American medicine. New York: Basic Books.
Stevens, R. (1971). American medicine and the public interest. New Haven, CT: Yale University Press.
Treatment of primary breast cancer -- Special Report. (1979). New England Journal of Medicine, 301, 340.
Zola, I. K. (1972a). Medicine as an institution of social control. Sociological Review, 20, 487-504.
Zola, I. K. (1972b). The concept of trouble and sources of medical assistance - to whom one can turn, with what, and why. Social Science and Medicine, 6, 673-679.
Zola, I. K. (1973). Pathways to the doctor - from person to patient. Social Science and Medicine, 7, 677-689.
Zola, I. K. (1975). In the name of health and illness: On some socio-political consequences of medical influence. Social Science and Medicine, 9, 83-87.
Zola, I. K. (1981). Structural constraints in the doctor-patient relationship: The case for non-compliance. In L. Eisenberg, & A. Kleinman (Eds.), The relevance of social science for medicine (pp. 241-252). Dordrecht, Holland: Reidel.
Zola, I. K. (1983). Socio-medical inquiries: Recollections, reflections and reconsiderations. Philadelphia: Temple University Press.

# PART V  COGNITIVE APPRAISAL PROCESSESS

# SYMPTOM REPORTING: A FOCUS ON PROCESS

Howard Leventhal

Department of Psychology
University of Wisconsin

## INTRODUCTION: THE IMPORTANCE OF SYMPTOMS

Why is symptom reporting important? This question can be answered from at least three perspectives: a) that of public health; b) that of medicine; and c) that of the lay person. From the public health perspective, symptom reports obtained in household surveys provide a major source of data on the incidence and prevalence of a variety of diseases (Dingle, 1973). Survey data is particularly valuable in tracking acute infectious and epidemic conditions such as the flu (Dingle, 1973), as well as chronic conditions for which there is no special reporting system or registry such as exist for cancer. These numbers can play a critical role in the detection and control of disease and are important for planning and public health policy.

For the practitioner, symptoms are typically the first line of contact with disease. The medical history and physical examination probe memory and body respectively to elicit symptom patterns. While today's high tech environment makes symptom reports seem inadequate for the diagnosis of underlying conditions, symptoms still guide the initial steps of hypothesis formation and the ordering of diagnostic tests. For many psychiatric conditions symptom reporting is still the only, if not the best, means of defining the underlying condition (Fabrega, 1975).

Finally, symptoms are important to the layman in their daily lives. They have an immediate effect on one's emotional states, generating anxiety, irritability and depressed mood; they alter one's actions, restricting work and social activity; and, they raise questions about one's underlying health and future well-being. Finally, they lead one to consider one's needs for medical care and for changes in life style. Thus, symptoms directly impact on everyday experience and current and future actions.

## THE PROBLEM: SYMPTOMS AS (UN)RELIABLE INDICATOR

Given their multiple functions, symptoms seem to be, and are, useful indicators. However, one must remain wary of their use. Why? First, while physician, public health worker, and layman may view symptoms as signs of disease, each is likely to have very different models of the disease process. These models dictate how to identify the disease, its causes, its consequences and its cure. Thus, each individual regards symptoms as

INDICATORS, but they do not necessarily agree on what is indicated (Kleinman, 1980). Because symptoms may be assigned different and conflicting meanings from lay and medical models, as well as within the medical model, questions can be raised about their sensitivity and specificity as indicators of particular, underlying conditions.

Second, symptoms are private, as are all conscious, perceptual events. But, unlike most perceptual events whose stimuli are public, the stimuli eliciting symptoms are typically unavailable for public examination. Thus, symptoms are not readily subject to shared experience, that is, social validation. A physician can never be certain as to the feel of their patients' symptoms nor can he/she be certain their reports are accurate or honest. Indeed, the physician's search for cause can be likened to a bio-feedback experiment in which elaborate instruments and tests are used to identify the bodily condition that has generated the perceptual experience of a symptom.

## Data Suggesting Symptoms are Unreliable Indicators of Disease

There are both theoretical and empirical grounds for suspicion that symptoms may be inaccurate indicators of underlying disease. A few key findings will be mentioned, and then, the dilemma they pose will be addressed.

Sex differences in symptom reporting. It is well documented that women are more likely to report symptoms than men, to spend more days on the disability list, and to record higher levels on other illness indicators (Nathanson, 1975; Verbrugge, 1985). Moreover, this sex difference persists even when gonadal and reproductive problems are removed from the symptom count (Verbrugge, 1985; Verbrugge & Steiner, 1981). It should come as no surprise, therefore, that this sex difference holds down to early ages: as early as second grade, females are more likely to engage in symptom reporting and other illness behaviours (e.g., worry about health, emotional upset about health, staying home with colds, etc.) and make use of a school nurse (Lewis, Lewis, and Lorimer, 1977). Multiple hypotheses have been offered to account for these sex differences. For example, it has suggested that women have more time to be ill and make use of services and that they experience more symptoms because they are more conflicted in their roles as mother, wife and wage earner (Gove and Hughes, 1979; Marcus and Seeman, 1981; Mechanic, 1976; see Kessler, this volume). Others have suggested that women are more emotional [surveys show women are more likely to express emotional distress (Kessler, Brown, and Broman, 1981)] and the difference in emotionality may reflect factors in their neurobiological development (Broverman, Klaiber, Kobayashi, and Vogel, 1968). One might seriously entertain the possibility that women are more sickly and more diseased until one realizes that women outlive their male counterparts (Nathanson, 1975; Verbrugge, 1981).

Psychological conditions and symptoms. Evidence for a substantial association between symptom reports and mental health or emotional status can be found in the psychiatric and psychological literatures. For example, many of the organic signs common to depression, such as lack of energy, constipation, weight loss, etc., (Katon, Kleinman, and Rosen, 1982a, 1982b) are related to more frequent use of health care (Cadoret, Widmer, and Troughton, 1980) and are found in chronic, "physical" diseases. Thus, these vegetative signs can indicate serious chronic disease or a disease of the emotional life.

Hypochondriasis is yet another condition marked by excessive attentiveness to the body and dwelling on symptomatology (Kenyon, 1964; Pilowsky, 1967). Hypochondriasis may be found in combination with both neurotic (depressive) and psychotic (schizophrenic) conditions (Pilowsky,

1967) or in isolation. Interest in this condition was intensified by the availability of an instrument for its demarcation: the Hs scale of the MMPI, and it would be futile to attempt a review of this vast and inchoate literature.

Finally, symptoms are a central component of illness behaviour (Pilowsky, 1978). A variety of practitioners have come to view illness behaviour as a generalized trait (Pilowsky, Bassett, Barrett, Petrovic, and Minniti, 1983) or as a readiness to report symptoms, to adopt the sick role, and to "use" illness to control their interpersonal environments by gaining attention from sympathetic listeners (Frankel and Nuttall, 1984; Ward, 1985) and manipulating unwary physicians and psychologists. These practitioners include psychiatrists and psychologists who must treat a broad range of symptomatic patients referred to them with no known organic disease (Wooley, Blackwell, and Winget, 1978) and psychologists coping with the chronic pain patient (Fordyce, 1976; Sternbach, 1968). They reject the hypothesis that their patients are well, an idea that is often explicit in the minds of the internist and surgeon who referred the patients to them. Thus, these psychiatrists and psychologists view illness behaviour as a syndrome that has become dissociated from its original physical source.

Environmental-Conditioning and symptoms. Symptoms and/or illness behaviour can be viewed as a product of environmental conditions. Examples of this hypothesis are the sociological analyses that relate reports of symptoms of physical and mental illness to social class (Syme and Berkman, 1976), means of production (Schnall and Kern, 1981) and socially induced economic and interpersonal stressors (Pearlin and Schooler, 1978). Psychological analyses that view symptoms as a form of operant or conditioned behaviour (Fordyce, 1976) rather than as a syndrome or a trait also fall into this category. From this perspective, the key to illness behaviour, to pain behaviour, or to symptom behaviour (a component of illness behaviour), is to identify and alter the environmental stimuli that reinforce and maintain pain and symptom reporting despite the removal of their initiating cause (injury or illness). By altering the social system, and/or by removing the reinforcing stimuli and rewarding new behaviours, the pain behaviour, symptom behaviour, and illness behaviour can be eliminated. Experimental and clinical work reveals this to be true (Wooley and Blackwell, 1975; Wooley, Blackwell, and Winget, 1978; Sternbach, 1968).

## Symptoms as Indicators of Mental, Social and Disease Status

This brief review suggests two alternatives to the hypothesis that symptoms are indicators of physical illness. Symptoms may be indicators of mental or psychological state and health, rather than of physical state; or symptoms may be indicators of social reinforcements rather than physical or mental state. Both hypotheses downgrade the role of symptoms as indicators of physical illness. If one wishes to continue to use symptoms as indicators of physical illness and hesitate to embrace either of these hypotheses, data can easily be supplied to support this inclination. For example, in their detailed analysis comparing lung cancer survival in the late 60's to that in the late 70's, Feinstein and his associates (1985) showed that a careful assessment of symptoms, which excluded information obtained from technological measures of disease status, was as powerful at predicting survival as were measures obtained with the best diagnostic technology available at that time. Symptoms are excellent indicators of survival and disease status!

These data and the data previously reviewed reveal two important features about symptoms: a) symptoms reflect both physical and mental disease and they reflect psychological or mental processes not typically classified as disease. Because symptoms reflect mental state, they are sensitive to a wide range of external and internal stimuli as well as to changes in the mechanism generating mental state, (e.g., social stimuli, which are important, if not the most important, stimuli affecting mental states); b) the influence on symptom reports of any single independent ("causal") variable such as disease, emotional response, sex role, operant stimuli, etc., will depend upon the variation and intensity of that variable and on the variation and intensity of other variables. Thus, symptoms were powerful predictors of survival for severely ill lung cancer patients because the intensity of the disease was likely to have restricted the influence of non-disease factors to symptom experience. Symptoms may do less well in predicting rate of recovery for less serious conditions where variation in other factors may contribute more to symptom load. For example, when one compares physically healthy normals to physically healthy hypochondriacs or physically healthy depressives, very substantial portions of the variance in symptom reporting will be attributable to variation in mental state.

While the above conclusions are likely to be true, they are not particularly satisfying, for they suggest that the utility of symptoms, whether for physical or mental diagnosis, is highly dependent upon context (Telles and Pollack, 1981). As there are a multitude of contexts and a multitude of symptoms, one is faced with a nearly infinite number of symptom-context combinations and therefore a nearly endless catalogue of symptom meanings. Moreover, the meaning of these combinations will vary across cultures (Fabrega, 1975; Kleinman, 1980), over time in the same culture, and over an individual's learning history (Chrisman, 1977).

There are at least two ways to approach the above complexity. First, one can undertake an empirical search for different patterns of symptoms associated with different determinants. If one is fortunate, one will discover that the patterns of cancer may differ from that for cardiovascular disease, that both these patterns may differ from those generated by emotional states, and that the symptom pattern for emotional states will differ for different emotions; e.g., the symptoms for depression may differ from those for anxiety and hostility (See Pennebaker, 1982, Chapter 5). The empirical approach has had some successes and will undoubtedly have more.

A second, complementary approach is to develop models of the bio-psychological processes involved in symptom production. This theoretical route can help order the empirical data and assist in understanding why similar symptom patterns may at times have very different underlying meanings. It is this latter route that will be considered. In the following section the basic assumptions and concepts of a model for the process by which body sensations become symptoms will be outlined. Once this is accomplished, the development of symptom processing and its interaction with emotional events will be addressed. The key hypothesis is that symptom emotion interactions are primarily, though, not entirely, responsible for differences in symptom reporting related to environmental reinforcement and the sex and psychological status of the respondent.

## TOWARD A THEORY OF SYMPTOM PROCESSING

### A Bio-Psychological System

This model of symptom processing is bio-psychological. It assumes that psychological events occur in a biological medium and that every psychological event can be described at a biological level. A complete understanding of symptom processing would elucidate the interconnection of the psychological and biological levels of analysis, something that may evolve at some future time. Although at present, the anatomic and physiological correlates of the psychological mechanisms underlying specific symptom experiences cannot be described, it is important to design our psychological constructs to maximize the possibility that they be parallel and susceptible to correlation with physiological and anatomical constructs.

## A Perceptual System

The second assumption is that symptom processing involves perceptual processes similar to the perceptual processing involved in other sensory modalities (Leventhal, 1970; 1975), an assumption shared by other investigators (Mechanic, 1972; Pennebaker, 1982). As is the case in describing other complex, sensory systems, it is convenient to begin at the sensory input and trace the signal through various steps of enrichment or "cognitive" and emotional elaborations. This process integrates the current sensory properties of a symptom with memories of past interpretations to create a representation of the current symptom episode. The representation of the episode has a variety of attributes including its presumed cause, identity (the symptom pattern and a "diagnostic" label), a time-line or expected duration, and consequences or expected outcome. These attributes of the representation elicit and guide the individual's coping responses.

The integration of sensations and memory codes to form illness representations is involved in all aspects of symptom experience. Thus, the perception of a symptom caused by a current physiological disorder (e.g. its strength, duration, etc.) may be modified by memories of similar, prior symptom episodes. Indeed, memories of prior illness may add symptoms to the present episode that are NOT a necessary consequence of the current physiological upset. The automatic emotional response to the symptom and the interpretation of its meaning are also partially determined by the activation of memory traces of prior illness and prior emotional episodes.

To deal with these complex interactions between present and past, a hierarchical enrichment mechanism is hypothesized that codes and elaborates sensory input at three levels: a) sensory motor, or innate perceptual structuring of the stimulus; b) schematic coding of the stimulus in perceptual memories, and c) an abstract or semantic coding. All three types of processing are simultaneously active in the integration of body sensations with prior memories that generates the experience of an illness or symptom episode.

A fourth, procedural, memory code is important for the acquisition of motor responses and procedures involved in action. This will be set aside for the moment. [There are alternative ways of organizing memory codes (Tulving, 1985).]

Sensory-motor processing. All sensory stimuli are elaborated upon by anatomical and neurochemical mechanisms that make up an individual's innate processing machinery. For example, the basic machinery in vision integrates each eye's somewhat separate view of the textures and surfaces of the world to form the perception of depth (See Gibson, 1950; Julesz, 1968). It also organizes perception into objects in a surrounding environment. Systems of this type operate in all modalities (e.g., vision, audition) including somatic perception, which is of direct concern to symptom perception. [Observation of the neonate suggests that innate mechanisms are also at work in cross modality integrations (Brazelton, Koslowski, and Main, 1974).]

Although in general the sensory motor machinery for the experience of symptoms has not been well defined, the important symptom of pain is an exception. The pain system can be divided roughly into two parts: a set of sensory pathways and central mechanisms for generating the quality of the pain sensation [e.g., as burning or sharp, or at a specific location] and a second set of pathways and central mechanisms involved primarily in activating the individual's emotional and coping responses (Beecher, 1959; Casey, 1973; Mountcastle, 1980; Snyder, 1977). The sensory-mechanical properties of pain, the emotional response accompanying it, and the reactions caused by the interpretation or meaning assigned the pain symptom will also provoke a variety of autonomic and endocrine reactions (heart rate increase, cortisol output, etc.). A key hypothesis in the bio-psychological model of symptom processing is that some of these reactions are conditioned responses, specifically, they are part of the memory traces of prior symptom episodes.

Schematic processing. It is hypothesized that classical conditioning forms memory codes or schemata of the symptoms, emotional reactions, and environmental events associated with illness episodes. These schemata associate events contiguous in time and space. The pain in the gut is associated with the facial reactions and vocal cry of pain, the autonomic responses associated with both, and all three with environmental cues, such as mother's worried face and the smells and sights of the doctor's office. These associations are formed automatically. Thus, if a child or an adult notices the medicinal smell of the doctor's office at the same time he or she experiences abdominal pains and cries, the pains and cries will be conditioned to (associated with) the contiguous smell, even though there is no objective, causal connection between them. [Conditioned events of this sort are a common occurrence for patients in cancer chemotherapy: e.g., Nerenz, Leventhal, Easterling, and Love (1986).]

Once formed, a schema (and its component parts) will be reactivated by the occurrence of any component that is similar to an attribute of the schema (e.g., a new symptom similar to old ones). The new symptoms need not be identical to those experienced in the past since schematic memories of illness will be general or prototypic because they are updated and represent a memory that reflects multiple episodes (Posner and Keele, 1970).

An important characteristic of schematic processing is that it gives perceptions structure and meaning. Allport and Pettigrew (1957) provided an excellent example of this type of structuring in visual perception. They compared the perception of a rotating trapezoid in a sample of tribesman from a bush culture who had no exposure to Western buildings and windows, and a sample of tribesman from the same culture who were raised in a South African city. Those raised in the city and therefore having perceptual (i.e., schematic) memories of windows, saw the trapezoid oscillate, although it was physically rotating, a result identical to that obtained with subjects raised in urban areas in the United States and Canada. Those raised in the bush lacked a perceptual schema of window and saw the trapezoid rotate. The word 'saw' is emphasized as there is every reason to believe this was a difference in immediate perception, and NOT a difference in thought or reasoning. A central hypothesis in this model is that body sensations undergo an identical process of schematic enrichment in becoming symptoms (Leventhal, 1975; 1982).

Semantic or conceptual processing. Semantic or conceptual codes make up a second memory record of illness episodes and symptoms. Conceptual or semantic coding is a more abstract code of illness experience that is propositional in form. Its propositional form reflects the fact that semantic memories are derived from observations and "reflections" or thoughts about experience. Propositional codes are abstracted from all forms of experience, visual and auditory perception as well as somatic perception, and can represent complex causal sequences spanning long periods of time. Conceptual or propositional memory codes are also particularly important in extracting and generating the meaning of verbal and written communications. These codes are the storehouse for the descriptions of the symptoms, causes, consequences and duration of illness and the probable outcome of various preventive and curative actions.

Conceptual codes appear to play an especially important role in establishing the context within which an individual experiences and interprets more concrete perceptions of symptoms. For example, a lump in the breast will generate a quite different reaction if interpreted and/or diagnosed as cancer rather than as a benign cyst. Similarly, the very same side effects of chemotherapy (e.g., nausea and tiredness) arouse more distress in patients with disseminated or metastatic disease than in patients whose adjuvant treatment follows successful removal of all detectable tumor (Leventhal, Easterling, Coons, Luchterhand, and Love, in press).

In summary, whereas conceptual or propositional processing of body states is highly abstract and generates meanings that bridge causes and consequences over long periods of time, schematic processing involves the immediate structuring of concrete experience and reflects the overlap between current symptoms and schema elicitors with patterns of prior, concrete symptom experience. As shall be seen in a moment, schemata can also be formed from direct observation and vicarious response to the experience of illness in others (Bandura, 1977).

### A Response System

The hierarchical memory system plays a key role in defining or representing health threat. Once the threat is defined, the second stage of response processes begins (Leventhal, 1970; Sternberg, 1969). Response processes are also hierarchically organized and the levels of their hierarchy are likely to be accessed by similar levels of stimulus organization. Thus, at the lowest reflexive level, a specific and fairly rigid set of response processes are accessed by sensory attributes, while the schematic or perceptual level accesses responses automatically by conditioned association or contiguity. The control of responses at the conceptual level involves active planning and execution of responses with respect to the longer term causes and consequences of an illness episode.

These levels of responding differ in the degree to which they are subject to voluntary control. Thus, reflex responses are difficult to regulate with verbal or other volitional processes. Similarly, control of conditioned, schematic reactions is often indirect: the individual minimizing stimulus control over behaviour by redirecting attention, by focusing on or imagining alternative stimuli, or by the voluntary production of competing responses. Finally, responding at the conceptual level is clearly open to control by self-instructions or instructions from others. But, because conceptual control is particularly effortful, making demands on attention and requiring effort, it is unlikely to sustain complex, long-term behavioural plans for cure or prevention unless portions of the plan are schematized and made automatic. A patient may make use of conditioning principles to establish an automatic reminder for the very first response of a more complex set of responses that comprise a treatment regimen. Once the beginning reaction is conditioned and automatic, the remainder of the reactions will be more reliably produced. For example, a diabetic who wants to reduce the frequency with which he fails to test blood sugar levels and use insulin could analyze his daily patterns, discover he always washes his hands after rising in the morning and after eating, and position his testing apparatus on the wall near his towel so as to condition himself to think of and take the first step to assess blood sugar levels upon drying his hands. Once automatically reminded, the remaining responses will be controlled by voluntary, conceptual codes. Finding time for regular exercise would be another example.

## DEVELOPMENT AND INTEGRATION OF EMOTION - SYMPTOM PROCESSES

The hierarchical processing system hypothesized to be involved in connecting new somatic sensations to past memories for the construction of symptomatology in current illness episodes has been outlined. Little has been said, however, about the activation of emotional responses by this system and the way in which emotion becomes part of illness memory. These ideas will be elaborated in this section through disussion of the development of illness and emotion cognition. A first, basic assumption is that the very same hierarchical and response systems involved in representing and guiding coping responses to illness are involved in the generation of emotion and in guiding coping with emotional reactions (Leventhal, 1982). A second basic assumption is that memory for the subjective, expressive and autonomic components of emotional reactions is also schematic, and the schemata for emotion can be fused with the schematic memory representations of illness (Leventhal, 1982). It is the overlap of function in the systems and the commonality in structure and content of the schematic (and also conceptual) memories that creates complex interactions between illness and emotion experiences. It is hypothesized that both of these factors are partially responsible for the complex effects of sex, psychiatric trait, psychological states and situational conditions upon symptom experience and symptom reports.

## The Development of Emotion-Illness Cognition

While it takes but a little imagination to describe a plausible sequence for the development of illness-emotion cognition, it is all too easy to focus on the disease part and forget the interpersonal context. Both will be included in the discussion.

The disease component of emotion-illness cognitions. Consider for a moment a typical 2- or 3- year-old child who contracts a severe case of gastrointestinal flu. The physiological problems, bowel distension, fever, and retching, etc., will generate a host of sensory experiences including dull aching pain, nausea, and retching sensations. In addition, the disease may activate a variety of autonomic, endocrine, and overt effector and subjective/cognitive reactions. The autonomic and endocrine reactions would include responses such as cardiovascular speeding, blood pressure changes, cortisol output, motor irritability, and trembling. The overt and subjective reactions would include the focusing of attention on the source of distress, rubbing and holding the abdomen, cries of distress, calls for help, and so on. These sensory-motor events will be recorded as a schematic memory of the illness episode. Those motor reactions, particularly the attentional and self-manipulating responses (feeling and rubbing), that are contiguous with the sensory events, will be conditioned to them and become part of the schema and its coding of temporal contiguity (b follows a: see Blass, Ganchrow and Steiner, 1984).

As the underlying physiological disease clears, the child will experience and observe a moderation of its associated symptomatic upset, and a conceptual code will be formed of this temporal contingency. These temporal expectations generate an implicit (and eventually explicit) awareness that illnesses have a "natural history" comprised of an early set of sensory-symptomatic features that change at a given rate, followed by a more severe period that lasts its prototypical 24 to 72 hours, and tapering off with residual symptomatology (fatigue, etc.) that may persist for 1 to 2 weeks. The schematic code with its symptomatic component, its contiguity-based time rules, and its attentional and self-manipulative motor reactions, and the conceptual code with its longer term temporal contingencies making up the history of the disorder and its associated consequences (disruption of play, social relationships, diet, etc.) function as a unit to establish memories for the experience and interpretation of future illness episodes. These codes both interpret and add to ongoing sensory experiences.

Interpersonal context and emotion-illness cognition. It is the rare and unfortunate 3-year-old who experiences a disease episode alone. In virtually all cases, someone is present; it can be mother, father, grandparent, housekeeper, sibling, or any combination of the above. The response of these persons to unfolding disease will be coded in both schema and concept. For example, if mother is unfamiliar with the fever and vomiting that accompany gastrointestinal flu, she may become anxious and display agitated facial and vocal behaviours, be less sure and perhaps more abrupt in holding the child, and provoke anxiety and fear in the youngster. These fear reactions, perceptual, cognitive, expressive, autonomic and endocrine, will be coded with both the schematic and conceptual codes formed during specific illness episodes. They will affect the experience and thoughts (interpretation) of subsequent episodes, in this case enhancing their perception as dangerous and threatening events.

If the mother is agitated and frightened solely during the peak of the symptom episode, interpersonally stimulated emotional reactions will only be added to the schemata and concepts for this specific period of time. On the other hand, if the mother remains anxious and distressed during the declining phase of the disease episode and/or continues to be wary and anxious after its termination, there are the makings of a chronically vigilant youngster. The mother can communicate her worry and fear by asking how the child feels, taking temperatures, controlling activities, fearfully scanning the child's eating, etc. Emotional reactions and chronic attentional and fearful interpretations of this sort can be linked to virtually any body experiences.

If the two types of episodes mentioned above are repeated over years for two different youngsters, one might expect quite different patterns of illness behaviour to subsequent disease. The first might lead to an adult pattern of excessive displays of pain and distress and seeking of emotional support during the height of illness episodes, a pattern characteristic of "Mediterranean" cultures (Zborowski, 1969). The latter would likely generate a pattern of chronic illness behaviour. If the social context responds even-handedly and moderately, one might anticipate a "matter of fact" response to disease episodes such as that shown by Irish- and English-American families (Zborowski, 1969; Zola, 1973).

It is important to note that direct experience is not the only way in which an individual's learning history can form both schematic and conceptual illness cognitions. Much can be learned by observation of others. How parents, friends, and media models attend to their bodies, self-treat, and express emotional distress during illness episodes can condition emotional reactions to the contextual factors that will enter into illness schemata and concepts. How these episodes are modeled and alter personal experience is unknown, although data suggest that the mother's behaviour may serve as an important model or shaper of the child's illness behaviour (Mechanic, 1979).

## Interaction of Emotion and Symptoms in Illness Episodes

It is clear that illness and emotion schemata and concepts share many properties because of their overlapping developmental histories. However, even when they lack an intimate, overlapping developmental history such as that outlined above, illness and emotion cognitions are similar because they are generated by a common underlying machinery and they have common subjective, emotional cognitive attributes. For example, the bodily experiences produced by emotional reactions to life stressors feel similar to those of many illnesses, that is, they have common autonomic, endocrine and subjective properties and last for similar periods of time. Thus, it may be difficult to distinguish episodes of emotional stress from episodes of illness. Both the developmental overlap and the similarity in features permit cataloguing a number of ways in which illness and emotion may interact.

1. Sensory elicitation. Physical or sensory properties of disease stimuli, such as pain, will not only elicit illness schemata and concepts,

they will also directly elicit emotional responses. These responses can be independent of the meaning of the pain sensation. For example, intense sharp pain and/or intense burning pain, whether due to an acute transient event or a chronic death-dealing one, will rouse subjective experience, facial expressions, and vocal cries of distress, and these emotional reactions can amplify the sensory pain experience. (This is NOT to deny that meaning may add to the experience!). Relatively simple, stimulus provoked interactions of this sort are probably rare because an individual's storehouse of schematic and conceptual codes will intervene and add to the complexity of such responses.

2. Illness and emotion schemata. Because disease and interpersonal stress situations may produce similar expressive, autonomic, and endocrine reactions, occurrence of these bodily sensations at a later point in time, regardless of their origin, can elicit the traces of both types of prior experience. The consequence will be the elicitation of the full complement of attributes of the illness or emotion schemata formed over prior interpersonal and illness episodes. Thus, interpersonal emotional stress can evoke the conditioned symptomatic, autonomic, endocrine, attentional and self-manipulative reactions, and the behavioural and temporal expectations associated with illness schemata and illness concepts. Because schemata are evoked automatically by current, matching body sensations, it is unlikely that the individual will be able to distinguish body sensations and symptoms due to a current medical condition from those elicited by the schemata of prior illnesses or prior emotional reactions.

Just as shared sensory attributes can evoke illness and emotion schemata, so too can the responses used to cope with illness and emotion. Thus, touching the body, examining oneself in the mirror, and other minimal and often undetected responses, can trigger illness schemata and evoke apprehension and other negative emotional states.

It is believed there will be a substantial amount of symmetry between emotion and illness schemata. Thus, emotionally provocative situations, at least those that are stressful and negative, can be expected to provoke symptoms and expectations related to illness. The more frequent and intense the emotional provocation from interpersonal sources during prior illness episodes, the more likely it is that new interpersonal stressors will evoke illness schemata and concepts along with emotions of depression and/or anxiety. However, all negative emotional episodes are expected to evoke illness schemata. An ongoing emotional episode is unlikely to evoke a schema of an illness that has very distinct and specific symptoms (e.g., a streptococcal throat or glandular swelling), and the episode may be less likely to evoke even a vague illness schemata (e.g., the onset of a cold) if the emotional response itself has clear, causal features. The opportunity to compare and share subjective feelings may also limit the possibility that an emotional state will evoke an illness schemata. One would also predict different durations in which specific emotions will generate illness schemata: anxiety and anger would operate over the short-term, (e.g., one to two days), while severe depression would operate over the long-term (e.g., one or more months).

3. Conceptual interpretation. Life events, such as the death of a friend or exposure to disasters, can activate conceptual or semantic codes which then prime and increase the availability of illness schemata. Once primed, the individual will be sensitized to monitor and interpret a particular set of body sensations. Thus, following a friend's death from cancer, an individual may notice and continually monitor various benign physical blemishes, pains, irritable bowel symptoms, etc., and experience them as potential signs of cancer. These automatic interpretations and their associated imagery may provoke fear and initiate a variety of appropriate and inappropriate diagnostic and preventive actions.

4. <u>Activation through central neural activity</u>. Finally, activity in the central nervous system, including changes in neurotransmitter levels due to tumors, drugs, dietary factors, aging and cell death, etc., can lead to changes in mood, and emotional state. These changes can influence illness experiences by generating or blunting the visceral and endocrine components of emotional reactions that can activate illness schemata.

<u>Conceptual-Schematic Interaction</u>

The interaction of conceptual or semantic codes with more concrete perceptual schemata deserves more attention than has been given in the previous discussion as it is a critical aspect of the construction of illness representations and the generation of coping responses. In a prior section, schemata were defined as concrete memory codes which are automatically combined with body sensations to enrich and structure the perception of new symptoms. This enrichment may depend upon a process in which the sensory properties of a symptom are compared and then matched to properties of the most similar underlying memory schemata. Conceptual codes, on the other hand, are more abstract rules or theories that define disease on the basis of an underlying property of the disease process (Murphy and Medin, 1985). Because people's conceptions or theories of specific diseases may neither be well structured (See Meyer, Leventhal, and Gutmann, 1985) nor accurate (Baumann and Leventhal, 1985) it will be difficult to obtain verbal reports that will clarify the interaction of concepts and schemata in the construction of representations and coping, although behaviours might be observed that clearly reflect this interaction. A clue to what might be observed comes from the suggestion that the symptomatic component of an illness representations is likely to be stored as a schemata while the attributes of cause, time-line, and consequence, are likely stored as conceptual rules. If this is true, one can readily hypothesize a number of ways in which the two types of code may interact.

First, as mentioned in the prior section, conceptual or theoretical concepts may prime schemata and increase the likelihood that specific concrete events are perceived as indicators of particular diseases. Second, the conceptual rules may guide a form of coping or <u>appraisal response</u>, that can be best described as hypothesis testing. If I am sensitized to view symptoms as signs of cancer, my perception of a symptom will elicit both an emotional response and a set of conceptual expectations related to my theoretical notion of the essential nature of cancer. This latter notion will be used to evaluate or test my perception.

For example, let's assume I've learned that my former college room-mate has unexpectedly died of cancer at the age of 35. This knowledge primes emotionally enriched schemata of lumps, sores, etc., which I had previously feared to be signs of cancer. If I notice a tender lump under my arm, I will immediately perceive or feel it as a cancer and respond with fear. My theory of cancer, that it slowly but inexorably gets worse (extended time-line and expected consequences of pain), will then come into play and generate a number of expectations or hypotheses than can be used to test or validate my automatically generated perception. If by the next morning or subsequent to using medication, the lump has receded, I am likely to conclude it is an infection and not a cancer. Indeed, this conclusion is likely even if by the next morning the lump becomes more painful and doubles in size. Both outcomes are inconsistent with my temporal conception of cancer.

The process of evaluation involved diagnostic, appraisal reactions of medicating and/or waiting to observe fluctuations in the symptom. Appraisal responses are likely to be rapid, relatively non-conscious, and under-reported, hence it may be exceptionally difficult to obtain data that makes public the process of checking schema to concept. One might guess that such a check process was present by observing certain consequences of hypothesis testing. For example, assume I had engaged in such checking, concluded a rapidly worsening and annoying sore an infection, but decided to seek medical care because it was painful. Assume next that my physician (expert) told me the infection is actually a cancer; I am likely to be stunned by this information, but more tellingly, I may be convinced that my cancer is dissimilar to the way cancer is typically experienced. The conviction that my cancer had a unique presentation may be the only evidence that I had checked the concrete experience against a prior set of abstract assumptions about the nature (form and time-line) of this disease.

### Sequence of System Operation

The preceding discussion of symptom processing may give the impression that the construction of a symptom experience always goes from a body sensation to a process of enrichment. However, this is NOT so. The system can be brought into action at any number of points, for example, by direct action on schemata or by the organism's own responses. Sensory and perceptual construction is at the service of responding and responses feed back to and alter sensory and perceptual events. Thus, a person who has been successfully managing a minor injury may become emotionally distraught upon learning that his or her self-treatment was ineffective and the injury became gangrenous. Interaction is the order of the day.

## EMPIRICAL EXAMPLE OF ILLNESS AND COPING REPRESENTATIONS

A number of data bases support the hypotheses that schematic and conceptual codes of emotion and illness play a crucial role in the construction of illness episodes. Data from three areas will be discussed briefly, each selected because of its importance in illustrating the various ways these codes impact on behaviour during illness episodes.

### Schemata and the Experience of Pain

Two types of studies provide vivid illustrations of the importance of emotion-illness schemata in the experience of pain, the key illness symptom: data on phantom pain and data on the effects of sensation monitoring in facilitating coping with painful medical episodes.

Phantom pain. Phantom pain phenomena provide dramatic evidence in support of the hypothesis that illness/emotion schemata integrate concrete symptomatic experience with autonomic, expressive, attentional and self-exploratory behaviours. Following the amputation of a body part (either by surgery or accident), an individual may come to experience a phantom limb replete with the sensations and pain that were present prior to the loss (Melzack, 1971, 1973; Simmel, 1962). The imagery can be exceptionally vivid, and the pain intense. It can be accompanied by subjective distress and anxiety, autonomic arousal (sweating and heart racing), and complete facial motor displays. It is not clear whether these latter (emotional and autonomic reactions) are part of the memory structure or elicited by the pain memory.

A memory interpretation is necessary for phantom pain because peripheral explanations are inadequate (e.g., Morgenstern, 1970). There are also cases where the phantom process selects one of several possible pains on the basis of its emotional significance rather than its severity. For example, Henderson and Smyth (1948) report a case of a soldier who became emotionally distraught during combat when he sprained his ankle: he was fearful the injury would limit his mobility and lead to more serious consequences. As fate would have it, a shrapnel wound in that same leg led to gangrene and several days of severe pain followed by amputation. Following the amputation a phantom appeared in which he experienced the pain of the sprained ankle, and not that of the subsequent, more severe injury. Cases have also been reported in which a dormant phantom has been rearoused by emotionally distressing life experiences (Melzack, 1973).

The above examples illustrate the importance of emotional reactions in the formation and arousal of memory for body parts and symptoms. Gross and Melzack (1978) have conducted several laboratory studies where they have generated short-lived experiences of phantom limbs, but the author is aware of only one report of a study on the formation of a painful memory. Hutchins and Reynolds (reported in Nathan, 1962) applied a nonpainful electrical stimulus to the trigeminal nerve of patients who had had dental work weeks earlier under either novocaine, which blocked transmission of sensory cues to the central nervous system (CNS), or nitrous oxide, which did not block sensory cues to the CNS. The mild electrical stimulus to the nerve recreated the pain of tooth drilling for the patients who had received the nitrous oxide but not for the patients who had received novocaine. There is good reason to believe, therefore, that body regions, symptoms, pain and emotion can be integrated in the type of memory codes we have labelled schemata.

Preparation and sensation monitoring. Several experimental studies have compared levels of emotional distress and effective coping in control subjects with subjects who were prepared with prior information on the sensations accompanying noxious events or were instructed to monitor the physical sensations created by these noxious events. Preparation and monitoring are assumed to create a neutral (non-emotion provoking) schema of the noxious stimulus, thereby reducing distress and enhancing effective coping. The subjects and/or patients instructed to monitor sensations and those receiving information describing the sensations showed lower levels of distress and more effective coping than did uninstructed control groups. This held whether the noxious stimuli were produced in the lab, such as ischemia induced by a blood pressure cuff (Johnson, 1973) and immersion of the hand for 6 minutes in ice water (Leventhal, Brown, Shacham, and Engquist, 1979) or by medical procedures such as endoscopy (Johnson and Leventhal, 1974), cast removal (Johnson, Kirchoff, and Endress, 1975), and surgery (Johnson, Rice, Fuller, and Endress, 1978). When subjects using the sensation monitoring strategies were compared to those using distraction, the latter showed more immediate reductions in distress than did the subjects monitoring sensations. But, the distraction subjects did not experience continued reductions in distress unless they actively continued to distract themselves from the noxious event. By contrast, subjects who monitored the sensations showed a gradual reduction in distress (an habituation process) and the reduction persisted even when they ceased to monitor the stimulus sensations (Ahles, Blanchard, and Leventhal, 1983). The results suggest that preparation and monitoring allow the individual to "get to know" the stressor, to form a schema of its "objective features", and to respond to it as an objective event rather than a threat. The durability of the effects and other memory changes (Dar, 1983) support a memory-schema interpretation of the effects.

## Schemata and Concepts in the Representation of Chronic Illness

Though the phantom pain studies provide vivid examples and the preparation studies practical examples of the operation of schemata in the construction of symptomatic experience, neither tells us about the schematic and conceptual processes involved in the representations of chronic illnesses such as hypertension and cancer. These diseases, with their long and complex histories, encourage the formation of multi-attribute representations integrated with emotional reactions. The illness models for these diseases are developed from the ongoing integration of body sensations and diverse social information with existent schematic and conceptual structures. Their representation can thus be expected to be complex in content and to reflect, respectively, the concrete and abstract qualities and the short-and long-term expectancies of schematic and conceptual codes. Our studies of patients with hypertension and cancer have supported these hypotheses.

Representations of chronic illnesses include at least four types of attribute: (1) a possible cause; (2) an identity (label and symptoms); (3) a set of possible consequences (physical, social, economic, etc.); and (4) a set of time-lines (the duration of the illness, time of onset, and duration of its consequences, etc.). There is also abundant evidence that at least one of the attributes of diseases such as hypertension and cancer has both abstract and concrete components: they are identified both conceptually, by labels, and concretely, by symptom complexes. The behavioural or action component of these illness episodes also include attributes and expectations regarding their control, including preventive and treatment responses, effectiveness of these responses, self-effectance or ability to perform these responses, and self-maintenance or ability to sustain effort. Both the representation of the illness and the action component may provoke emotional reactions.

Studies of hypertension. Interviews with hypertensives have shown that their representations had multiple attributes and were both concrete and abstract. Thus, we found that 71% of our patients who were new to treatment believed their symptoms (headache, face flushing, heart pounding) indicated blood pressure elevations, while this same belief was held by 92% of the patients who had been in treatment for 6 months or longer (Meyer, Leventhal, and Gutmann, 1985). A 6-month follow-up of the newly treated group showed the subset holding this belief increased from 71% to 92%. Only 46% of a control group of non-hypertensives in treatment for other conditions believed they could tell when their pressures were elevated. In this particular sample, therefore, the longer one is in treatment the stronger the belief that symptoms IDENTIFY blood pressure elevation and can be used to monitor one's physical condition.

Moreover, the symptomatic identity of hypertension was important for compliance: 70% of the continuing treatment patients who believed their symptoms were helped by the medication were taking it as prescribed, as compared to 31% compliance among those who did not detect a beneficial effect. In addition, 61% of the newly treated patients who said they reported their symptoms to the nurse or the doctor were lost to treatment 6 months later: only 24% were lost to treatment from among those who said they did not report these symptoms to their practitioner.

In addition to confirming that symptom processing can affect treatment behaviour, the results suggested that symptoms did not accurately detect blood pressure levels. Correlations were found between symptoms and blood pressure ranging from -.08 to +.11. In a second study of 43 persons, the association of their blood pressure readings with their predictions of their blood pressure and with their reports of symptoms and moods was assessed. These measures were recorded twice a day for a 10 day period (Baumann and Leventhal, 1985). The within-subject correlations between blood pressure and predictions of blood pressure levels (high, normal, or elevated) were modest (mean r=.14). There were substantial positive correlations, however, between subjects' predictions of their blood pressure and their symptom reports (mean r=.34) and moods (mean r=.22). Neither symptom reports nor moods were related to their blood pressure. Pennebaker has obtained new data that confirm these findings and suggest a more robust relationship between blood pressure and predictions of blood pressure among normotensives in comparison to hypertensives. He suggests hypertensives are inaccurate at estimating their pressure because they base their predictions on idiosyncratic symptoms that are unrelated to actual variations in blood pressure. The associations between blood pressure and symptoms are, however, quite modest (mean r = .14). (1)

The author's studies also show that symptom processing can be initiated by a verbal label and need not begin with a body sensation. In two laboratory studies half of the subjects were given false feedback indicating that their blood pressure was high; the other half received normal readings (Baumann, Leventhal, Zimmerman, and Linz) (2). In both instances subjects receiving the false feedback reported experiencing a greater number of symptoms during the prior weeks. Pennebaker and his colleagues (Pennebaker and Skelton, 1981) have shown similar effects: subjects led to believe it is flu season report more symptoms than those not so instructed, and subjects who fail on a task report more symptoms than subjects who had success. Moreover, the symptoms evoked by these experimental manipulations are in many cases identical to those reported by patients! There are mental representations or schemata that link disease labels and symptoms, and conceptual processes (false feedback) may activate these schematic traces of prior body sensations, which then evoke symptom reporting. Pennebaker (1982) has extensive data on this issue.

The representation of cancer and emotional distress. The author's studies of adaptation to cancer chemotherapy treatment have produced some understanding of the way in which both the abstract and concrete aspects of the representations of cancer influence the interpretation of body sensations and generate emotional distress. Over 400 women with breast cancer, who were either in adjuvant treatment or had metastatic disease, were interviewed in seven studies. In adjuvant treatment all signs of cancer have been removed by surgery, but because of evidence of cancer cells in axillary lymph nodes, combinations of cytotoxic and hormonal agents are given to increase the possibility of a disease-free interval. Treatment for metastatic disease involves similar therapeutic agents given with palliative intent in cases in which disease has spread to other organs. Approximately 70% of the metastatic women in the author's samples had recurrent disease, (i.e., their cancers had returned following successful surgery years earlier) although the majority were on chemotherapy for the first time (See Leventhal, et al., in press for a detailed report of the sample).

Because of the differences in their disease and treatment histories it was expected that adjuvant treatment and metastatic women would have different representations of cancer and would be distressed by somewhat different aspects of treatment. For example, by the 6th cycle of treatment, 89% of metastatic patients conceptualized their cancer as a cyclic or chronic condition, while 50% of the adjuvant treatment women conceptualized their cancer as an acute disease. This conceptual difference in the temporal representation of cancer appeared to be responsible for the increasingly strong correlation in the metastatic women between their reports of treatment side effects and distress about cancer: a relationship that did not appear for the adjuvant treatment women. Because metastatic patients conceptualized cancer as a recurrent and chronic disease, the context in which they

---

1. Pennebaker, J. W., and Watson, D. (Unpublished manuscript). Blood pressure perception among normotensives and hypertensives. Southern Methodist University, Dallas, Texas.

2. Baumann, L. J., Leventhal, H., Zimmerman, R., and Linz, D. (Unpublished manuscript). Effects of false blood pressure feedback on symptom reports. University of Wisconsin, Madison, Wisconsin.

perceived side effects was more likely to convert them into distressing reminders of cancer. Interestingly, adjuvant treatment women with similar cyclic and chronic views were also more distressed than their peers who viewed cancer as acute.

## THE MULTIVARIATE NATURE OF SYMPTOM PROCESSING

The original question posed was, "Why is symptom reporting important?". The evidence was reviewed for differences in the frequency of symptom reports as a function of sex, psychological status, or environmental reinforcement, and these findings were contrasted to evidence on the validity of symptoms as indicators of the severity of lung cancer. The contrast made clear that a complex process underlies the experience of symptoms and their reporting. It has been suggested that understanding of these differences has been advanced somewhat by descriptive approaches, that is, by linking symptom reporting to psychological traits and states and to specific environmental conditions. It is essential, however, to formulate a general model or framework of the processes underlying symptom experiences to increase understanding of the commonalities and differences between various descriptive phenomena. The hypothesis of a hierarchical processing system provides one such framework: conceptual and schematic memories elaborate an innate sensory base and integrate sensations and automatic reactions to disease with sensations and automatic reactions elicited by emotionally evocative interpersonal settings.

The value of this framework or model is twofold. First, it provides a synthetic view of otherwise disparate phenomena. Second, it provides a working model for generating specific hypotheses about the impact and the interaction of particular variables on symptom experience. The full value of the model cannot be realized, however, without further specification of its concepts and their mode of operation. It will also be necessary to stipulate the relationship between its "psychological" terms and concepts at the sociological and biological level, a step that could prove most fruitful. It is undoubtedly true that further specification may lead to modification or to rejection of several of the model's operating assumptions. But that is the price of a deeper understanding of these intriguing phenomena.

## ACKNOWLEDGEMENTS

Preparation of this chapter was supported by Grant Number DA03530, National Institute of Drug Abuse and Grant Number AG03501, National Institute on Aging.

## REFERENCES

Ahles, T., Blanchard, E., & Leventhal, H. (1983). Cognitive control of pain: Attention to the sensory aspects of the cold pressor stimulus. Cognitive Therapy and Research, 7, 159-178.

Allport, G., & Pettigrew, T. F. (1957). Cultural influence on the perception of movement: The trapezoidal illusion among Zulus. Journal of Abnormal and Social Psychology, 55, 104-113.

Bandura, A. (1977). Self-efficacy: Toward a unifying theory of behavioral change. Psychological Review, 84, 191-215.

Baumann, L. J., & Leventhal, H. (1985). "I can tell when my blood pressure is up: Can't I?" Health Psychology, 4, 203-218.

Beecher, H. K. (1959). Measurement of subjective responses. New York: Oxford University Press.

Blass, E. M., Ganchrow, J. R., & Steiner, J. E. (1984). Classical conditioning in newborn humans 2-48 hours of age. Infant Behavior and Development, 7, 223-235.

Brazelton, T. B., Koslowski, B., & Main, M. (1974). The origins of reciprocity: The early mother-infant interaction. In M. Lewis & L. A. Rosenblum (Eds.), The effect of the infant on its caretaker. (pp. 49-76). New York: Wiley.

Broverman, D. M., Klaiber, E. L., Kobayashi, Y., & Vogel, W. (1968). Roles of activation and inhibition in sex differences in cognitive abilities. Psychological Review, 75, 23-50.

Cadoret, R. J., Widmer, R. B., & Troughton, E. P. (1980). Somatic complaints: Harbinger of depression in primary care. Journal of Affective Disorders, 2, 61-70.

Casey, K. L. (1973). Pain: A current review of neural mechanisms. American Scientist, 61, 194-200.

Chrisman, N. J. (1977). The health seeking process: An approach to the natural history of illness. Culture, Medicine and Psychiatry, 1, 351-377.

Dar, R. (1983). Schematic processes in pain perception: Effects of sensation monitoring. Unpublished masters thesis, University of Wisconsin, Madison, WI.

Dingle, J. H. (1973). The ills of man. Scientific American, 229, 77-84

Fabrega, H. (1975). The need for an ethnomedical science. Science, 189, 969-976.

Feinstein, A. R., Sosin, D. M., & Wells, C. K. (1985). The Will Rogers Phenomenon's stage migration and new diagnostic techniques as a source of sleading statistics for survival in cancer. New England Journal of Medicine, 312, 1604-1608.

Fordyce, W. E. (1976). Behavior methods for chonic pain and illness. St. Louis: The C.V. Mosby Co.

Frankel, B. G., & Nuttall, S. (1984). Illness behaviour: An exploration of determinants. Social Science and Medicine, 19, 147-155.

Gibson, J. J. (1950). The perception of the visual world. Boston: Houghton-Mifflin.

Gove, W., & Hughes, M. (1979). Possible causes of the apparent sex differences in physical health: An empirical investigation. American Sociological Review, 44, 126-146.

Gross, Y. & Melzack, R. (1978). Body image: Dissociation of real and perceived limbs by pressure-cuff ischemia. Experimental Neurology, 61, 680-688.

Henderson, W. R., & Smyth, G. E. (1948). Phantom limbs. Journal of Neurology, Neurosurgery and Psychiatry, 11, 88-111.

Johnson, J. (1973). Effects of accurate expectations about sensations on sensory and distress components of pain. Journal of Personality and Social Psychology, 27, 261-275.

Johnson, J. E., Kirchoff, K. T., & Endress, M. P. (1975). Deferring children's distress behavior during orthopedic cast removal. Nursing Research, 75, 404-410.

Johnson, J., & Leventhal, H. (1974). The effects of accurate expectations and behavioral instructions on reactions during a noxious medical examination. Journal of Personality and Social Psychology, 29, 710-718.

Johnson, J. E., Rice, V. H., Fuller, S. S., & Endress, M. P. (1978). Sensory information, instruction in a coping strategy and recovery from surgery. Research in Nursing and Health, 1, 4-17.

Julesz, B. (1968). Experiment in perception. Psychology Today, 2, 16-23.

Katon, W., Kleinman, A., & Rosen, G. (1982a, January). Depression and somatization: A review. Part 1. The American Journal of Medicine, 72, 127-135.

Katon, W., Kleinman, A., & Rosen, G. (1982b, February). Depression and somatization: A review. Part 2. The American Journal of Medicine, 72, 241-247.

Kenyon, F. E. (1964). Hypochondriasis: A clinical study. British Journal of Psychiatry, 110, 478 - 488.

Kessler, R. C., Brown, R. L., and Broman, C. L. (1981). Sex differences in psychiatric help-seeking: Evidence from four large-scale surveys. Journal of Health and Social Behavior, 22, 49 - 64.
Kleinman, A. (1980). Patients and healers in the context of culture: An exploration of the borderland between anthropology, medicine and psychiatry. Berkley: University of California Press.
Leventhal, H. (1970). Findings and theory in the study of fear communications. Advances in Experimental Social Psychology, 5, 120-186.
Leventhal, H. (1975). The consequences of depersonalization during illness and treatment. In J. Howard & A. Strauss (Eds.), Humanizing health care. (pp. 119-160). New York: Wiley.
Leventhal, H. (1982). The integration of emotion and cognition: A view from the perceptual-motor theory of emotion. In M. S. Clark and S. T. Fiske (Eds.), Affect and cognition: The Seventeenth Annual Carnegie Symposium on Cognition (pp. 121-156). Hillsdale, NJ: Erlbaum.
Leventhal, H., Brown, D., Shacham, S., & Engquist, G. (1979). Effects of preparatory information about sensations, threat of pain, and attention on cold pressor distress. Journal of Personality and Social Psychology, 37, 688-714.
Leventhal, H., Easterling, D. V., Coons, H. L., Luchterhand, C. M., & Love, R.R. (in press). Adaptation to chemotherapy treatments. In B. L. Andersen (Ed.), Women with cancer: Psychological consequences. New York: Springer-Verlag.
Lewis, C. E., Lewis, M. A., & Lorimer, A. (1977). The use of school nursing services by children in an "adult free" system. Pediatrics, 60, 499-507.
Marcus, A. C., & Seeman, T. E. (1981). Sex differences in reports of illness disability: A preliminary test of the "fixed role obligations" hypothesis. Journal of Health and Social Behavior, 22, 174-182.
Mechanic, D. (1972). Social psychologic factors affecting the presentation of bodily complaints. New England Journal of Medicine, 286, 1132-1139.
Mechanic, D. (1976). Sex, illness, illness behavior, and the use of health services. Journal of Human Stress, 2, 29-40.
Mechanic, D. (1979). Development of psychological distress among young adults. Archives of General Psychiatry, 36, 1233-1239.
Melzack, R. (1971). Phantom limb pain. Anesthesiology, 35, 409-419.
Melzack, R. (1973). The puzzle of pain: Revolution in theory and treatment. New York: Basic Books.
Meyer, D., Leventhal, H., & Gutmann, M. (1985). Common sense models of illness: The example of hypertension. Health Psychology, 4, 115-135.
Morgenstern, F. S. (1970). Chronic pain. In O. U. Hill (Ed.), Modern trends in psychosomatic medicine. Nwe York: Appleton.
Mountcastle, V. B. (1980). Pain and temperature sensibilities. In V. B. Mountcastle (Ed.), Medical physiology. (pp. 391-427). St. Louis: C. V. Mosby.
Murphy, G. L. and Medin, D. L. (1985). The role of theories in conceptual coherence. Psychological Review, 92, 289-316.
Nathan, P. W. (1962). Pain traces left in the central nervous system. In C. A. Keele & R. Smith (Eds.), The assessment of pain in man and animals. Edinburgh: E. & S. Livingston.
Nathanson, C. A. (1975). Illness and the feminine role: A theoretical review. Social Science and Medicine, 9, 57-62.
Nerenz, D. R., Leventhal, H., Easterling, D. V., & Love, R. R. (in press). Anxiety and drug taste as predictors of anticipatory nausea in cancer chemotherapy. Journal of Clinical Oncology.
Pearlin, L. I., & Schooler, C. (1978). The structure of coping. Journal of Health and Social Behavior, 19, 2-21.
Pennebaker, J. W. (1982). The psychology of physical symptoms (pp. 81-102). New York: Springer-Verlag.
Pennebaker, J. W., & Skelton, J. A. (1981). Selective monitoring of bodily sensations. Journal of Personality and Social Psychology, 41, 213-223.
Pilowsky, I. (1967). Dimensions of hypochondriasis. British Journal of Psychiatry, 113, 89-93.

Pilowsky, I. (1978). A general classification of abnormal illness behaviours. British Journal of Medical Psychology, 51, 131-137.
Pilowsky, I., Bassett, D., Barrett, R., Petrovic, L., & Minniti, R. (1983-84). The illness behavior assessment schedule: Reliability and validity. International Journal of Psychiatry in Medicine, 13, 11-28.
Posner, M. I., & Keele, S. W. (1970). Retention of abstract ideas. Journal of Experimental Psychology, 83, 304-308.
Schnall, P. L. & Kern, R. (1981). Hypertension in American society: An introduction to historical materialist epidemiology. In P. Conrad & R. Kern, The sociology of health and illness: Critical perspectives (pp. 97-125). New York: St. Martin's Press.
Simmel, M. L. (1962). The reality of phantom sensations. Social Research, 29, 337-356.
Snyder, S. H. (1977). Opiate receptors and internal opiates. Scientific American, 236, 44-56.
Sternbach, R. A. (1968). Pain: A psychophysiological analysis. New York: Academic.
Sternberg, S. (1969). Memory-scanning: Mental processes revealed by reaction-time experiments. American Scientist, 57, 421-457.
Syme, S. L., & Berkman, L. F. (1976). Social class, susceptibility and sickness. American Journal of Epidemiology, 104, 1-8.
Telles, J. L., & Pollack, M. H. (1981). Feeling sick: The experience and legitimation of illness. Social Science and Medicine, 15A, 243-51.
Tulving, E. (1985). How many memory systems are there? American Psychologist, 40, 385-398.
Verbrugge, L. M. (1981). Sex differentials in health and mortality. In A. H. Stromberg (Ed.), Women, health and medicine. Palo Alto: Mayfield Publishing.
Verbrugge, L. M. (1985). Gender and health: An update on hypotheses and evidence. Journal of Health and Social Behavior, 26, 156-182.
Verbrugge, L. M. and Steiner, R. P. (1981). Physician treatment of men and women patients: Sex bias or appropriate care? Medical Care, 19, 609-632.
Ward, S. (1985). Social support: Reciprocity, the negatives and the person with cancer. Unpublished masters thesis, University of Wisconsin, Madison, WI.
Wooley, S., & Blackwell, B. (1975). A behavioral probe into social contingencies on a psychosomatic ward. Journal of Applied Behavior Analysis, 8, 337.
Wooley, S. C., Blackwell, B., & Winget, C. W. (1978). A learning theory model of chronic illness behavior: Theory, treatment, and research. Psychosomatic Medicine, 40, 379-401.
Zborowski, M. (1969). People in pain. San Francisco: Jossey-Bass.
Zola, I.K. (1973). Pathways to the doctor: From person to patient. Social Science and Medicine, 7, 677-689.

# COGNITION, EMOTION, AND ILLNESS

Peter Lang, Bruce Cuthbert and Barbara Melamed

Department of Clinical Psychology
University of Florida

Whenever general physicians are polled as to the source of their patients' complaints, they invariably respond that most symptoms are directly or indirectly related to emotional factors (Shapiro, 1959). However, excluding a vigorous neurohumoral and behavioural tradition in animal research, there is surprisingly little scientific work elucidating the role of human emotion in illness. Even among researchers, the study of emotions has in many ways remained in the domains of subjective conjecture, patient anecdotes, and armchair psychology.

When applied science fails to come to grips with a pressing social need, it is almost always attributable to a limitation in the basic disciplines on which the desired practical advance depends. Thus, man can go to the moon if the necessary resources are expended - because the fundamental physics of this task are well understood. However, we cannot now find a cure for cancer or even lay out an exact plan of experiments that will achieve this end, no matter how much money is spent or how many researchers directly address the task, because the underlying basic biochemistry, immunology, and/or genetics are not sufficiently advanced to guide the enterprise.

In an analogous way, our practical understanding of how emotions may instigate or modulate physical illness has been stymied. Cancer aside, the last several decades have seen enormous progress in understanding the biology and physiology of many illnesses. Nevertheless, there has been no parallel major advance in the basic behavioural science of emotion. In brief, psychological theory and research have not been at state of development that would support a direct attack on the problem.

A major reason for the slow progress of emotion research lies in the difficulty psychologists have in defining emotion independent of the introspective experience of affect, coupled with the impossibility of applying quantitative methods and scientific procedures to this private world of feeling. From the beginnings of psychological science, researchers have generally followed one of two paths in dealing with this dilemma: (1) They have ignored subjectivity, attending only to behavioural data, attempting to understand the function, origin, and organization of overt actions, while making few if any inferences about cognition or mental processes (e.g., the operant conditioning approach of B. F. Skinner). (2) They have accepted everyman's view that subjective experience determines behaviour, elevating it to the level of a theory, using the laboratory as a place to gather facts in its support. In this latter case, the key phenomena are "cognitions" which are very like the reports Western man makes about his mental life, i.e., that he behaves on the basis of felt needs and desires, after appraisal of his environment, physical capacity, and the consequences of his acts.

It is suggested here that neither of these paths has greatly advanced our understanding of the psychology of emotion. While the first approach has yielded a technology of behaviour modification (e.g., effective procedures for stress reduction and for promoting compliance with medical regimes (Melamed and Siegel, 1980)), it cannot be said that a narrow behavioural analysis has elucidated the basic mechanism of emotion or shown how emotion impacts on illness. Advocates of the second approach, the scientific phenomenologists, have promoted treatment methods based on self-talk (Ellis, 1962) and "cognitive restructuring" (Meichenbaum, 1977), but the specific effectiveness of these procedures in the context of physical illness is still being evaluated (Holroyd, Appel, and Andrasik, 1983). More pertinent to the present argument, the "cognitive appraisal" view has also failed to provide any very new insight into emotional processes, greater than that already achieved by epistemologically similar philosophical and literary analyses.

As this is currently the dominant viewpoint in studies of the psychology of illness, the following discussion will first review theory and research based on the "cognitive appraisal" approach. The arguments which lead to questioning of its heuristic value will be described. An alternative frame of reference is then presented, based on an integration of contemporary information processing theory and psychophysiology. This new view is not offered as a finished model of emotion, nor will it be argued that the approach provides immediate solutions to the problems of emotion and illness. However, it does represent the kind of major reconsideration of affective processing on which any significant progress may depend. Furthermore, it has already suggested a novel line of experimentation, yielding new knowledge about the nature of emotion and showing promise for practical application.

## Cognitive Appraisal and Cognitive Restructuring

An explanation of emotion based on "cognitive appraisal" was proposed by Schachter and associates in the early 1960's (Schachter and Singer, 1962; Schachter, 1964), and has since been developed and elaborated by several psychological theorists (most notably, Lazarus (see this volume) and George Mandler, (1975, 1984)). Following the lead of Cannon (1936) and Duffy (1962), they argue that different emotions share a similar underlying physiology - a viscerally active, "stirred-up" state of arousal. The quality, character, and organization of a specific emotional state depend on the individual's interpretation of the arousal. That is to say, emotions are determined by a need to explain the arousal's significance. This is achieved through "appraisal" of the immediate environmental circumstances and relevant past experience:

> "... given a state of physiological arousal for which an individual has no immediate explanation, he will "label" this state and describe his feelings in terms of the cognitions available to him. To the extent that cognitive factors are potent determiners of emotional states, it could be anticipated that precisely the same state of physiological arousal could be labeled "joy" or "fury" or any of a great diversity of emotional labels, depending on the cognitive aspects of the situation" (Schachter, 1964, p. 53).

The experiments presented in support of this theory often involve camouflaged induction of arousal, with various situational manipulations affecting the nature and degree of the subsequent reported emotion. The classic paradigm developed by Schachter and Singer (1962) involved the administration of epinephrine or a placebo, with a deceptive cover story that the drug was a vitamin or other arousal-irrelevant agent. Subjects receiving epinephrine were given either true information regarding its effects, or misleading or no information (misattribution). Subsequently, they were exposed to a situation in which an experimental confederate expressed anger or behaved euphorically. Schachter and Singer reported that as predicted, only epinephrine-injected subjects in the misattribution conditions showed increased emotionality in these situations on both behavioural and self-rating indices, compared to those subjects given placebo. This initial work has spawned numerous attempts at replication and extension (recently reviewed by Reisenzein, 1983), and further theoretical development by other investigators (e.g., Lazarus, 1984; Mandler, 1984).

While a review of all the experimental literature is outside the scope of the current chapter, several points regarding this theory deserve comment here. First, the arousal/appraisal theories all assume an undifferentiated arousal state, based upon elevated levels of sympathetic nervous system activity (Duffy, 1962). It is not clear, however, given the wide variety of effects associated with other catecholamines, that the pharmacologic manipulation in Schachter's studies produced the "normal" physiological substrate of emotion. Even within the domain of sympathetic activation, reports of the distinct distributions and gradations of response patterns associated with alpha and beta receptors call into question a simplistic approach employing a single agent. Finally, the consequences for the cardiovascular system are very different when drugs are ingested as a single bolus, in contrast to a slow infusion approximating glandular secretion rates (Keele and Neil, 1971).

Furthermore, developments in psychophysiological theory have served to modify our conceptions of arousal. Lacey's early demonstration (1967) of directional fractionation, for example, showed that different measurement systems may change in opposite directions under several conditions which all putatively involve arousal. More recently, Obrist and associates (Obrist, 1981) showed that the nature and patterning of physiological response vary as a function of whether subjects are actively versus passively coping with a stressful situation. Such data serve to mitigate against arguments based on unidimensional arousal theories.

In addition to these concerns with the physiological aspects of cognitive appraisal models, further considerations arise with respect to the fundamental theoretical orientation and definition of emotions. As mentioned earlier, Schachter's view is a theory of emotional <u>experience</u>, rather than of emotional behaviour or expression. This distinction can appear subtle, particularly since for many investigators, the phenomenological experience is the archetypical defining characteristic of emotion, which is to be understood or indexed by all other relevant assessment devices such as physiology. As Gellhorn and Loofbourrow stated some years ago, "... emotion is a fact upon which all introspection agrees. Anxiety, depression, elation, indifference, anger, fear, pleasurable anticipation and dread, for example, are undeniable because they are states which we have experienced personally" (1963, p. 41). However, phenomenological experience represents only one aspect of emotion. Furthermore, this emphasis narrows the focus of investigation. It fails to consider the broad range of emotional behaviours and their varied inter-relationships.

For nearly two decades (e.g., Lang, 1968), it has been generally agreed that emotions consist of behaviour in three output systems: physiological responses, overt or expressive behaviour, and verbal reports regarding subjective experience (Izard, 1984; Lazarus, 1984; Zajonc, 1980). The term "emotion" is actually a construct used to denote activity observed to various degrees of all three of these systems, rather than some central event <u>indexed</u>

by these measures. Indeed, the lack of consistency among these various response systems is one of the most striking features in conducting research on emotion (Lang, 1978; Rachman and Hodgson, 1974); the commonality of response seldom accounts for more that ten to 15 percent of the variance (e.g., Lacey, 1959). Individuals frequently are much more responsive in one system than another; also, during behaviour therapies it is common to find the systems changing at different rates over the course of treatment (Lang, 1978; Rachman, 1974). While verbal report is unarguably one datum in studying emotion, an emphasis only on reports of experience overlooks the massive amounts of data regarding physiological and behavioural responding, with great theoretical and practical import (Levin, Cook, and Lang, 1982; Levi, 1975; Fenz and Jones, 1972; Rachman, 1978).

A related point concerns the relatively slow nature of the cognitions involved. Experiencing some state of physiological upheaval, one must ask where such feelings are coming from and execute a dialogue of various lengths to search for the answer. Sometimes this is fairly forthcoming - "I just ran up a flight of stairs" - but at other times, may be more complex - "I wonder what it is about that person that seems to bother me?" It is argued here, however, that the timing of such theories is much too slow to account for the rapidity with which emotion is frequently experienced. Zajonc, (1980), e.g., has reviewed evidence that emotional reactions and behaviour can be determined within milliseconds following a stimulus.

This problem has led theorists sympathetic to Schachter's position to espouse a variety of solutions. In particular, it is posited that the cognitive appraisal process can be very rapid and unconscious (Mandler, 1975; Lazarus, 1982). Mandler (1984) also proposed that immediate responses to stimuli of an emotional nature can themselves be evaluated, thus satisfying the appraisal requirement: "These actions, often occur rapidly and sometimes long before autonomic arousal can be activated or an evaluative analysis performed. Under these conditions, the evaluated (perceived) actions themselves become objects of a meaning analysis and determine the evaluative state. In other words, the emotional 'behaviour' determines the evaluative state that, subsequently, defines the subjective emotional experience" (Mandler, 1984, p. 121). Except for some loss of parsimony, this analysis is little changed from that of William James (1890), writing at the end of the nineteenth century. It is consistent with a theory directed toward explaining emotional experience; however, it explicitly ignores consideration of the initiating emotional behaviour itself. Finally, if it is held that cognitions _must_ precede the occurrence of any emotional response, then the theory becomes essentially untestable, because it would be impossible ever to prove beyond doubt that some appraisal had not taken place.

Alternative theories which accept the possibility of specific stimuli and specifiable response patterns in emotional response - either through hard-wired connections (Seligman and Hager, 1972; Ohman, 1986) or associative learning (Eysenck, 1979) - are much more parsimonious and heuristic in evaluating the entire temporal range of emotional behaviour. In contrast to the appraisal theories which emphasize an understanding of phenomenological experience, considerations such as these lead to the view that the central problem lies in predicting and controlling emotional _behaviour_, in all of its manifestations. The approach taken here is that it is precisely these relatively focused, rapidly occurring episodes of organismic response that come at the crux of how emotions are organized and expressed. While the model to be presented below is cognitive in nature, it is concerned with those programs which support emotional expression directly, rather than with secondary appraisal processes.

Emotion, Language, and Memory

One of the striking things abut human emotional reactions is the great extent to which they can be triggered indirectly, by the most brief descriptions or references to emotion-related matters. Accordingly, much of our interest in emotion and language, rather than secondary appraisal and elaboration of experience, has been directed toward an understanding of how language can control the behavioural, verbal, and physiological events occurring during emotional expression. To describe this approach, it is best to distinguish the theory of emotion employed here from the experiential models referred to above. As these ideas have been elaborated at length elsewhere (Lang, 1984, 1985), only a brief description will be given here. An emotion is conceived to be an action set, i.e., a tendency to respond with a given set of behaviours (verbal, motoric, and physiological) in a specified situation. The metaphor adopted is that of modern information processing theory, in which cognitive operations reflect processes roughly similar to those performed by a computer in running a program. The brain program is stored in long-term memory; when accessed by appropriate stimuli, it is loaded into the brain's work space and run.

Affective programs are presumed to be associative networks of the type originally formulated for semantic knowledge (Quillian, 1966), and later adapted for the representation of other kinds of information (Anderson, 1976; Johnson-Laird, Herrmann, and Chaffin, 1984). Knowledge is stored in these networks as basic nodes of information connected by links specifying the relationship between them; each such assertion is referred to as a proposition. For example, the phrase "boy hits ball" is a simple proposition in which the word "hits" indicates the relation of "boy" and "ball". Affective networks are seen as comprised of three kinds of propositions. Stimulus propositions convey elements of the stimulus setting for the emotion, and are the usual elements that we think of in recalling an episodic event. Response propositions represent physiological outputs which occur in the situation, and are important to an understanding of emotional response. These elements are seen as doubly coded: not only are they stored as linguistic nodes in the network, they are also connected to actual efferent systems leading to the periphery. Finally, meaning propositions provide information about the context not otherwise apparent in the stimulus setting, such as elaborative information about persons or objects. Within this model, these latter propositions correspond to the cognitive appraisal processes emphasized by Schachter, Lazarus, and others. While their role in emotion has been the focus of such investigators, in the current model meaning possesses no special salience for emotional expression.

Activation of individual nodes occurs when inputs match propositions in the network; when some sufficient number of nodes is so activated, the entire network is loaded into the work space and run as a unit. Inputs matching any of the three types of propositions are all seen as potentially effective in this process, a hypothesis supported by data from the laboratory (Lang, Kozak, Miller, Levin, and McLean, 1980; McLean, 1981; Kozak, 1982).

In sum, emotions are seen as action sets based upon brain associative networks, which may be based to varying degrees upon innate and learned programs. In this, they do not differ in principle from other, non-emotional associative networks. The chief distinction between emotional and non-emotional action sets would seem to be the intensity of the former, and the fact that they reflect situations of relative salience in a survival or phylogenetic sense, e.g., fear, eating, reproduction, etc. In fact, it has been argued that all behaviour can be construed as emotional to some degree, varying in its intensity. For example, the British neuroscientist J. Z. Young has stated, "the symbolic systems that we use to describe our perceptions and handle our problems are a combination of positional concepts and emotional responses to the objects perceived ... even the simplest act of comparison involves emotional factors" (Young, 1978, p. 194; italics in original).

As mentioned above, the presence of response concepts is a crucial aspect of the network. The composition of the particular representations in a network must determine which kinds of activity are observed in the three measurement systems described initially. A major goal of our research program has been to discover how these response programs are stored in memory and accessed, and how they may be changed under various circumstances. The procedure for testing this has relied heavily upon emotional imagery. Like many other situations in everday life, imagery involves the evocation of physiological and other efferents in response to a language stimulus; thus, it is a useful and heuristic method for the study of network organization.

Imagery and Action

The rationale for the presence of response outputs in imagery is not limited to emotion, and in fact has a long history. Shaw (1940) e.g., presented subjects with a series of weights, varing in heaviness, to be lifted in succession. After the actual lifting of the weights, subjects were asked to imagine lifting each weight while electromyographic activity was recorded from the arm. Thus, a language instruction was used to provide a stimulus to a previous episodic event. The results showed a roughly linear relationship between the mass of the imagined weight and the amplitude of the EMG response, even though subjects were not instructed to generate any muscle activity in imagery; further, EMG oscillations were higher when the images were reported as vivid. The inference is that the efferents to the arm were coded in memory at the time of the original lift, and then regenerated at the time of imagery. Although the final overt action was gated out, some "efferent leakage" occurred to the periphery which was proportional to the magnitude of the effort coded in memory.

Similar results were observed from a study from our laboratory, in which subjects observed a display on a CRT screen with rapidly flashing numbers and letters. The letters, detected in sequence, spelled out a word which was to be remembered as the second half of a word pair. (The first word was presented in its entirety immediately preceding this display). On half the trials the characters in the display slowly traversed the screen horizontally in two directions, while the characters were presented at a single point on the screen for the remaining trials. Following the detection of the words, subjects were presented the first word of each pair and requested to recall the second. One group of each subjects was instructed to imagine performing the tracking task during recall, while the other group was simply told to recall the word without any reference to the tracking task. Fast Fourier Transforms (FFT's) of eye movement potentials from this paradigm revealed very high power in the frequency band of the original display during the tracking trials. During recall, FFT power was significantly higher in the frequency bands near the display frequency for trials where the original display had involved horizontal traversing, as opposed to fixed character trials. However, this effect was observed equally whether or not subjects had been told to imagine performing the detection task during recall. As in Shaw's study, such activity was apparently coded in memory and regenerated during reactivation of the relevant network, even in the absence of specific instructions to do so.

Other experiments in the laboratory have specifically involved emotional imagery. In one recent study, subjects imagined single sentences of two different types (Vrana, Cuthbert, and Lang, in press). One set of sentences were fear sentences, while the other set comprised neutral sentences. The fear sentences involved giving a speech and sitting in the dentist's office, while the neutral sentences depicted relaxing in one's living room or porch. Subjects memorized the sentences in advance, and were cued over a CRT screen as to which sentence to imagine at each trial. Imagery was cued by a set of tones ten seconds apart, and the subject self-initiated the trial by choosing the tone at which he/she began the imagery sequence. Subjects performed two different operations with each sentence in successive ten-second periods. One was to "think" the sentence, which was defined as silent repetition of the words of the sentence. The other was imagery, in which the subject imagined the situation as vividly as possible, as though actually present in the imagined situation. One group of subjects performed these tasks in the order "think-image," while the other group carried out the reverse sequence.

Figure 1 shows the change in heart rate (from pre-trial baselines) for subjects during the think and image periods. No differences were apparent betweeen fear and neutral sentences for the think periods; however, significant effects were observed for imagery, particularly during the last five seconds. Even though the effects are subtle - two to three beats per minute - they nevertheless indicate that the imagery task can generate a physiology consonant with the fear situation, and once again support the hypothesis of efferent leakage.

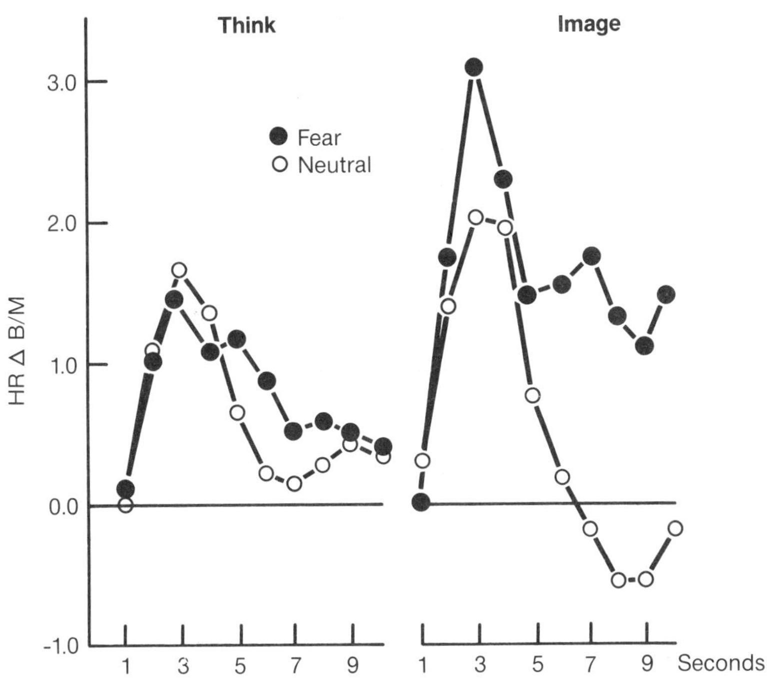


**FIGURE 1**

Figure 1. Heart rate change from the average heart rate in the two seconds before each processing period ("Think" and "Image"), averaged across think-first and image-first subjects. Tones occur in the first 250 ms. of the seconds marked "1". From Vrana et al., in press.

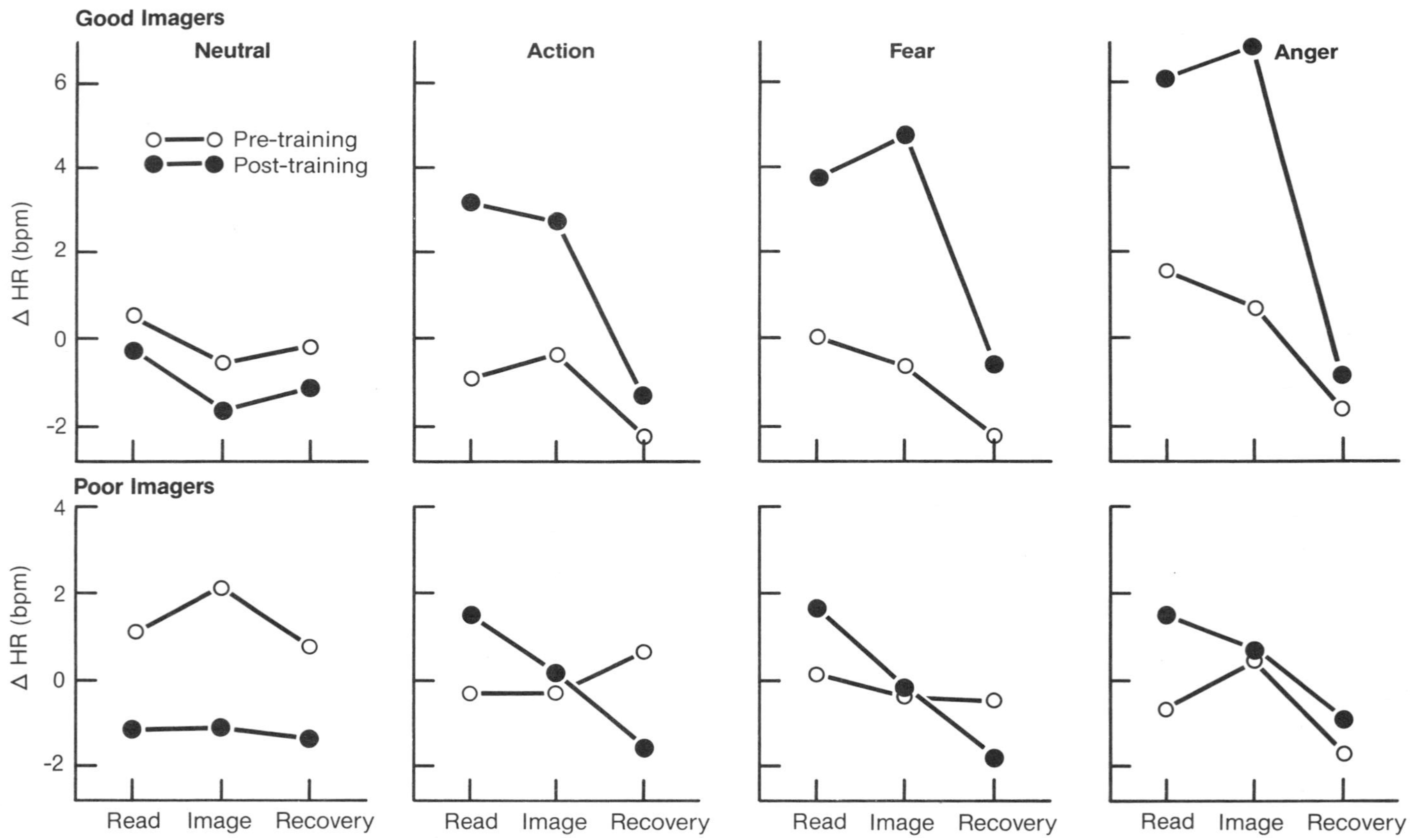

Good Imagers
Neutral
Action
Fear
Anger
Pre-training
Post-training
Δ HR (bpm)
6
4
2
0
-2
Poor Imagers
4
2
0
-2
Read
Image
Recovery

More elaborate experiments have been carried out to explore some of the variables involved in such imagery processing. One such variable was the inclusion of response propositions in imagery processing. Because most common-sense notions of imagery involve a perceptual or stimulus orientation, there were concerns that subjects might not process imagery texts adequately for response propositions. Accordingly, a response training procedure was developed. Small groups of subjects were presented with vivid imagery texts, and asked to report on their imagery. The experimenter shaped, by combinations of direct solicitation and verbal approval, the inclusion of autonomic and skeletal responses in subjects' reports of their imagery. Control groups were given stimulus-oriented training, in which the experimenter encouraged and reinforced the elaboration of the stimulus aspects of the training scenes. The result was two groups of subjects who both reported greatly enhanced imagery, but with markedly disparate content. Initial studies revealed that this response training was a powerful variable in eliciting substantial response during emotional imagery in unselected subjects imagining a variety of scenes (Lang et al., 1980). Further experiments confirmed the efficacy of the response training procedure for amplifying basic differences among scenes and subject groups, in samples selected for specific fears (Lang, Levin, Miller, and Kozak, 1983).

In addition to the two variables reviewed above - image processing and response proposition training - a third, individual difference variable has been studied. If imagery is in fact a somewhat different way of processing material, then subjects who report themselves to be good imagers should show more recruitment of the physiology as a function of imagery instructions than other kinds of subjects. In a recent experiment, subjects scoring high and low on the Questionnaire on Mental Imagery (QMI; Sheehan, 1967) were selected from an undergraduate population, and given a variety of fear, anger, action, and neutral scenes (Miller et al, 1986). All subjects were given a response training session intervening between two identical psychophysiological imagery sessions. As in the previous study, there was little effect of scene type or group at the first imagery session. However, following training, good imagery subjects demonstrated significantly higher physiological response for the fear and anger scenes (Figure 2). That these were not non-specific arousal or artifactual effects is indicated by the lack of difference for neutral scenes between the two groups. Thus, there seem to exist differences among subjects in the extent to which they recruit physiological efferent systems during imagery.

In terms of our model, the nature of this individual difference variable is not yet clear - whether poor imagers simply do not have response propositions coded in memory, or whether the information is present but not accessed during imagery. The fact that subjects seem to be different in the extent to which language processing controls their physiology may be a very important distinction as far as psychopathology and illness behaviour are concerned. In behaviour therapy for phobias, e.g., patients showing deficits in physiological response during fear-related imagery have a poorer outcome prognosis (Lang, Melamed, and Hart, 1970; Levin et al, 1982; McNeil, Melamed, Cuthbert, and Lang, 1983). This factor may be equally important in considering the extent to which illness behaviour is determined by the emotional processing that a subject does. That is, those subjects that

Figure 2. (see previous page) Median heart rate change scores from pre-trial resting levels for standard imagery scripts, according to group, training, content, and period. READ = 30-second period during which the pre-recorded script was played; IMAGE = 30-second imagery period; RECOV = 30-second recovery period, with subjects instructed to stop imagining and relax. (from Miller et al, 1986).

recruit or fail to recruit appropriate efferents may have very different kinds of illness behaviours and very different kinds of prognoses. Such phenomena, for example, could include alexithymia (Sifneos, 1972), in which the patient is reported not to have good language description of his emotional responding. Such a person could be one of the poor imagers as identified in our experiments.

## Imagery and Illness

Thus, the research program described here is basic in terms of addressing current practical problems of illness behaviour. However, potential ramifications for several applied lines of research are reflected in the current literature; although most such studies were not generated by the model presented here, they represent areas that could well be explored further in terms of this theoretical framework. First, many studies have shown the utility of imagery in ameliorating various pathophysiological functions associated with disease processes. For example, Varni (1981, 1983) used imagery procedures alone and in conjunction with thermal biofeedback and progressive relaxation in reducing arthritic pain in children with hemophilia. The guided imagery training involved images of warmth, gentle flowing of blood into joints, and suggestions of reduced pain. Zeltzer, Dash, and Holland (1979) reported the success of imagery techniques associated with self-hypnosis in reducing pain crises and analgesic intake in sickle-cell anemia patients; following an induction comprised of eye fixation and progressive relaxation, patients were instructed in guided imagery focussing on pleasant, pain-free scenes, and suggestions of increased body warmth and vasodilation.

From the current theoretical perspective, such reduction in symptomatology associated with imagery could come about due to an interference with the associative emotional networks normally loaded into the brain's work space. Replacing the usual maladaptive efferents (which exacerbate pain or lead to abnormal organ system functioning) with a quiescent physiology leads both to directly observable reductions in symptomatology (as in psychosomatic disorders) and to alterations of related verbal reports (as in pain).

Conversely, the potential for the generation of ultimately pathological efferents through imagery has also been demonstated. In a series of classic studies by Graham and associates, imagery of an attitude previously hypothesized to be associated with a given psychosomatic symptom resulted in increases in activity in the relevant organ system. For instance, imagery associated with a hypertensive attitude resulted in elevations in blood pressure, while imagery of the attitude linked to hives was followed by increases in hand temperature (Graham, Kabler, and Graham, 1962).

Other studies have shown that emotion-related imagery of various types can affect pathologically relevant responding in a variety of disorders. For instance, Tal and Miklich (1976) asked ten to 15-year-old children with chronic asthma to imagine neutral, fearful, and anger arousing situations. Increased heart rate and decreased expiratory flow rates occurred for the fear and anger scenes, contrasted to decreased heart rate and increased expiratory flow rates for neutral scenes. Melamed and Johnson (1979) reported significant differences in blood, urine, and glucose values for juvenile and adult diabetics when they imagined a recent stressor as opposed to positive or neutral affective memories. More recent studies have begun to examine systematically the nature of the imagery variable itself. For example, Hermecz and Melamed (1982) studied the effects of stimulus and response imagery training, as described above, in six to 12-year-old dental patients. Their results indicated a greater concordance between behavioural and physiological measures during subsequent dental restorations, in the group given response-oriented imagery training.

These studies indicate that specific efferents can occur when certain brain programs are processed, depending, in our framework, on the propositional composition of the associative structure so accessed. Although imagery was employed to study these effects in the examples cited above, we see the processes involved as highly similar for actual situations. Thus, while further research must determine exactly how these changes come about, issues of both etiology and treatment are addressed by the model presented here.

## CONCLUSIONS

Two points may be noted in conclusion. First, the current theory does not ignore the role of semantic knowledge and conscious (controlled) processing in the emotional response complex. The category of meaning information includes much that is called "cognitive appraisal" and efforts to interpret this material in the present framework have already begun (Foa and Kozak, 1986). However, we have argued here that emotional responses generally occur too quickly, and depend too heavily upon automatic stimulus and response associations for an appraisal explanation. The "rationalist" view cannot account for the majority of emotional responding, which often persists despite the presence of non-affective explanations of the affect (e.g., irritability and anger are often present in pre-menstrual syndrome, even though the woman "knows" its physiological basis). On the other hand, processing of afferent data may act to sustain emotional reactions that might otherwise be shorter and/or less debilitating in effect. Attitudes towards physiological sensations can set the individual for a particular emotional reaction. For example, the anxious patient's distress is augmented by the perception of his/her anxious behaviours. Thus, a trembling chin can itself be a further stimulus to anxiety, perhaps related to social concerns about the reactions of others. Such positive feedback loops could, of course, occur with or without conscious awareness.

Second, the view of emotion described here is framed in terms of the brain's programs. Cognition is construed to be the <u>software</u> of the metaphorical brain/computer. We have shown the value of this approach in working out the functional relationships among the imagery, individual difference, and emotional response variables discussed earlier. Obviously, however, the running of these programs is implemented in the <u>hardware</u> of the brain, and some attention to anatomical and physiological architecture is warranted, particularly for the study of medical disorders. For instance, the importance to emotional behaviour of the hypothalamic and paleocortical structures of the limbic system is well known (Usdin, Kvetnansky, and Kopin, 1980). The way in which persistent activation of these structures may ultimately result in peripheral disease is of considerable current research interest. A theory such as ours, explicitly addressing the presence and nature of efferent outputs in emotional brain memories, is certainly compatible with this line of investigation. In addition, by linking to current work regarding the modulation of recall by the emotional and/or physiological states present at learning (e.g., Bower, 1981; Clark, Milberg, and Ross, 1983; Zillmann, 1983), the theory meshes well with neurophysiological data such as Kety's (1970) indicating that processes associated with emotional responses may modulate memory storage. In summary, the model of emotional processing developed here has already proved useful in organizing a variety of research findings, and appears well suited for application to the difficult problems of disease and illness behaviour.

REFERENCES


Anderson, J. R. (1976). Language, memory, and thought. Hillsdale, NJ: Erlbaum.

Bower, G. H. (1981). Mood and memory. American Psychologist, 36, 129-148.

Cannon, W. B. (1936). Bodily changes in pain, hunger, fear, and rage (2nd ed.). New York: Appleton-Century-Crofts.

Clark, M. S., Milberg, S., & Ross, J. (1983). Arousal cues, arousal-related material in memory: Implications for understanding effect of mood on memory. Journal of Verbal Learning and Verbal Behavior, 22, 633-649.

Duffy, E. (1962). Activation and behavior. New York: Wiley.

Ellis, A. (1962). Reason and emotion in psychotherapy. New York: Lyle Stuart.

Eysenck, H. J. (1979). The conditioning model of neurosis. The Behavioral and Brain Sciences, 2, 155-199.

Fenz, W. D., & Jones, G. B. (1972). Individual differences in physiologic arousal and performance in sport parachutists. Psychosomatic Medicine, 34, 1-8.

Foa, E. B., & Kozak, M. J. (1986). Emotional processing of fear: Exposure to corrective information. Psychological Bulletin, 99, 20-35.

Gellhorn, E., & Loofbourrow, G. N. (1963). Emotions and emotional disorders. New York: Harper and Row.

Graham, D. T., Kabler, J. D., & Graham, F. K. (1962). Physiological response to the suggestion of attitudes specific for hives and hypertension. Psychosomatic Medicine, 24, 159-169.

Hermecz, D. A., & Melamed, B. G. (1984). Emotional imagery as an influence in children's affective responses to stress. Behavior Therapy, 15, 156-172.

Holroyd, K. A., Appel, M. A., & Andrasik, F. (1983). A cognitive-behavioral approach to psychophysiological disorders. In D. Meichenbaum & M. E. Jaremko (Eds.), Stress reduction and prevention (pp. 219-259). New York: Plenum Press.

Izard, C. E. (1984). Emotion-cognition relationships and human development. In C. E. Izard, J. Kagan, & R. B. Zajonc, (Eds.), Emotions, cognition, and behavior (pp. 17-37). New York: Cambridge University Press.

James, W. (1890). Principles of psychology. New York: Holt, Rinehart, & Winston.

Johnson-Laird, P. N., Herrmann, D. J., & Chaffin, R. (1984). Only connections: A critique of semantic networks. Psychological Bulletin, 96, 292-315.

Keele, C. A., & Neil, E. (1971). Samson Wright's applied physiology (12th ed.). New York: Oxford University Press.

Kety, S. S. (1970). The biogenic amines in the central nervous system: Their possible roles in arousal, emotion, and learning. In F. O. Schmitt (Ed.), The neurosciences. New York: Rockefeller University Press.

Kozak, M. J. (1982). The psychophysiological effects of training of variously elicited imaginings. Unpublished doctoral dissertation. University of Wisconsin, Madison.

Lacey, J. I. (1959). Psychophysiological approaches to the evaluation of psychotherapeutic process and outcome. In E. A. Rubinstein & M. B. Parloff (Eds.), Research in Psychotherapy, (Vol. 1). Washington, D. C.: American Psychological Association.

Lacey, J. I. (1967). Somatic response patterning and stress. Some revisions of activation theory. In M. H. Appley & R. Trumbull (Eds.), Psychological stress: Issues in research. New York: Appleton-Century-Crofts.

Lang, P. J. (1968). Fear reduction and fear behavior: Problems in treating a construct. In J. M. Shlien (Ed.), Research in Psychotherapy (Vol. III, pp. 90-103). Washington, D. C.: American Psychological Association.

Lang, P. J. (1978). Anxiety: Toward a psychophysiological definition. In H. S. Akiskal & W. L. Webb (Eds.), Psychiatric diagnosis: Exploration of biological predictors (pp. 365-389). New York: Spectrum.

Lang, P. J. (1984). Cognition in emotion: Concept and action. In C. Izard, J. Kagan, & R. Zajonc (Eds.), Emotion, cognition and behavior (pp. 192-225). New York: Cambridge University Press.

Lang, P. J. (1985). The cognitive psychophysiology of emotion: Fear and anxiety. In A. H. Tuma and J. A. Maser (Eds.), Anxiety and the anxiety disorders (pp. 131-170). Hillsdale, NJ: Lawrence Erlbaum.

Lang, P. J., Kozak, M. J., Miller, G. A., Levin, D. N., & McLean, A., Jr. (1980). Emotional imagery: Conceptual structure and pattern of somato-visceral response. Psychophysiology, 17, 179-192.

Lang, P. J., Levin, D. N., Miller, G. A., & Kozak, M. H. (1983). Fear behavior, fear imagery, and the psychophysiology of emotion: The problem of affective response integration. Journal of Abnormal Psychology, 92, 276-306.

Lang, P. J., Melamed, B. G., & Hart, J. D. (1970). A psychophysiological analysis of fear modification using an automated desensitization procedure. Journal of Abnormal Psychology, 76, 220-234.

Lazarus, R. S. (1982). Thoughts on the relations between emotion and cognition. American Psychologist, 37, 1019-1024.

Lazarus, R. S. (1984). On the primacy of cognition. American Psychologist, 39, 124-129.

Levin, D. N., Cook, E. W. III, & Lang, P. J. (1982). Fear imagery and fear behavior: Psychophysiological analysis of clients receiving treatment for anxiety disorders. Psychophysiology, 19, 571-572. (Abstract).

Levi, L. (Ed.). (1975). Emotions: Their parameters and measurement. New York: Raven Press.

Mandler, G. (1975). Mind and emotion. New York: John Wiley.

Mandler, G. (1984). Mind and body: Psychology of emotion and stress. New York: W. W. Norton.

Melamed, B., & Johnson, S. (1979). Assessment of chronic illness: Asthma and diabetes. In E. Mash & L. Terdal (Eds.), Behavioral assessment of childhood disorders. New York: Guilford Press.

Melamed, B. G., & Siegel, L. J. (1980). Behavioral medicine: Practical applications in health care. New York: Springer Publishing.

McLean, A., Jr. (1981). Emotional imagery: Stimulus information, imagery ability and patterns of physiological response. Unpublished doctoral dissertation. University of Wisconsin, Madison.

McNeil, D. W., Melamed, B. G., Cuthbert, B. N., & Lang, P. J. (1983). Emotional imagery and psychophysiological responsivity in simple phobia and agoraphobia. Psychophysiology, 20, 459. (Abstract).

Meichenbaum, D. (1977). Cognitive-behavior modification: An integrative approach. New York: Plenum Press.

Miller, G. A., Levin, D. N., Kozak, M. J., Cook, E. W. III, McLean, A., & Lang, P. J. (1986). Emotional imagery: Effects of individual differences in perceptual imagery on physiological response. (Manuscript submitted for publication).

Obrist, P. A. (1981). Cardiovascular psychophysiology: A perspective. New York: Plenum Press.

Ohman, A. (1986). The psychophysiology of emotion: An evolutionary-cognitive perspective. In P. K. Ackles, J. R. Jennings, & M. G. H. Coles (Eds.), Advances in psychophysiology. (Vol. 2). Greenwich, CT: JAI Press.

Quillian, M. R. (1966). Semantic memory. In M. L. Minsky (Ed.), Semantic information processing. Cambridge, MA: MIT Press.

Rachman, S. (1974). The meaning of fear. Middlesex: Penguin Books.

Rachman, S. (1978). Fear and courage. San Francisco: W. H. Freeman.

Rachman, S., & Hodgson, R. I. (1974). Synchrony and desynchrony in fear and avoidance. Behavior Research and Therapy, 12, 311-318.

Reisenzein, R. (1983). The Schachter theory of emotion: Two decades later. Psychological Bulletin, 94, 239-264.

Schachter, S. (1964). The interaction of cognitive and physiological determinants of emotional state. In L. Berkowitz (Ed.), Advances in experimental social psychology (Vol. 1, pp. 48-80). New York: Academic Press.

Schachter, S., & Singer, J. E. (1962). Cognitive, social, and psychological determinants of emotional state. Psychological Review, 69, 379-399.

Seligman, M. E. P., & Hager, J. E. (Eds.). (1972). Biological boundaries of learning. New York: Appleton-Century-Crofts.

Shapiro, A. K. (1959). The placebo effect in the history of medical treatment: Implications for psychiatry. American Journal of Psychiatry, 116, 298-304.

Shaw, W. A. (1940). The relation of muscular action potentials to imaginal weight lifting. Archives of Psychology, 23, 380-389.

Sheehan, P. Q. (1967). A shortened form of Betts' questionnaire upon mental imagery. Journal of Clinical Psychology, 23, 386-389.

Sifneos, P. E. (1972). The prevalence of "alexithymic" characteristics in psychosomatic patients. In H. Freyberger (Ed.), Topics of psychosomatic research. Basle, Switzerland: Karger.

Tal, A., & Miklich, D. R. (1976). Emotionally induced decreases in pulmonary flow rates in asthmatic children. Psychosomatic Medicine, 38, 190-200.

Usdin, E., Kvetnansky, R., & Kopin, I. J. (Eds.). (1980). Catecholamines and stress: Recent advances. New York: Elsevier/North-Holland.

Varni, J. W. (1981). Self-regulation techniques in the management of chronic arthritic pain in hemophilia. Behavior Therapy, 12, 185.

Varni, J. W. (1983). Acute and chronic pain. In J. W. Varni (Ed.), Clinical behavioral pediatrics: An interdisciplinary approach. New York: Pergamon Press.

Vrana, S. R., Cuthbert, B. N., & Lang, P. J. (in press). Fear imagery and text processing. Psychophysiology.

Young, J. Z. (1978). Programs of the brain. London: Oxford University Press.

Zajonc, R. B. (1980). Feeling and thinking: Preferences need no inferences. American Psychologist, 35, 151-175.

Zeltzer, L., Dash, J., & Holland, J. (1979). Hypnotically induced pain control in sickle cell anemia. Pediatrics, 64, 533.

Zillmann, D. (1983). Treatment of excitation in emotional behavior. In J. T. Cacioppo & R. E. Petty (Eds.), Social Psychophysiology. New York: Guilford Press.

# THE SOCIALIZATION OF INTROSPECTION AND ILLNESS BEHAVIOUR

Stephen Hansell and David Mechanic

Institute for Health, Health Care Policy, and Aging Research
Rutgers University

The decision to seek medical care depends on the process through which individuals become aware of symptoms and interpret their significance, as well as the severity of an illness. Many social and psychological factors affect this process (Mechanic, 1978), but it has its roots in one of the most fundamental human characteristics - the capacity to think about oneself and one's feelings. Because a symptom must first be perceived by an individual before it can be interpreted and dealt with, a reasonable hypothesis is that people who spend more time and energy introspecting will recognize and report more symptoms than less introspective individuals.

Although philosophers and poets have long noted that introspectiveness can be a burden as well as a source of inspiration, its relationship to illness behaviour has not been investigated until relatively recently. However, evidence is now accumulating that generally supports the basic hypothesis. Individuals high on introspectiveness have been shown to report more physical symptoms and psychological distress and to use more medical care services than less introspective people (e.g. Mechanic, 1983; Hansell and Mechanic, 1985).

This chapter reviews what is known about the relationship between introspectiveness and illness behaviour and describes some new research directions. The goal is to identify socialization processes and life experiences, embedded in social-structural contexts, that shape the capacity for introspectiveness, and that have implications for subsequent illness behaviour.

## THE CONCEPT OF INTROSPECTIVENESS

The personality disposition of introspectiveness involves the degree to which diffuse attention is focused either inward on oneself or toward the outside world. This concept reflects several assumptions about the nature of attention common to research in this area. First, it is assumed that an individual usually focuses attention on one thing at a time (Duval and Wicklund, 1972; Carver and Scheier, 1981). Second, attention is assumed to be focused either on self-related thoughts, feelings, and bodily states, on non-self related thoughts (Carver and Scheier, 1981) or the environment (Duval and Wicklund, 1972). Third, it is assumed that over a long period of time, relatively stable individual differences in average amounts of time spent attending to the self will emerge although transient, situationally-induced changes in the focus of attention occur frequently (Mechanic, 1983; Mechanic and Hansell, 1983; Fenigstein, Scheier, and Buss, 1975; Buss, 1980; Carver and Scheier, 1981).

The word "diffuse" is emphasized in the conceptualization of introspectiveness because it is thought the highly introspective person habitually monitors a wide variety of thoughts, feelings, and bodily states with no specific goal or task in mind (Mechanic, 1983). Thus, introspectiveness is not necessarily contingent on situational factors, although self-attention can be triggered by events in the environment and by changes in internal physical, emotional, and cognitive states. Finally, this concept refers only to the focus of attention and not to the content of thoughts about the self or the environment. Thus, introspection can involve both good and bad thoughts and feelings, although existing literature supports the hypothesis that it more often leads to non-specific feelings of malaise than to feelings of well-being.

As part of our efforts to develop reliable survey measures of introspectiveness, college students, younger adolescents, and older adults were interviewed intensively about their experience of thinking about themselves and their feelings. Interviews with college students, for example, who scored at the extremes of introspectiveness revealed that nearly all of them thought about age-specific issues dealing with peer relationships, family relationships, schoolwork, sports and other activities, their appearance, and the future. The content of thoughts and feelings did not differentiate between college students high and low on measured introspectiveness. However, they differed markedly in their styles of thinking and feeling (Hansell and Mechanic, 1985).

Highly introspective college students clearly directed their thinking inward on these topics and tended to evaluate themselves in the context of each issue. They more often thought about their feelings and motivations, and searched for underlying significance in routine life events. Highly introspective students valued self-attention because it increased their understanding of themselves and others, and they reported that their thinking patterns were mysterious, complex, and fascinating. However, the experience of self-attention also could be very intense and absorbing, and sometimes difficult to control. Highly introspective students said things like:

> I've always been like that, I always think [about myself]. Sometimes thinking is a negative thing because you can think too much and really screw things up. Sometimes my mind doesn't relax and I get tense, and I get really down. And sometimes when you get down it's really hard to get back up again.

In contrast, students low on introspectiveness were less interested in their own thought processes or feelings, and rarely analyzed the implications of issues for their self-systems. They were oriented more toward what they were doing, and tended to evaluate environmental conditions and constraints rather than themselves. They tended to focus on the present, and as a group, were much less aware of their own motivations and had less complex inner lives than highly introspective students. Students low on introspectiveness said things like:

> I don't have time to think [about myself]. I just live one day at a time, just enjoy life as it comes. I just take it day by day. I don't like thinking too much.

Evidence about the relationship between self-attention and illness behaviour comes from several types of studies. Laboratory studies of college students have shown that experimentally-induced self-attention can cause psychological distress and physical symptoms. Duval and Wicklund (1972) and Wicklund (1975) focused subjects' attention on themselves using mirrors, TV cameras, and other means, and asked them to evaluate their abilities. Self-awareness lead most frequently to negative self-evaluations. They explained this in terms of the potentially large number of negative social comparisons subjects can make.

Pennebaker and Skelton (1978) and Pennebaker (1982) have demonstrated that focusing sujects' attention on some aspect of body functioning causes them to report more physical symptoms on a subsequent illness inventory. Carver (1978) and Carver and Scheier (1981) also found that attention focused on the self increased the intensity of reported emotions. Finally, Buss (1980) has concluded that experimentally manipulated private self-awareness provides better knowledge of monitored dimensions of the self, and an intensification of affect.

Buss and his colleagues (Fenigstein et al., 1975; Buss, 1980; Carver and Scheier, 1981) have also created a measure of the personality disposition of private self-consciousness, which is similar to the concept of introspectiveness, and which has been used primarily as an individual difference factor in experimental studies of transient self-attention. Results generally indicated that individuals high on private self-consciousness paid more attention to internal cues than those low on this measure, and tended to experience stronger emotions in experimental situations. However, this measure has not often been used in studies of symptom reporting outside of the laboratory.

Mechanic and his colleagues have investigated the relationship between introspectiveness and illness behaviour among relatively normal community populations using a simple three-item survey measure of introspectiveness (Mechanic and Greenley, 1976; Greenley and Mechanic, 1976; Mechanic, 1979, 1980; Mechanic and Cleary, 1980). For example, in a study of a community sample of children who were followed up as young adults, individuals with high introspectiveness scores were more likely to report psychological distress and common physical symptoms than others (Mechanic 1979, 1980).

In more recent work, better measures of introspectiveness have been used to investigate their association with illness behaviour in samples of college students, younger adolescents, and older adults. Cross-sectional data from all three studies support the basic hypothesis. The college study, for example, involved a random sample of 1,014 freshmen (Hansell and Mechanic, 1985). Results showed that introspectiveness was positively associated with self-reports of psychological distress (r=.41) and common physical symptoms (r=.27), and was also the best predictor of these variables when other demographic characteristics, discontinuities and life stresses, and parental factors were controlled. In addition, introspectiveness correlated negatively with self-esteem (r=-.23), and happiness (r=-.19), but was not significantly correlated with social desirability, internal versus external control or academic achievement.

A second study involved 1,236 younger adolescents aged 12 through 18 (Hansell, Mechanic and Brondolo, in press) in a three-year longitudinal study of the relationship between introspectiveness and symptom reporting. Preliminary results indicate that introspectiveness was positively correlated with measures of depression (r=.25), anxiety (r=.30), and common physical symptoms (r=.15). However, introspectiveness was not associated with a measure of verbal intelligence. One advantage of this study is that independent data were also collected directly from one parent, usually the mother, of 842 of the adolescents. Similar to the case for adolescents, parents' introspectiveness was positively correlated with measures of their depression (r=.29), psychological distress (r=.25), neuroticism (r=.31), and common physical symptoms (r=.17).

A third project that is just beginning is a longitudinal study of the determinants of symptom reporting and medical care utilization among older adults of age 60 and over. Preliminary results from a pilot study of 48 older adults recruited from two senior nutrition centres indicated that introspectiveness was significantly correlated with psychological distress (r=.45), physical symptoms (r=.26), and concern about health (r=.51).

Taken together, these results show that introspectiveness is positively associated with symptoms in samples varying widely in age and other characteristics. Of course, key questions about causation remain unresolved. Although the hypothesis that introspectiveness predisposes individuals toward symptom reporting is plausible, the alternative hypothesis that distress and symptoms cause higher levels of introspectiveness cannot be ignored. (Nor can the likely possibility that there are reciprocal causal relationships among these variables).

## THE SOCIALIZATION OF INTROSPECTIVENESS

Relatively little research has investigated explicitly how introspectiveness develops. One speculation is that introspectiveness develops through the kind of socialization process described by symbolic interactionists (Mead, 1934; Sullivan, 1953; Rosenberg, 1979). As pre-adolescents gradually differentiate themselves from parents and other care-givers, they learn to view themselves as abstract objects. This enables them to focus attention on themselves, as well to think about their thoughts, feelings, and bodily states. This capacity for introspectiveness is presumed to develop during pre-adolescence, and then to increase during the adolescent years. This hypothesis is supported from the cited data from the study of adolescents. Age and introspectiveness were positively correlated (r=.18), indicating that older adolescents tended to be more introspective.

Individuals probably learn the disposition of introspectiveness in part from significant others in their lives such as parents. Highly introspective parents may communicate their interest in their own thoughts and feelings, and as role models may teach the growing child that introspectiveness is useful and valuable. Moreover, such parents may interact with their child in ways that explicitly cause self-attention. Also, parents may encourage their children to participate in the arts, social sciences, literature, or other self-oriented activities that have been shown to be preferred by highly introspective individuals (Hansell et al., in press).

The independent measures of introspectiveness and health outcomes obtained directly from both adolescents and one of their parents in the Hansell et al. study allows examination of the influence of socialization on these variables. Adolescent introspectiveness was positively associated with parental introspectiveness (r=.12), and the degree to which parents actively encouraged their adolescents to think about themselves and their feelings (r=.09). Also, highly introspective adolescents had parents who encouraged them to participate in artistic activities (r=.08). Finally, parents of highly introspective adolescents felt that they mattered more to their children than other parents (r=.13). Of course, most adolescents had two parents living at home, and the strength of these associations might have been greater if data had been collected from both parents. Moreover, there was a weak tendency for adolescents and parents of the same sex to show greater similarity in their characteristics, which will be examined in more detail in future analyses.

The linkage between adolescent introspectiveness and symptoms is quite complex, and may be partly mediated or caused by parental symptomatology. Witnessing the psychological or physical deterioration or crisis of a parent may be an upsetting experience for a child, and the resulting sense of loss or uncertainty may focus attention on the self as well as generate feelings of helplessness and insecurity. The data show that adolescent introspectiveness was positively associated with parental depression (r=.12), neuroticism (r-.10), and distress (r=.08).

Additional significant others may contribute to the socialization process, or may help maintain existing levels of introspectiveness. A study by Greenley and Mechanic (1976), for example, found that introspectiveness was associated with the structure of social networks among college students. Some students belonged to an "introspective subculture" of friends who shared interests in self-oriented activities. Students who identified most strongly with this subculture reported more psychological distress and were more likely to seek psychiatric help than other students (Greenley and Mechanic, 1976). Current interviews with highly introspective adolescents indicated that their friendship groups spend a lot of time talking about self-oriented issues and exchanging opportunities for self-attention. For some of these students, introspectiveness tends to be a criterion of friendship choice.

## INTROSPECTIVENESS AND LIFE EXPERIENCES

A major hypothesis is that socio-environmental discontinuities and life events induce introspectiveness. Discontinuities include any events that are problematic, that require appraisal of the self, or that significantly alter relationships to the environment or other people. Such events usually stimulate social comparisons and mental imagery. Although most people have problems on which they can focus (White, Williams, and Greenberg, 1961), the routine of most activities and everyday interactions is non-problematic, and people are usually distracted from self-attention. In contrast, significant discontinuity stimulates thought about what has occurred, and in particular, re-evaluations of oneself in the context of work and social relationships. Discontinuities with negative implications for the self probably stimulate more self-attention because they require more complex and detailed reappraisals.

The experiences of individuals in these samples can be examined for clues about how discontinuities relate to introspectiveness. All adolescents experience age-related discontinuities such as biological maturation, which may add to confusion in identifying and labeling sensations and feelings. The degree of pubertal development was positively associated with introspectiveness, controlling for age (partial r=.11), and was also associated with depression (partial r=.08) and anxiety (partial r=.11). Similarly, all older adults experience discontinuities such as physical deterioration and changes in social networks and living arrangements. Thus, discontinuities that induce introspectiveness are built into specific life stages and transitions.

Other discontinuities are less uniformly experienced by individuals. These include deaths or serious illnesses among friends or family members, separation and divorce of parents or children, problems with peers, or large changes in the social and economic fortunes of the family. For adolescents, a measure of life events was positively correlated with introspectiveness (r=.16), as well as depression (r=.31) and physical symptoms (r=.16). For parents, a measure of life events was also associated with their introspectiveness (r=.14), depression (r=.19), physical symptoms (r=.22), and neuroticism (r=.20). Thus, both developmental discontinuities and life events may provoke introspection and contribute to emotional distress.

Discontinuities may trigger introspectiveness by overwhelming an individual's coping abilities, but a lack of stimulation may also lead to introspectiveness. Although adolescents and older adults obviously are different, they share some problems of living caused by their marginal status in society and some uncertainty about the future. Of particular theoretical interest is the extensive amount of free time that adolescents and older adults have. Adolescents are not yet caught up in work and family lives, while many older adults have retired and must develop new patterns of activity. Many adolescents and older adults participate in hobbies, part-time employment, sports, or cultural activities that engage their time and attention, and provide a source of enjoyment and self-esteem. Other members of these age groups are relatively inactive, and may have more occasion for self-attention.

For adolescents, being alone tends to be especially unpleasant, and is almost always associated with negative feelings (Csikszentmihalyi and Larson, 1984). It is hypothesized that time alone encourages self-attention, which in turn contributes to distress. In the college study cited above, time spent alone was positively correlated with introspectiveness (r=.25), psychological distress (r=.31), and physical symptoms (r=.10). Similar results were also obtained in the adolescent study, in which time alone was positively correlated with introspectiveness (r=.11), depression (r=.24), and anxiety (r=.18). Although the relationship among these variables needs to be analyzed further, these data may indicate that introspectiveness and the experience of being alone are closely related for some adolescents.

Research on older adults has emphasized the importance of activity and continued participation for maintaining well-being and perceived health, and has shown that inactivity, however measured, tends to be associated with poorer health. However, research has not yet clarified causal relationships among well-being, perceived health, and activity levels. Inactivity may provide opportunities for self-attention which may then contribute to subjective awareness of distress and symptoms. Preliminary results from the pilot study of older adults cited above has shown that the number of hours spent sitting and doing nothing was positively correlated with introspectiveness (r=.41), psychological distress (r=.29), and physical symptoms (r=.23). These results suggest the potential value of exploring causal relationships among these variables in future research.

## CONCLUSION

Although there are many questions yet to be answered about the role of introspectiveness in illness behaviour processes, the accumulating cross-sectional evidence strongly suggests that it may be important. Introspectiveness was positively associated with a variety of physical and mental symptoms in widely varying samples. Moreover, the evidence suggests that introspectiveness may be learned in part from parents and significant-others, and transmitted from generation to generation in much the same way as other personal characteristics and habits. However, because only one parent was interviewed, tests of possible concordance between adolescent and parents were relatively crude. Also, introspectiveness clearly varies within families because of the unique discontinuities and life events that individuals experience.

A substantial minority of the highly introspective individuals in the three samples did not complain of distress or symptoms, and described how introspectiveness contributed to positive self-knowledge, interpersonal skills, and creativity. The introspectiveness scale seems to tap an undirected tendency to attend to the self that is often associated with intense affect as well as cognition. Self-attention that is goal-directed may facilitate understanding of the self on a cognitive level without increasing the emotional reactivity usually associated with diffuse self-attention. An important topic for further research is to investigate the relationship between varying types of self-attention and effective coping strategies. Eventually, it may be possible to discover the conditions under which introspectiveness can contribute to postive as well as negative health outcomes.

ACKNOWLEDGEMENTS

This research was supported by the William T. Grant Foundation, the Robert Wood Johnson Foundation, and NIMH Grant No. MN 39590.

REFERENCES

Buss, A. H. (1980). Self-consciousness and social anxiety. San Francisco: W. H. Freeman.

Carver, C. (1978). A cybernetic model of self-attention processes. Journal of Personality and Social Psychology, 37, 1251-1281.

Carver, C. S., & Scheier, M. F. (1981). Attention and self-regulation: A control theory approach to human behavior. New York: Springer-Verlag.

Csikszentmihalyi, M., & Larson, R. (1984). Being adolescent: Conflict and growth in the teenage years. New York: Basic Books.

Duval, S., & Wicklund, R. A. (1972). A theory of objective self-awareness. New York: Academic Press.

Fenigstein, A., Scheier, M. F., & Buss, A. H. (1975). Public and private self-consciousness: Asssessment and theory. Journal of Consulting and Clinical Psychology, 43, 522-527.

Greenley, J. R., & Mechanic, D. (1976). Social selection in seeking help for psychological problems. Journal of Health and Social Behavior, 17, 249-262.

Hansell, S., Mechanic, D., & Brondolo, E. (in press). Introspectiveness and adolescent development. In Journal of Youth and Adolescence.

Hansell, S., & Mechanic, D. (1985). Social structure, introspectiveness, and adolescent symptom reporting. Journal of Human Stress.

Mead, G. H. (1934). Mind, self and society. Chicago: University of Chicago Press.

Mechanic, D. (1978). Medical Sociology (2nd ed.). New York: The Free Press.

Mechanic, D. (1979). Development of psychological distress among young adults. Archives of General Psychiatry, 36, 1233-1239.

Mechanic, D. (1980). The experience and reporting of common physical complaints. Journal of Health and Social Behavior, 21, 146-155.

Mechanic, D. (1983). Adolescent health and illness behaviour: Hypotheses for the study of distress in youth. Journal of Human Stress, 9, 4-13.

Mechanic, D., & Cleary, P. (1980). Factors associated with the maintenance of positive health behaviour. Preventive Medicine, 9, 805-814.

Mechanic, D., & Greenley, J. R. (1976). The prevalence of psychological distress and help-seeking in a college student population. Social Psychiatry, 11, 1-14.

Mechanic, D., & Hansell, S. (1983). Adolescent introspection, psychological distress, and physical symptoms. Paper presented at the 78th Annual Meeting of the American Sociological Association, Detroit, MI.
Pennebaker, J. W. (1982). The psychology of physical symptoms. New York: Springer-Verlag.
Pennebaker, J. W., & Skelton, J. A. (1978). Psychological parameters of physical symptoms. Personality and Social Psychology Bulletin, 4, 524-530.
Rosenberg, M. (1979). Conceiving the self. New York: Basic Books.
Sullivan, H. S. (1953). The interpersonal theory of psychiatry. New York: W. W. Norton & Company.
White, K. L., Williams, T. F., & Greenberg, B. G. (1961). The ecology of medical care. New England Journal of Medicine, 265, 885-892.
Wicklund, R. (1975). Objective self-awareness. In L. Berkowitz (Ed.), Advances in experimental social psychology (Vol. 8). New York: Academic Press.

# ASSESSMENT OF COGNITIVE PROCESSES

Zindel Segal

Cognitive and Behaviour Therapies Section
Clarke Institute of Psychiatry
University of Toronto

With the broadening of the traditional biomedical model of disease to include behavioural, psychological and social aspects of health and illness (Lipowski, 1977) an increased need has arisen for the assessment of these components as part of the evaluation of health-related outcomes and predictors. This chapter will focus on the assessment of cognitive processes in illness behaviour and will present a number of issues which are current concerns in the field and which relate in a direct manner to any endeavour associated with the measurement of cognitive processes. These are questions regarding which types of thoughts or cognitive contents we are interested in knowing about, what type of framework, if any, exists for the organization of cognitive assessment procedures and how true a reflection is cognitive assessment of what subjects or patients are really thinking.

By way of historical introduction, it is important to stress that the emergent focus on cognitive processes in illness behaviour stems from concurrent developments in the fields of personality research and cognitive behaviour therapy (Bradley and Kay, 1985, Lamping, 1985). Cognition in personality research was accorded respectful status, due in part to the work of Bandura (1977; 1982), O'Leary, (1985) and Lazarus (1981; Lazarus, Averill, and Opton, 1970) who helped bring mediational models of the individual in from the cold after years of behaviourist imposed exile. In a parallel fashion, the recognition that behaviour is critically affected by the manner in which persons appraise environmental challenges and their ability to meet these challenges, had led to the development of cognitively oriented interventions for behaviour change (Kendall and Hollon, 1979; Turk, Meichenbaum and Genest, 1983). Perhaps the best articulated of these is Meichenbaum's (Meichenbaum and Cameron, 1981) stress inoculation training. Given the profileration of cognitive strategies for both intervention and prevention in the illness behaviour domain, an obvious question becomes how can these processes best be monitored. Kendall (1982) has identified four purposes which such assessment can serve, addressing both theoretical and practical issues (see Table 1). The decision directing assessment of a

---

Some material in this chapter is abridged from Z.V. Segal and B.F. Shaw. (in press). Cognitive Assessment: Issues and Methods. In K.S. Dobson (Ed.), Handbook of Cognitive-Behavioral Therapies. New York: Guilford Press.

Table 1

PURPOSES OF COGNITIVE ASSESSMENT

1) To study the relationships among cognitive phenomena and their relationship to patterns of behaviour and expressions of emotion.

2) To study the role of cognitive processes in the development of distinct psychopathologies and to examine their role in the behavioural patterns associated with coping.

3) To confirm the effects of treatment and to study the mechanism of change.

4) To check studies where cognitive factors have either been manipulated or implicated in the effects of the manipulation.

(Kendall, 1981)

particular cognitive content is often grounded in the theory which specifies the mediational role this content is thought to play (Segal and Shaw, in press). For example, Hollon and Bemis, (1981) provide a taxonomy of cognitive contents which exemplifies self-statements or self-referent speech. In this type of speech, the individual places himself/herself as the object of the statement (e.g., I am clumsy. I guess I didn't do that too well). Used more broadly, the term self-referent suggests that the audience, for certain comments is primarily the person himself/herself. Starting with Hollon and Bemis' taxonomy, examples of research in health psychology have been appended which include each type of cognitive content as a specific assessment focus in the studies described (see Table 2).

While the examples listed above are primarily propositional in nature, other classes of cognition should not be excluded from consideration. Imagery, for instance, represents a case where reported cognitive experience mirrors a distinctly different sensory channel than the auditory or verbal modes associated with self-talk (Anderson, 1980; Lyles, Burish, Krozely, and Oldham, 1982).

The actual task of cognitive assessment can be accomplished through a number of methods. Each method has its advantages and drawbacks as can be seen in Table 3. Some authors have suggested that an organizational framework for procedures would facilitate the matching of assessment needs with available methods (Kendall and Korgeski, 1979). One such approach has been advocated by Glass and Arnkoff (1982) and Genest and Turk (1981) and organizes cognitive assessment procedures temporally according to when they were administered relative to the occurrence of the thoughts one is interested in studying. The resulting scheme yields a continuum of assessment procedures ranging from those concurrently to retrospectively linked to the thoughts of interest, as is shown in Table 4. A brief discussion of each method follows.

Recordings of spontaneous speech have been employed in a number of studies assessing subjects's self-talk. These recordings can be taken unobtrusively or following specific instructions and are thought to represent verbal behaviour which can then be transcribed and coded into categories

Table 2

TAXONOMY OF COGNITIVE CONTENTS

| Propositions (Beliefs) | Example |
|---|---|
| ATTRIBUTION:<br>X causes Y | Taylor, Lichtman and Wood (1984)<br><br>Attributions of perceived control significatnly predicted adjustment in patients with breast cancer. |
| ATTRIBUTE:<br>X is an aspect of Y | Newton, Barbaree and Segal (1983)<br><br>Evaluation of headache attributes significantly predicted headache duration and headache activity. |
| EXPECTATION:<br>X predicts Y | Alagna and Reddy (1984)<br><br>Self-efficacy significantly predicted proficient technique and successful lesion detection in breast self-examination. |
| SELF-REFERENCE:<br>$X_1$ .... $X_n$ are aspects of Y<br>OR<br>X values Y | Reda, Carpiniello, Secchiaroli and Blanco (1985)<br><br>Dysfunctional attitudes toward the self were significantly related to post-hospital outcome in depressed patients at 1-year follow-up. |

(Adapted from Hollon and Bemis, 1981)

(Kendall and Hollon, 1981). This format is one of the most concurrent methods for assessing private speech, yet the investigator is limited to the subject's verbalizations and can never be fully certain that silences are synonomous with the lack of cognitive processing. The free association method as used in psychoanalysis also meets the concurrence criterion since patients are asked to verbalize their thoughts as they experience them throughout the therapy session (Bowers and Meichenbaum, 1984).

Think aloud procedures require subjects to provide a continuous monologue of their thoughts during the performance of a specific task. The exact wording of the think aloud instructions may well influence the content of the protocol (Ericsson and Simon, 1984) yet most instructions capture the spirit of this sample request by Duncker to his subjects in 1926:

"I am not primarily interested in your final solution, still less in your reaction time, but in your thinking behaviour, in all your attempts, in whatever comes to your mind, no matter whether it is a good or less good idea or a question. Be bold. I do not count your wrong attempts, therefore speak them all out".

At the next level we find random sampling of thoughts and self-monitoring procedures. The former procedure attempts to provide an unbiased estimate of cognitive frequencies by requesting subjects to record their current thoughts when cued (either in person or by a portable mechanical device) at random intervals. Its advantages include enabling data to be gathered over relatively long periods of time in the subject's own milieu, at intervals which are not contingent on the occurrence of any particular environmental events (Hurlburt, 1979). Newton (1984) for example, utilized in vivo random sampling to assess pain related thoughts in a population of chronic headache sufferers. He reports a significant shift in appraisal processes and coping strategies following a cognitive-behavioural treatment program for headaches. Genest and Turk (1981) offer the analogy that thinking aloud provides a motion picture of conscious events, while thought sampling provides repeated snapshots.

With self-monitoring procedures, the individual is asked to record the occurrence of specific thoughts in a particular stimulus situation or at a particular time. Their utility lies in the fact that they maximize the probability of gathering clinically relevant information concerning important but possibly infrequent situations. In headache research, for example, the experience of pain is a salient event which serves as an internal signal to begin self-monitoring, therefore cognitive samples are collected during the period of interest (Newton, 1984). However, a number of problems inherent to self-monitoring procedures in general exist and reflect concerns regarding reactivity, social desirability and evaluation apprehension (Nelson, 1977).

Table 3

GENERAL COGNITIVE ASSESSMENT FORMATS

| | PRO | CON |
|---|---|---|
| Inventory approach | economical | open to fabrication |
| | easy to administer/ score | limited to inventory content |
| | standardization across studies | |
| Open ended format | richer data source | scoring problematic |
| | less open to fabrication | difficult to standardize |

(from Meichenbaum and Cameron, 1981)

Table 4

SPECIFIC TECHNIQUES

| | | CONCURRENT | UNSTRUCTURED |
|---|---|---|---|
| 1) | Recording spontaneous private speech<br>Free association<br>Thinking aloud | ↑ | ↑ |
| 2) | Random sampling of thoughts<br>Self-monitoring procedures | ¦ | ¦ |
| 3) | Videotape thought reconstruction<br>Self-statement inventories<br>Thought-listings | ↓ | ↓ |
| 4) | Clinical interview | RETROSPECTIVE | STRUCTURED |

(from Glass and Arnkoff, 1982)

Videotape thought reconstruction allows subjects to reconstruct their train of cognitions by viewing a videotape of an actual or role-played problematic situation, often immediately after it is recorded. Subjects may be asked to think aloud while watching themselves, or to record the occurrence of specific cognitive events (Genest and Turk, 1981). With respect to temporality, this procedure is classified as more retrospective than techniques discussed earlier since its aim is to facilitate subjects' 'reliving' and reporting of a prior experience, as opposed to reporting on the original experience while it is occurring. A methodology related to videotape thought reconstruction is thought listing, where subjects are asked to report what thoughts they experienced while being in a particular stimulus situation. This procedure is more constrained than think aloud methods since the assessment takes place once the subject is out of the situation and can be likened to videotape thought reconstruction without the videotape. Cacioppo and Petty (1981) distinguish between listings which examine 1) thoughts elicited by the stimulus situation, 2) general thoughts about the situation or problems and 3) all thoughts which occurred while subjects anticipated and/or attended to the stimulus. Thoughts can then be coded and scored on a number of dimensions which are of interest to the investigator. Segal and Marshall (1985) using such a procedure in a study of incarcerated sex offenders found that negative self-evaluative thoughts bore a stronger relation to poor heterosexual social skill than did task-referent thoughts, regardless of their valence.

Endorsement methods such as self-report inventories or questionnaires contain a predetermined set of thoughts which subjects are asked to rate with respect to whether or not they had experienced the specific thought in the assessment situation, as well as its frequency of occurrence (Kendall and Hollon, 1981). Such instruments have been developed to assess cognitive contents particular to a number of domains such as depression (Hollon and Kendall, 1980), social anxiety (Glass, Merluzzi, Biever, and Larson, 1982), chronic headaches (Newton, 1984) and stressful medical procedures (Kendall et al., 1979). Finally, the clinical interview can be used as a retrospective cognitive assessment tool, in the case where a therapist will ask the client to recall a recently upsetting situation and then recount what he or she was thinking and feeling at the time (Glass and Arnkoff, 1982).

Cognitive assessment procedures may also be organized on the basis of structure, wherein the extent to which the assessment imposes its own limits or format on the individual, determines its placement on this continuum (see Table 4). Structured assessments offer the benefits of economy, ease of scoring and administration, as well as a greater potential for standardization across studies (Meichenbaum and Cameron, 1981). The trade-off, however, is against a potentially richer data source and the investigators ability to uncover unexpected information or unpredicted relationships (Genest and Turk, 1981). Deciding on how structured an assessment will be often requires specifying to what extent the individual's ongoing cognitive activity can be "punctuated" and still be considered to provide an accurate picture of its flow. This concern is echoed by Glass and Arnkoff (1982) who point out that as structure is added, the demand characteristics of the assessment also increases.

For example, while think aloud procedures have an appeal due to their provision of the unaltered flow of subjects' thoughts, the instruction given to subjects to "think aloud" are consequential (Cacioppo and Petty, 1981) and can result in the reporting of varying contents. The rationale for videotape thought reconstruction is that providing subjects with a record of their performance will yield a richer description of what the person was thinking at the time, due to the enhancement of memory functions (Genest and Turk, 1981). Yet, it is also possible that subjects are reporting what they guess they could have been thinking in the situation, rather than reporting on the basis of a visual and auditory aided re-experience of the event (Meichenbaum, 1977)

With respect to psychometrics the focus turns to questions about threats to the validity of the assessment process. The proliferation of research aimed at explicating cognitive factors in various populations has led to the development of numerous new assessment tools for this express purpose. It is therefore doubly important not to lose sight of the fact that methodology is no substitute for validity. Lacking a direct check on the accuracy of self-reported information we tend to be at the respondent's mercy. Such accuracy has been shown to be affected by a host of variables, some of which also affect the accuracy or self-monitored observable events (e.g., value of the target, temporal schedule, concurrent activities (Kanfer, 1980; Nelson, 1977). It is equally important to distinguish between errors (subject misperceives or distorts) and dissimulations (self-report contradicts observation) (Hollon and Kriss, 1984).

At a theoretical level, cognitive assessment endeavours to demonstrate that the self-report of cognitive experience generated by the subject is the result of a patterned and consistent model, albeit idiosyncratic, of information processing. This is in contrast to the same self-report generated by an essentially random, individual process which tells us nothing about the way in which an individual's cognitive experience is patterned, much less about the utility of our assessment.

Ericsson and Simon (1984, p. 172) suggest three criteria which verbal reports should meet if they are to be used to infer underlying cognitive processes. The relevance criterion specifies that verbalizations should be relevant to the given task or performance. To be considered pertinent, verbalizations should be logically consistent with those that just preceded them. The memory criterion states simply that some of the information attended to during the situation will be remembered. The authors then go on to illustrate how these criteria can be used as validity checks on verbal protocols. First, "if a verbalization describes a situation that the subject can perceive directly, its correspondence with the stimulus can be checked. Second, its relevance to the task and to plausible steps toward a solution (as determined by task analysis) can be assessed. Third, its consistency with just previously verbalized information presumed to be in short-term memory can be checked. Finally, whenever there is reason to believe that verbalized information will be committed to memory, its presence in memory can be tested by subsequent demands for recall or recognition".

Assumptions regarding the temporal and situational stability of cognitive contents impacts on the validity of the assessment process by portraying these contents according to models which do not capture their inherent variability (Kendall, 1982). Arguing against the notion of cognitive intransience (the belief that people think the same things in the same situation at all times), Hollon and Bemis (1981) point out that the burden of proof falls on the assessor to demonstrate that this in fact is the case. By way of illustration, consider the case of self-efficacy versus attribution assessment. The assessment of self-efficacy expectations dictates that the rating of the particular behavioural item be taken just prior to performance, in this way providing the investigator with a measure of self-efficacy specific to the assessment session. Measuring attributions involves asking individuals to provide their explanations for the causes of events in their lives usually at a point further removed in time from the actual event.

While in the case of self-efficacy ratings we have access to the individual's beliefs at the time of performance, applying this same model to measuring attributions would require that "a retrospectively recalled attribution of job loss to bad luck was indeed the attribution made at the time the job was actually lost" (Hollon and Bemis, 1981, p. 150). This type of verification is rarely performed.

Situational stability is another reason why the assumption of cognitive intransience seems to be ill-founded. Perhaps the best illustration of this phenomenon can be seen in the differences between thoughts elicited by imagining a stressful situation in the therapist's office as opposed to the thoughts elicited by the situation in vivo (Hollon and Bemis, 1981, Kendall, 1982). Data from a study by Last, Barlow, and O'Brien (1985) makes this point more forcefully. In an attempt to assess the congruence between three cognitive measures of anxiety these authors compared an in vivo think aloud procedure performed with subjects in a shopping mall to a thought-listing procedure which was administered after the in vivo assessment. Their final measure was an imaginal cognitive assessment task. Last et al. (1985) found little congruence between the in vivo think aloud procedure and the thought-listing protocol which was taken when subjects were no longer in the situation they dreaded. Their conclusions that there was little evidence of a direct one-to-one correspondence between these two measures, underlines the need to take situational induced variance into account when deciding at what point in time, and where the assessment process will take place.

Questions regarding the construct validity of cognitive assessment focus not on the prediction of a criterion or the match between the content of a test and a specific domain, but rather on the ability of the test itself to measure the cognitive processes of interest (Ghiselli, Campbell, and Zedeck, 1981). This issue applies, perhaps most strongly, to questionnaire or self-report formats which supply the subject with a particular content which he/she is then asked to rate on metrics such as presence or absence, frequency, degree of belief. The best example of this format is the self-statement inventory, which as Kendall (1984) points out is one of the most popular formats for assessing self-talk. The question of content validity should not be confused with concerns regarding construct validity, for while one can establish that the self-statements of which the inventory is composed are a representative sample of what people in general think in the assessment situation, it is less clear of what actual meaning an endorsement of one of these statements carries for the individual. Furthermore, meaning checks or inquiries are rarely conducted in conjunction with the administration of self-statement inventories (Arnkoff and Glass, 1982, Kendall, 1982), leaving one with the assumption that self-statements have the same personal meanings for all individuals involved. One step towards remediation can be found in the "degree of belief" ratings which some inventories require in addition to the usual frequency tallies (e.g., Automatic Thoughts Questionnaire; Hollon and Kendall, 1980).

Glass and Arnkoff (1982) provide a cogent critique of the assumption of an isomorphic relationship between cognition and its representation on self-statement inventories (Table 5 provides an illustrative example). They list four possibilities which would reflect different processes underlying item endorsement. One possibility is that subjects who report having a thought "very frequently" may be indicating the impact or the importance of the thought to themselves, and not necessarily its frequency. This is problematic for most self-statement inventories, as scores usually reflect a simple tally of items endorsed. The second possibility is that a translation process is occurring on the part of the subjects, whereby the idiosyncratic or fragmented thoughts the subject experiences in the situation are translated into grammatically correct sentences as they appear on the inventory. Alternatively, a decision to endorse a thought may reflect the view that the thoughts match one's view of oneself, rather than the actual experience of that specific thought. For example, a woman who sees herself as poorly skilled at solving math problems may endorse an item such as "I'm no good at math so why even try" on an exam anxiety questionnaire, because it corresponds to her self-image rather than because she necessarily had the thought.

Table 5

SELF-STATEMENT INVENTORY - COPING WITH STRESSFUL MEDICAL PROCEDURES

| | HARDLY EVER | | | | VERY OFTEN |
|---|---|---|---|---|---|
| I was thinking that the procedure could save my life. | 1 | 2 | 3 | 4 | 5 |
| I kept reminding myself to just think about pleasant things and take my mind off the procedure. | 1 | 2 | 3 | 4 | 5 |
| I was thinking about the catheter breaking off and sticking into my heart. | 1 | 2 | 3 | 4 | 5 |
| I kept thinking how much I disliked the smell of being in the hospital. | 1 | 2 | 3 | 4 | 5 |

(Kendall, 1983)

A final possibility is that endorsement may reflect the translation of affective experiences into a language-based format. While a subject who is in a highly aroused state may or may not be aware of any ongoing cognitive activity, self-statement inventories may provide the opportunity for converting this experience into a linguistic representation of the event. In this sense, the subject may endorse a thought such as "I'm really getting worked up about this" without necessarily having experienced it at the time (Glass and Arnkoff, 1982).

To conclude the discussion at this point would run the risk of imparting a message which is unwarrantedly pessimistic and certainly premature. As Glass and Arnkoff (1982) point out, it may not be possible to have 100 percent accuracy in identifying the exact sequence of a person's thoughts, but it is still important that they chose to report them in that order. Similarly, while the reporting of self-statements has its flaws, people are still telling us something meaningful about themselves which may reflect differences in their information processing styles. This chapter has tried to demonstrate that each cognitive assessment approach has strengths and weaknesses and so the use of several complementary strategies may serve to minimize individual deficits. This type of reliance on converging sources of information also allows for the integration of cognitive assessment with other modes of measurement (Meichenbaum and Cameron, 1981; Webb et al., 1966). While the eventual goal is to map out the complex interactions among cognitive affective and behavioural change (Greenberg and Safran, 1984) the current state of affairs is that these three domains exist in isolation.

To conclude, if the past five to ten years were spent building cognitive assessment up into a content area in its own right, the next five to ten years ought to be spent building bridges to link cognitive assessment to behavioural change and the influence of emotion.

## REFERENCES


Alagna, S. W., & Reddy, D. M. (1984). Predictors of proficient technique and successful lesion detection in breast self-examination. Health Psychology, 3, 113-127.

Anderson, M. P. (1980). Imaginal processes. In M. J. Mahoney (Ed.), Psychotherapy Process: Current issues and future directions (pp. 211-253). New York: Plenum.

Arnkoff, D. B., & Glass, C. R. (1982). Clinical cognitive constructs: Examination, evaluation, and elaboration. Advances in cognitive-behavioral research and therapy, (Vol. 1). New York: Academic Press.

Bardura, A. (1977). Self-efficacy: Toward a unifying theory of behavioral change. Psychological Review, 84, 191-215.

Bardura, A. (1982). Self-efficacy mechanisms in human agency. American Psychologist, 37, 122-147.

Bowers, K. S., & Meichenbaum, D. (1984). The unconscious reconsidered. New York: John Wiley & Sons.

Bradley, L. A., & Kay, R. (1985). The role of cognition in behavioral medicine. In P.C. Kendall (Ed.), Advances in cognitive-behavioral research and therapy (Vol. 4, 137-213). New York: Academic Press.

Cacioppo, J. T., & Petty, R. E. (1981). Social psychological procedures for cognitive response assessment: The thought listing technique. In C. R. Glass, T. V. Merluzzi, & M. Gerest (Eds.), Cognitive assessment (pp. 309-342). New York: Guilford Press.

Duncker, K. (1926). A qualitative (experimental and theoretical) study of productive thinking (solving of comprehensible problems). Pedagogical Seminary, 33, 642-708.

Ericsson, A. K., & Simon, H. A. (1984). Protocol analysis. Massachusetts: The M.I.T. Press.

Genest, M., & Turk, D. C. (1981). Think-aloud approaches to cognitive assessment. In T. V. Merluzzi, C. R. Glass, & M. Genest (Eds.), Cognitive assessment (pp. 233-269). New York: Guilford Press.
Ghiselli, E. E., Campbell, J. P., & Zedeck, S. (1981). Measurement theory for the behavioral sciences. San Francisco: W. H. Freeman and Company.
Glass, C. R., & Arnkoff, D. B. (1982). Think cognitively: Selected issues in cognitive assessment and therapy. In P. C. Kendall (Ed.), Advances in cognitive-behavioral research and therapy (Vol. 1). New York: Academic Press.
Glass, C. R., Merluzzi, T. V., Biever, J.L., & Larsen, K. H. (1982). Cognitive assessment of social anxiety: Development and validation of a self-statement questionnaire. Cognitive Therapy and Research, 6, 37-55.
Greenberg, L. S., & Safran, J. D. (1984). Integrating affect and cognition: A perspective on the process of therapeutic change. Cognitive Therapy and Research, 8(6), 559-578.
Hollon, S. D., & Bemis, K. M. (1981). Self-report and the assessment of cognitive functions. In M. Hersen & A. S. Bellack (Eds.), Behavioral assessment: A practical handbook (pp. 125-174). New York: Pergamon Press.
Hollon, S. D., & Kendall, P. C. (1980). Cognitive self-statements in depression: Development of an automatic thought questionniare. Cognitive Therapy and Research, 4, 383-396.
Hollon, S. D., & Kriss, M. R. (1984). Cognitive factors in clinical research and practice. Clinical Psychology Review, 4, 35-76.
Hurlburt, R. T. (1979). Random sampling of cognitions and behavior. Journal of Research in Personality, 13, 103-111.
Kanfer, F. H. (1980). Self-management methods. In F. H. Kanfer & A. P. Goldstein (Eds.), Helping people change (pp. 334-389). New York: Pergamon Press.
Kendall, P. C. (1981). Assessment and cognitive-behavioural interventions: Purposes, proposals, and problems. In P. C. Kendall & S. D. Hollon (Eds.), Assessment strategies for cognitive-behavioral intervention. New York: Academic Press.
Kendall, P. C. (1982). Behavioral assessment and methodology. In C. M. Franks, G. T. Wilson, P. C. Kendall, & K. D. Brownell (Eds.), Annual Review of Behavior Therapy (Vol. 8, pp. 39-81). New York: The Guilford Press.
Kendall, P. C. (1983). Stressful medical procedures: Cognitive-behavioral strategies for stress management and prevention. In D. A. Meichenbaum, & M. E. Jaremko (Eds.), Stress reduction and prevention. New York: Plenum.
Kendall, P. C., & Hollon, S. D. (1981). Assessing self-referent speech: Methods in the measurement of self-statements. In P. C. Kendall & S. D. Hollon (Ed.), Assessment strategies for cognitive-behavioral interventions (pp. 85-118). New York: Academic Press.
Kendall, P. C., & Korgeski, G. P. (1979). Assessment and cognitive-behavioral interventions. Cognitive Therapy and Research, 3, 1-21.
Kendall, P. C., Williams, L., Pechacek, T. F., Graham, L. G., Shisslak, C., & Herzoff, N. (1979). Cognitive-behavioral and patient education interventions in cardiac catheterization procedures: The Palo Alto medical psychology project. Journal of Consulting and Clinical Psychology, 47, 49-58.
Lamping, D. L. (1985). Assessment in health psychology. Canadian Psychology, 26(2), 121-139.
Last, C. G., Barlow, D. H., & O'Brien, G. T. (1985). Assessing cognitive aspects of anxiety: Stability over time and agreement between several methods. Behavior Modification, 9(1), 72-93.
Lazarus, R. S. (1981). The stress and coping paradigm. In C. Eisdorfer, D. Cohen, A. Kleinman, & P. Maxim (Eds.), Models for clinical psychopathology (pp. 177-214). New York: Spectrum.
Lazarus, R. S., Averill, J., & Opton, E. (1970). Towards a cognitive

theory of emotion. In M. Arnold (Ed.), Personality and psychopathology. New York: Academic Press.
Lipowski, S. J. (1977). Psychosomatic medicine in the seventies: An overview. American Journal of Psychiatry, 134, 233-244.
Lyles, J. N., Burish, T. G., Krozely, M. G., & Oldham, R. K. (1982). Efficacy of relaxation training and guided imagery in reducing the aversiveness of cancer chemotherapy. Journal of Consulting and Clinical Psychology, 50, 509-521.
Meichenbaum, D. (1977). Cognitive-behavior modification: An integrative approach. New York: Plenum.
Meichenbaum, D., & Cameron, R. (1981). Issues in cognitive assessment: An overview. In T. V. Merluzzi, C. R. Glass, & M. Genest (Eds.), Cognitive assessment (pp. 3-15). New York: Guilford Press.
Nelson, R. C. (1977). Methodological issues in assessment via self-monitoring. In J. D. Cone & R. P. Hawkins (Eds.), Behavioral assessment: New directions in clinical psychology. New York: Brunner/Mazel.
Newton, C. R. (1984). The use of a thought-sampling procedure in the cognitive assessment and treatment of chronic headache. Unpublished doctoral dissertation, Queen's University, Kingston.
Newton, C., Barbaree, H., & Segal, Z. (1983). Cognitive assessment in chronic headache: A preliminary investigation. Paper presented at the World Congress of Behavior Therapy, Washington.
O'Leary, A. (1985). Self-efficacy and health. Behavior Research and Therapy, 23(4), 437-451.
Reda, M. A., Carpiniello, B., Secchiaroli, L., & Blanco, S. (1985). Thinking, depression, and antidepressants: Modified and unmodified depressive beliefs during treatment with amitroptyline. Cognitive Therapy and Research, 9(2), 135-143.
Segal, Z. V., & Marshall, W. L. (1985). Heterosexual social skills in a population of rapists and child molesters. Journal of Consulting and Clinical Psychology, 53(1), 55-63.
Segal, Z. V., & Shaw, B. F. (in press). The role of cognition in depression: A reappraisal of Coyne and Gotlib's critique. Cognitive Therapy and Research.
Taylor, S. E., Lichtman, R., & Wood, J. V. (1984). Attributions, beliefs about control, and adjustment to breast cancer. Journal of Personality and Social Psychology, 46, 489-502.
Turk, D. C., Meichenbaum, D. H., & Genest, M. (1983). Pain and behavioral medicine: A cognitive-behavioral perspective. New York: Guilford Press.
Webb, E. F., Campbell, D. T., Schwartz, R. D., & Sechrest, L. (1966). Unobtrusive measures: Non-reactive research in the social sciences. Chicago: Rand McNally.

# PERSONALITY, CARDIOVASCULAR DISORDERS, AND ILLNESS BEHAVIOUR

David Krantz and Victoria Leu

Department of Medical Psychology
Uniformed Services University of the Health Sciences

The idea that personality traits and psychological characteristics play a role in the etiology of physical disease has its roots in medicine and philosophy before Descartes. Early physicians believed that intense emotions could produce imbalances in bodily function, culminating in various forms of physical pathology. In the first half of this century, the role of chronic emotional conflicts in the etiology of physical disorders was emphasized. Based on observations of clinical groups, correlations between particular diseases and personality types were reported, and striking psychological similarities among patients suffering from the same organic disease were described. These similarities were formulated into personality profiles, and characteristic personality types were linked to specific disorders, such as coronary heart disease (CHD), peptic ulcer, and asthma (Alexander, 1939). Later trait approaches suggested that certain dispositions, such as giving up, depression, and inability to express feelings, were related to general susceptibility to illness.

Much of the early psychosomatic work can be criticized for over-emphasizing the role of traits without taking into account physiological, genetic, and situational factors that interact to predispose an individual to a particular disorder (Weiner, 1977). Psychological variables were often poorly defined. Specific emotions were presumed to produce specific physiologic responses, but little evidence supported this assertion. Until recently, few attempts were made to advance understanding beyond the correlational level by exploring basic mechanisms linking behavioural processes to disease states. As a result, the contribution of these early approaches to clinical medicine was limited.

This chapter will provide a brief overview of several general conceptual approaches to the study of the role of personality traits and behaviour patterns in the etiology and progression of disease. Since research on psychological factors is particularly well-developed in regard to coronary heart disease, this discussion will focus on this area of study.

## Personality as a Causal Factor in Disease

Research assuming that personality plays a causal role in disease can be divided into three general approaches (Krantz and Glass, 1984). The first assumes that personality is causally involved in the etiology of disease before symptoms are manifest. Usually this implies that traits produce pathogenic alterations in tissue function via neuroendocrine or other physiological mechanisms. Most research on the Type A behaviour pattern as a risk factor for CHD fits into this category.

The second approach emphasizes the influence of psychological factors on the course and outcome of illness once disease is manifest. Most research in this category views illness as a stressor and presumes that the way in which an individual appraises and reacts to illness can affect the subsequent clinical course of disease. Central to this notion is the assumption that the adequacy of coping can influence the course of illness by altering physiological processes involved in the progression of disease or recovery. However, psychological attributes may also influence the course of illness by altering behavioural reactions to disease such as medical compliance.

One example of this approach is a study relating coping mechanisms to survival from breast cancer. Derogatis, Abeloff, and Melisaratos (1979) tested 35 women undergoing treatment for metastatic breast cancer on symptom reporting and illness adjustment measures. One year later, the 22 long-term survivors were compared with the 13 patients who had died. Those who had died exhibited less hostility and had more positive attitudes toward their physicians, whereas long-term survivors showed more negative affect and had poorer attitudes toward their physicians.

### Alternatives to a Causal Role for Personality

In contrast to viewing personality characteristics as causal factors in the etiology and/or clinical course of illness, a third general approach minimizes the causal role of personality. In one version of this approach, factors associated with illness, such as characteristics of the treatment received or experience with the health-care system, are thought to alter psychological or behavioural attributes. The notion that treatment experiences can affect personality is plausible, since much of the research linking traits and illness consists of cross-sectional and retrospective studies. For example, in the Derogatis et al. (1979) study of breast cancer, although no initial differences in clinical status between those who survived and those who died were reported, a higher percentage of short-term survivors had received chemotherapy prior to testing. It is possible that the dramatic trait differences between the groups resulted from differential exposure to chemotherapy.

Another version of this perspective presumes that a set of traits characterizes those individuals who are most likely to notice symptoms and seek medical care. Associations between personality and certain illness categories are seen as resulting from factors involving symptom perception or the tendency to use health-care facilities. This view contrasts with approaches presuming that personality directly influences biological disease states.

There apparently are enduring individual differences in the perception, interpretation, and reporting of bodily symptoms. (Hansell and Mechanic, this volume). For instance, neuroticism seems to be associated with somatic complaints for normal individuals (Costa and McCrae, 1985). Neuroticism is a broad dimension of normal personality that includes such traits as the tendency to experience anxiety, hostility, and depression, as well as vulnerability to stress. Costa and McCrae have reported a positive linear relationship between neuroticism scores and somatic complaints on the Cornell Medical Index in 1,038 men aged 17 to 97.

Finally, since research linking personality and disease is inherently correlational, a third factor, such as physiologic reactivity to stress, may influence both the development of disease and the expression of certain behavioural characteristics. This approach will be discussed later in relation to research on Type A behaviour and CHD.

To demonstrate that traits are involved in the etiology and/or progression of disease, consistency of traits across different situations and over time is necessary. While traits are defined as consistent and enduring individual differences in the style or content of behaviour (Willerman, 1979), the existence of traits is controversial. Mischel (1968) has argued that the behaviour of an individual is not consistent across situations and that the situation is a better predictor of behaviour than are personality traits. Bowers (1973) and others have challenged Mischel's emphasis on the role of situations to the exclusion of traits in predicting behaviour. Bowers argues that behaviour is determined by an interaction between traits and situations rather than by traits or situations alone. The Type A behaviour pattern is an example of an interaction between situations and personality predispositions; it is a tendency to respond in a particular way to challenging situations.

## Behaviour Patterns and Coronary Heart Disease

The failure of the standard physical risk factors such as cholesterol, hypertension, and smoking, to predict many new cases of CHD (Jenkins, 1971) has prompted the study of a variety of psychosocial risk factors. Considerable attention has been devoted to the study of "coronary-prone" behaviour patterns, and two general patterns have been identified. The first consists of negative, disturbing emotions such as life dissatisfaction, anxiety, and depression. Given generally fairly high correlations between these dysphoric characteristics, it seems reasonable to incorporate them into the broad rubric of "neuroticism". A second example of a "coronary prone behaviour" conceptualization is the Type A behaviour pattern, which is the most extensively researched psychosocial risk factor for CHD. Individuals with the Type A behaviour pattern are intensely ambitious, competitive, impatient, and hostile. In contrast, Type B individuals are relatively relaxed and easy-going.

In this chapter it will be argued from existing data, (cf. Costa, in press) that characteristics such as anxiety, depression, and neuroticism are primarily related to symptom experience of coronary disease such as so-called "soft" events of chest pain, whereas certain elements of Type A, including hostility, appear to be antedecents of physical, as opposed to purely subjective manifestations of CHD.

Type A is typically assessed by the Structured Interview (Rosenman, 1978) in which individuals are asked to indicate how they usually respond in situations that are likely to elicit competitiveness, impatience, and hostility in certain individuals. The evaluation of Type A is primarily based on speech stylistics, such as loudness and explosiveness, associated with responding, and to a lesser extent on the content of the answers. A number of questionnaires for assessing Type A exist; the Jenkins Activity Survey (JAS) (Jenkins, Rosenman, and Friedman, 1967) is the most commonly used. Studies that have correlated various Type A measures with other psychological scales (e.g., Chesney, Black, Chadwick, and Rosenman, 1981) have found that the stylistic dimensions of the interview are relatively independent of dysphoric emotional states such as anxiety and depression, whereas the self-report measures correlate more highly with those negative emotional states.

The Western Collaborative Group study (Rosenman, Brand, Jenkins, Friedman, Straus, and Wurm, 1975), begun in 1959, assessed over 3,500 men using the Structured Interview. This study found that 8 1/2 years after the initial assessment, Type A individuals were more likely to develop virtually all manifestations of coronary heart disease than Type B individuals, including symptomatic and asymptomatic myocardial infarction and angina. The Framingham Heart Study (Haynes, Feinleib and Kannel, 1980) used an ad hoc scale to measure Type A behaviour. Individuals who were classified as Type A were more likely to have developed CHD at the follow-up eight years later than were Type B subjects. The Framingham scale predicted the development of myocardial infarction alone, angina pectoris alone, and myocardial infarction with angina.

Recent studies suggest that epidemiological evidence for a link between Type A and CHD is no longer unequivocal. A number of studies have quantified the degree of coronary artery disease present in patients undergoing coronary angiography and have correlated disease severity with measures of Type A behaviour. (see Matthews and Haynes, in press, for a review). In general, initial studies showed that Type A patients were more likely to have severe coronary artery disease documented by coronary angiography than Type B patients. However, 12 of 15 subsequent studies found that Type A was not associated with extensive coronary artery disease. These findings may be due to differences in referral patterns for coronary angiography; nonetheless, the preponderance of evidence in these cross-sectional studies indicates that Type A is not associated with the degree of coronary artery disease.

The Multiple Risk Factor Intervention Trial (MRFIT) was conducted to determine whether intervention directed at modifying coronary risk factors could reduce incidence of a first coronary event among men at high risk for heart disease based on a variety of criteria, including high cholesterol level, smoking, and hypertension. Measures of Type A were obtained for 3,110 subjects who were followed for an average of seven years (Shekelle et al., 1985). Type A behaviour, assessed by Structured Interview and by JAS in this high risk group, was unrelated to the incidence of a first heart attack. This study, then, failed to support the existence of a relationship between Type A and heart disease.

Although in a number of studies (e.g., Dembroski, MacDougall, Williams, Haney, and Blumenthal, 1985) global Type A was not associated with coronary artery disease, certain components of Type A such as hostility and anger were significantly associated with the degree of disease determined by coronary angiography.

Consistent with the possibility that characteristics such as anxiety, life dissatisfaction, and depression do not predict actual disease but do predict symptoms are the results of a study conducted by Elias and associates (1982). They studied patients undergoing coronary angiography and compared those with angina symptoms only to those with both angina symptoms and significant coronary artery disease (CAD). Depression and anxiety were more strongly associated with angina symptoms in patients with clear coronary arteries than in patients with occluded arteries. Similarly, Costa and co-workers (Costa, Fleg, McCrae, and Lakatta, 1982) found that emotional instability predicted the development of angina in patients without CAD, but did not predict the development of CAD. The Belgian-French Pooling Project (1984) found that neuroticism scores were only predictive of soft coronary events, that is, angina documented by reports of chest pain, but not corroborated by electrocardiographic or enzymatic changes indicative of myocardial infarction. These studies support the hypothesis that neuroticism is related to symptoms associated with coronary disease, but unrelated to occurrence of actual disease.

<u>Type A and Physiologic Reactivity</u>

Since associations between Type A and ischemic heart disease cannot be explained solely by the standard coronary risk factors (Rosenman et al.,

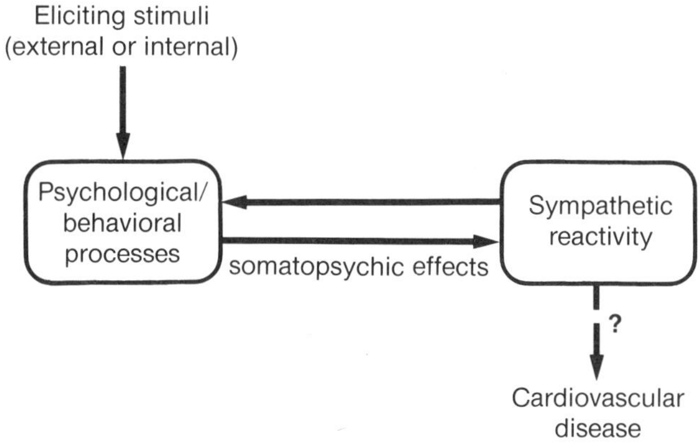


**FIGURE 1.** Two-way relationship between reactivity and behavior

1975), research has attempted to determine physiologic mechanisms linking Type A to disease. Most explanations for this link suggest that behaviours exhibited by Type A individuals are accompanied by sympathetic neuroendocrine and cardiovascular responses which might promote the development of coronary atherosclerosis or precipitate its clinical symptoms of ischemic heart disease. As indicated in Figure 1, experimental situations perceived as psychologically stressful or challenging evoke heightened cardiovascular and endocrine response in Type A individuals (Krantz and Manuck, 1984).

It should be noted, however, that the correlation between Type A behaviour and hyper-reactivity appears to be only moderate, with some components of Type A behaviour, such as anger and hostility, showing stronger relationships with physiologic responses than others (Krantz and Manuck, 1984). In addition, there is no doubt that the individual's interpretation of stressful situations influences certain components of behaviour and physiologic correlates (Krantz and Manuck, 1984). However, there is some evidence that aspects of physiological reactivity can be an antecedent as well as consequent to Type A characteristics/behaviour.

Although most studies have found that Type A physiologic correlates emerge in situations viewed by an individual as stressful or challenging, two recent studies examined cardiac patients under general anesthesia for coronary artery bypass surgery - a situation in which conscious awareness is minimized. In these studies (Kahn, Kornfeld, Frank, Heller, and Hoar, 1980; Krantz, Arabian, Davia and Parker, 1982), Type A patients with manifest disease showed greater intraoperative systolic blood pressure increases than did Type B patients.

The results of the above studies suggest that there may be an underlying psychobiological or "constitutional" basis for Type A behaviour (see Figure 1) in cardiac patients, since increased cardiovascular responses were observed in patients under general anesthesia - a condition where conscious awareness, and hence, perceptions of a stressful situation are minimized. Therefore, the impatience, hostility, and speech patterns exhibited by Type A patients with manifest disease may, in part, reflect an underlying sympathetic nervous system hyperreactivity (Krantz and Durel, 1983). This view is different from, but not necessarily contradictory with, the idea that Type A appraisals or behaviours produce elevated sympathetic responses. If Type A is a consequence of sympathetic hyperreactivity, then Type A behaviour might be suppressed by treatment techniques that decrease sympathetic responsiveness. Beta-blockers such as propranolol are commonly used to treat cardiovascular disorders. These drugs antagonize certain sympathetic nervous system responses that would otherwise be activated by epinephrine or norepinephrine. These responses occur primarily in organs such as the heart, and in smooth muscle of the blood vessels and lungs.

Krantz, Durel and colleagues (1982) conducted a correlational analysis comparing behavioural and psychophysiological characteristics of coronary patients receiving propranolol as part of their medical program with characteristics of patients not receiving beta-blockers. Propranolol-treated patients displayed less interview-rated Type A behaviour than patients not taking propranolol. No such effects were found among patients receiving diuretics, nitrates, or various other central nervous system active drugs (such as valium), thus suggesting an effect specific to the beta-blocker. Several components of Type A were lower in propranolol-treated patients, specifically speech stylistics such as loud/explosive, rapid/accelerated, and potential-for-hostility. The correlational nature of these data do not permit concluding that the beta-blocker caused the decrease in Type A behaviour. Nevertheless, the data are very suggestive, since the effects persisted after controlling for a variety of possibly confounding factors such as age, presence of symptoms, and severity of disease.

Additional evidence that chronic beta-blocker therapy might decrease Type A behaviour comes from a recent experiment by Schmieder, Friedrich, Neus, Rudel and von Eiff (1983). In this study, seven hypertensive patients received the beta-blocker atenolol and nine patients received a thiazide diuretic. After four to ten weeks, only the atenolol-treated group showed a decrease in intensity of interview-rated Type A behaviour. Speech stylistics associated with Type A appeared to be lessened by attenuation of beta-adrenergic reactivity with atenolol. These data are particularly interesting since the behavioural effects were obtained with the hydrophilic beta-blocker atenolol, which is believed to poorly penetrate the brain.

Despite the suggestive nature of these findings, a placebo-controlled study of the effects of beta-blockers on Type A behaviour has not been conducted. Such studies comparing placebo with atenolol and the lipophilic propranolol are currently being conducted by the authors.

## Reduction of Type A Behaviour with Beta-blockers: Implications for Cardiovascular Disorders

An understanding of the mechanisms responsible for the presumed effects of beta-blockers on Type A must take into account what is known about the psychological effects of these drugs. This area is particularly relevant to the domain of illness behaviour. Since beta-blockers were introduced and have come to be widely used in the treatment of cardiovascular disorders, a variety of behavioural and psychological effects has been observed. One of the most commonly noted beneficial effects is the reduction of anxiety among certain patient groups (Frishman, Razin, Swencionis, and Sonnenblick, 1981). For example, when given to patients who characterize their anxiety in somatic terms, such as palpitation and tremor, beta-blockers are effective anxiolytic agents. Among patients with predominantly cognitive symptoms, such as worry or mental tension, beta-blockers seem to be relatively ineffective. In addition, beta-blockers appear to be useful for decreasing the anxiety of healthy subjects in acutely stressful situations such as public speaking, examinations, or stage fright, where bodily symptoms of anxiety might interfere with performance (Frishman et al., 1981).

Recent animal model data in this area is available from a study of the behavioural effects of beta-blockers (Durel, Krantz, and Barrett, 1985), which used a conflict paradigm. In this paradigm, which is commonly used to study the anti-anxiety effects of benzodiazepines, responses are simultaneously reinforced and punished. A study with pigeons showed that suppression of responding by punishment is released by several types of beta-blockers - an effect that occurs with benzodiazepines. Propranolol produced a considerably larger effect on punished responding than did atenolol.

Decreases in heart rate and contractility are the effects of beta-blockers believed to be most relevant to cardiac treatment and anxiety reduction. To determine whether heart rate could be related to the behavioural effects obtained, following the beta-blocker conflict study just reported, pilot EKG's were recorded during the experimental session at a sampling of drug doses in the same birds. Under control conditions, heart rate increases during punished responding exceeded increases during unpunished responding. Although heart rate tended to be positively related to response rate, during punished responding high heart rate usually accompanies low response rate. Under effective doses of propranolol, heart rate increases associated with both types of behaviour were substantially limited. Thus, a peripheral feedback mechanism may be involved in the behavioural effects of beta-blockers in pigeons.

The precise means by which beta-blockers reduce anxiety are not clear. Although all of the commonly used beta-blockers penetrate the blood-brain barrier to some extent, they vary widely in this characteristic. However, it is widely believed that the peripheral actions of beta-blockers can explain many of their anxiolytic effects (Frishman et al., 1981). This mechanism may involve the role of bodily changes in the subjective experience of emotion.

TABLE 1

COMPARATIVE FREQUENCIES OF SOMATIC AND PSYCHOLOGIC SYMPTOMS

IN PATIENTS WITH CARDIAC AND PSYCHIATRIC DISEASE

(Adapted from Frishman et al., 1981)

| SYMPTOM | CARDIOLOGY PATIENTS (% with symptoms) | ANXIETY NEUROTICS (% with symptoms) |
|---|---|---|
| Palpitations | 97 | 90 |
| Tires easily | 95 | 78 |
| Breathlessness | 90 | 75 |
| Nervousness | 88 | 99 |
| Sighing | 79 | 20 |
| Dizziness | 78 | 55 |
| Faintness | 70 | 20 |
| Apprehension | 61 | 80 |
| Headache | 58 | 65 |
| Paresthesias | 58 | 25 |
| Weakness | 56 | 65 |
| Trembling | 54 | 70 |
| Breath unsatisfactory | 53 | 73 |
| Insomnia | 53 | 48 |
| Shakiness | 47 | 70 |
| Fatigued all the time | 45 | 76 |
| Sweating | 45 | 62 |

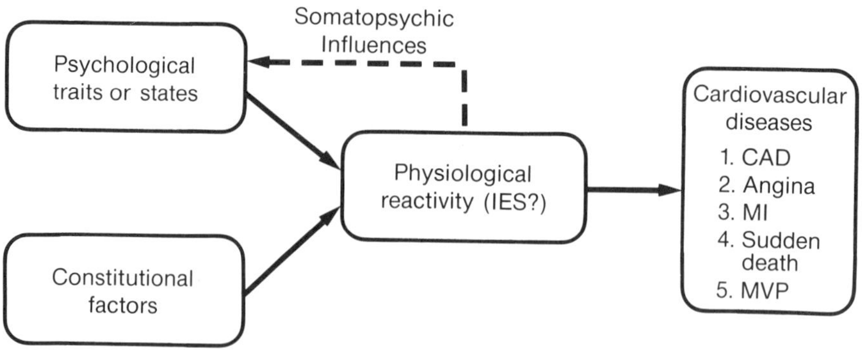


**FIGURE 2.** General model linking traits, physiological reactivity, and cardiovascular disorders

Specifically, the experience of anxiety or other related emotion can be intensified by a sequence of events beginning with increased sympathetic activity, with subsequent manifestations of arousal such as palpitations and trembling. The individual's perception and cognitive interpretation of these bodily responses reinforces the experience of anxiety (see Figure 1). Beta-blockers, by inhibiting selected physiologic responses, may interrupt the feedback loop from bodily responses to psychological reactions, thereby reducing the emotional intensity of anxiety.

Particularly relevant to illness behaviour is the fact that beta-blockers are currently indicated for a wide variety of conditions with suspected autonomic nervous system involvement. This suggests that sympathetic reactivity to stress may play a role in the symptomatology of many of these disorders. Studies comparing the symptoms of patients with coronary disease and patients with anxiety disorders indicate that these two types of disorders share a considerable commonality of symptoms (see Table 1). Thus, medical treatment of these disorders and patients' views of the nature of their illness may depend on the manner in which patients or their physicians label and interpret these symptoms.

## Summary and Future Directions

To summarize, the purpose of presenting these data is to illustrate ways in which pharmacologic techniques have been used to tease apart psychophysiological research issues relating to reactivity. Despite some very suggestive findings, the existing literature indicates that cardiovascular reactivity _per se_ should _not_ yet be regarded as a _proven_ risk factor. The types of direct evidence that an epidemiologist or critical scientist would demand in order to establish reactivity as a risk factor for either coronary heart disease or hypertension do not yet exist. As in any developing field, early assumptions tend to be oversimplified, and excessive claims are made. The extent to which acute physiologic changes produced in a controlled lab setting generalize to naturalistic settings is unknown. Furthermore, different tasks and situations produce different patterns of physiologic responses. In addition, the findings in the Type A and anxiety literatures illustrate the complex, two-way relationship between reactivity and behaviour shown in Figure 1.

A general model linking traits to physiologic reactivity and several cardiovascular disorders - for example, mitral valve prolapse (MVP) can be proposed (see Figure 2). The individual's interpretation of events can heighten sympathetic reactivity which in turn influences symptoms, while the interpretation of these physiologic responses affects both the diagnosis and the emotional state of the patient.

## ACKNOWLEDGEMENTS

Preparation of this chapter was supported by National Institutes of Health grant HL31514 and USUHS grant R07233. The opinions or assertions contained herein are the private ones of the authors and are not to be construed as official or reflecting the views of the DoD or the USUHS.

## REFERENCES

Alexander, F. (1939) Psychoanalytic study of a case of essential hypertension. Psychosomatic Medicine, 1, 139-152.

Belgian-French Pooling Project. (1984). Assessment of Type A behaviour by the Bortner scale and ischaemic heart disease. European Heart Journal, 5, 440-446.

Bowers, K. S. (1973). Situationism in psychology: An analysis and a critique. Psychological Review, 80, 307-336.

Chesney, M. A., Black, G. W., Chadwick, J. H., & Rosenman, R. H. (1981). Psychological correlates of the Type A behaviour pattern. Journal of Behavioral Medicine, 4, 217-229.

Costa, P. T. (in press). Is neuroticism a risk factor for CAD? Is Type A a measure of neuroticism? In T. Schmidt, T. Dembroski, & G. Blumchen (Eds.), Biological and psychological factors in cardiovascular disease.

Costa, P. T., Fleg, J. L., McCrae, R. R., & Lakatta, E. G. (1982). Neuroticism, coronary artery disease, and chest pain complaints: Cross-sectional and longitudinal studies. Experimental Aging Research, 8, 37-44.

Costa, P. T., & McCrae, R. R. (1985). Hypochondriasis, neuroticism, and aging. When are somatic complaints unfounded? American Psychologist, 40, 19-28.

Dembroski, T. M., MacDougall, J. M., Williams, R. B., Haney, T. L., & Blumenthal, J. A. (1985). Components of Type A, hostility, and anger-in: Relationship to angiographic findings. Psychosomatic Medicine, 47, 219-233.

Derogatis, C. F., Abeloff, M. D., & Melisaratos, N. (1979). Psychological coping mechanisms and survival time in metastatic breast cancer. Journal of the American Medical Association, 242, 1504-1508.

Durel, L. A., Krantz, D. S., & Barrett, J. E. (1985). The antianxiety effect of beta-blockers on punished responding. Psychosomatic Medicine, 47, 78, (Abstract).

Elias, M. F., Robbins, M. A., Blow, F. C., Rice, A. P., & Edgecomb, J. L., (1982). A behavioral study of middle-aged chest pain patients: Physical symptom reporting, anxiety, and depression. Experimental Aging Research, 8, 45-51.

Frishman, W. H., Razin, A., Swencionis, C., & Sonnenblick, E. H. (1981). Beta-adrenoreceptor blockade in anxiety states: A new approach to therapy? Cardiovascular Reviews & Reports, 2, 447-458.

Haynes, S. G., Feinleib, M., & Kannel, W. B. (1980). The relationship of psychosocial factors to coronary heart disease in the Framingham study. III. Eight-year incidence of coronary heart disease. American Journal of Epidemiology, 111, 37-58.

Jenkins, C. D. (1971). Psychologic and social precursors of coronary disease. New England Journal of Medicine, 284, 244-255, 307-317.

Jenkins, C. D., Rosenman, R. H., & Friedman, M. (1967). Development of an objective psychological test for the determination of the coronary-prone behavior pattern in employed men. Journal of Chronic Diseases, 20, 371-379.

Kahn, J. P., Kornfeld, D. S., Frank, K. A., Heller, S. S., & Hoar, P. F. (1980). Type A behavior and blood pressure during coronary artery bypass surgery. Psychosomatic Medicine, 42, 407-414.

Krantz, D. S., Arabian, J. M., Davia, J. E., & Parker, J. S. (1982). Type A behavior and coronary artery bypass surgery: Intraoperative blood pressure and perioperative complications. Psychosomatic Medicine, 44, 273-284.

Krantz, D. S., & Durel, L. A. (1983). Psychobiological substrates of the Type A behavior pattern. Health Psychology, 2, 393-411.

Krantz, D. S., Durel, L. A., Davia, J. E., Shaffer, R. T., Arabian, J. M., Dembroski, T. M., & MacDougall, J. M. (1982). Propranolol medication among coronary patients: Relationship to Type A behavior and cardiovascular response. Journal of Human Stress, 8, 4-12.

Krantz, D. S., & Glass, D. C. (1984). Personality, behavior patterns, and physical illness: Conceptual and methodological issues. In W. D. Gentry (Ed.), Handbook of Behavioral Medicine. New York: Guilford.

Krantz, D. S., & Manuck, S. B. (1984). Acute psychophysiologic reactivity and risk of cardiovascular disease: A review and methodologic critique. Psychological Bulletin, 96, 435-464.

Matthews, K. A., & Haynes, S. G. (in press). Type A behavior pattern and coronary risk: Update and critical evaluation. American Journal of Epidemiology.

Mischel, W. (1968). Personality and Assessment. New York: Wiley.

Rosenman, R. H. (1978). The interview method of assessment of the coronary-prone behavior pattern. In T. M. Dembroski, S. M. Weiss, J. L. Shields, S. G. Haynes, & M. Feinleib (Eds.), Coronary-Prone Behavior (pp. 55-69). New York: Springer-Verlag.

Rosenman, R. H., Brand, R. J., Jenkins, C. D., Friedman, M., Straus, R., & Wurm, M. (1975). Coronary heart disease in the Western Collaborative Group study: Final follow-up experience of 8 1/2 years. Journal of the American Medical Association, 233, 872-877.

Schmieder, R., Friedrich, G., Neus, H., Rudel, H., & von Eiff, A. W. (1983). The influence of beta blockers on cardiovascular reactivity and Type A behavior pattern in hypertensives. Psychosomatic Medicine, 45, 417-423.

Shekelle, R. B., Hulley, S. B., Neaton, J. D., Billings, J. H., Borhani, N. O., Gerace, T. A., Jacobs, D. R., Lasser, N. L., Mittlemark, M. B., & Stamler, J. (1985). The MRFIT behavior pattern study. II. Type A behavior and incidence of cornonary heart disease. American Journal of Epidemiology, 122(4), 559-570.

Weiner, H. (1977). Psychobiology and human disease. New York: Elsevier.

Willerman, L. (1979). The psychology of individual and group differences. San Francisco: Freeman.

# ILLNESS COGNITION, SYMPTOM REPORTING AND SOMATIZATION IN FAMILY MEDICINE

James Robbins and Laurence Kirmayer

Institute of Community and Family Psychiatry
McGill University

Biomedical practitioners hope for a simple correspondence between clinical presentation and organic pathology. Unfortunately, illness behaviour supervenes to make the relationship between illness and disease exceedingly complex. Style of symptom presentation interacts with the structure of the health-care system to determine whether patients' distress is accurately recognized and alleviated. From 20 to 84 percent of patient visits to primary care are for somatic complaints that receive no organic diagnosis (Kellner, 1985). When psychosocial factors are noted as part of their presentations, patients with obscure somatic symptoms may be described as somatizing or hypochondriacal and referred for psychiatric evaluation of "abnormal illness behaviour" (Pilowsky, 1969). When psychosocial factors are not recognized, these patients may be exposed to lengthy diagnostic and therapeutic intervention and, when no organic explanation is forthcoming, casually reassured or abruptly told their problems are imaginary.

Far from being dictated by pathobiology, human suffering takes shape through thought and action. The translation of inchoate distress into symptom reports and presenting complaints is mediated by cognitive processes. As an outcome of the cognitive mediation of distress, people may amplify or minimize symptoms while emphasizing somatic or emotional aspects of suffering. Variations in these processes may help account for the observed clinical and sociodemographic differences in symptom reporting.

The research outlined in this chapter focuses on the cognitive components of illness behaviour. Measures of several distinct cognitive styles that may be involved in the translation of distress into somatic or psychosocial symptoms are proposed. The ability to measure multiple cognitive styles that make independent contributions to the outcomes of illness experience has application to the study of everyday symptom reporting as well as to primary care patient populations who appear to somatize or psychologize their distress.

## Illness Cognition and Symptom Presentation

While specific pathophysiological disturbances account for many of the complaints presented to physicians and much of the variation in reports of distress gathered by self-report symptom inventories, the presentation and declaration of symptoms may also be influenced by the patient's illness cognition (Leventhal, Nerenz and Strauss, 1982; Pennebaker, 1982). As the term is used in this chapter, illness cognition refers to the outcomes of cognitive processes that accompany each illness experience and is hypothesized to include: (1) focusing on unusual bodily sensations and feeling states; (2) recognizing these sensations or states as symptoms of a physical illness or emotional problem; and (3) attributing symptoms to physical or psychosocial cause. (1)

Self-focus. An illness episode typically begins when an individual becomes aware of a change in bodily sensation or feeling state. Recognition of unusual bodily sensations is a function of attention focused on those sensations. Laboratory subjects instructed to focus on their bodies have been shown to report more somatic symptoms than subjects instructed to attend to external stimuli (Pennebaker, 1982). Similarly, scales devised to measure individual differences in self-consciousness, body focus, and introspection are correlated with reports of both affective and somatic symptoms (Fenigstein, Scheier, and Buss, 1975; Miller, Murphy, and Buss, 1981; Mechanic, 1980; Hansell and Mechanic, this volume).

Symptom recognition. Once unusual sensations are noticed they must then be recognized as symptoms, that is, as evidence that something is wrong before they are likely to be declared on a self-report inventory or reported to a physician. Barsky and Klerman (1983) have proposed that hypochondriacal or somatizing patients may tend to amplify normal bodily sensations and to view them as evidence of serious disease. The chronic tendency to worry about illness and to evaluate trivial or transitory sensations as signs of illness, as measured, for example by the hypochondriasis scale of Pilowsky (1967), is related to increased symptom reports on somatic symptom checklists (Fava, Pilowsky, Pierfederici, et al., 1982; Pilowsky and Spence, 1975) and on the Center for Epidemiological Studies Depression scale (Radloff, 1977). Factorial studies by Pilowsky (1967; Pilowsky, Murrel, and Gordon, 1979) suggest that this tendency to interpret sensations as abnormal and hence view them as symptoms might be activated by such factors as worry or fear about illness, sensitivity to sensations, perceived vulnerability to illness, and the conviction that one is sick.

Symptom interpretation. Given the recognition that sensations or feelings indicate an illness, expression of distress is determined by the cause attributed to the discomfort. Causal attribution, not necessarily a direct reflection of pathology, becomes increasingly subject to interpretive biases as discomforting sensations increase in vagueness, ambiguity, and location in parts of the body not directly observable (Barsky and Klerman, 1983). In the laboratory, manipulation of suggested labels can result in misattribution of identical internal sensations to feelings of hunger, need for smoking, sexual aggression, or crowding (Pennebaker, 1982). A more limited repertoire of classifications may exist for sensations clearly suspected as being symptoms of an illness. An upset stomach for example, may be interpreted psychologically as a sign of anxiety, somatically as evidence of an ulcer, or environmentally as the result of dietary indiscretion.

Attributing a cause to symptoms depends on the familiarity of the condition, the illness experiences and suggestions of significant others,

---

1. Our use of the term illness cognition should be distinguished from that of Leventhal and colleagues (Leventhal and Nerenz, 1985; Leventhal, Nerenz, and Steele, 1985). While they propose a self-regulatory illness cognition model including common sense representations of the attributes of a symptom, plans to cope with a symptom, and appraisal of the outcomes of coping efforts, our use is restricted to the perceptual and evaluative steps leading up to and including the expression of distress as a discrete symptom.

previous contact with the medical profession, and social and cultural restrictions on the appropriate expression of distress (Kleinman, 1980; McKinlay, 1973; Meyer, Leventhal, and Gutmann, 1985). An outcome of these influences may be a general tendency to interpret sensations and feelings as somatic in origin, psychosocial in origin, or environmental in origin.

Interpretations of symptoms in turn determine the objectification of the condition as a complaint offered to a physician. Distress, open to alternative interpretations, may also be open to alternative modes of expression. Weakness, tiredness and fatigue, for example, may be expressions of distress that have a common origin with feelings of hopelessness and worthlessness, varying only in the manner in which meaning is assigned.

To summarize, symptom reporting and presenting complaints should be influenced by self-focus, symptom recognition and symptom interpretation. Heightened awareness of bodily sensations, the tendency to believe that sensations represent serious illness, and a bias toward interpreting symptoms as physical in origin should be related to increased somatic symptom reporting and the declaration of somatic symptoms to the physician. In contrast, heightened awareness of thoughts and feelings, the conviction that emotional changes are abnormal and thus reflect a serious emotional problem, and the tendency to employ psychological concepts when attributing origin to symptoms should contribute to increased psychological symptom reporting and the presentation of psychosocial symptoms to the physician. A study designed to investigate these hypotheses among family medicine patients is presented below.

## Measuring Illness Cognition in Family Medicine

Patients attending a hospital-based family medicine teaching unit of McGill University were recruited for the study. Patients able to speak and read English and for whom their current visit was not a follow-up for a previously diagnosed problem were eligible. Subjects were sampled on varying days of the week over five months. Interviews were completed with a total of 100 patients who were visiting one of 23 staff or resident family physicians.

The average age of the sample was 44.2 years; 58 percent were women; and 42 percent were currently married. The patients in the sample had an average of 12.3 years of schooling; 45 percent were working at a job for pay; and they had visited a doctor an average of 4.2 times over the last 12 months. Slightly over a quarter (27 percent) were Jewish; 13 percent French Canadian; 19 percent non-Jewish English Canadian; and 17 percent were of other non-Jewish European background. Patients of West Indian, Asian, Southeast Asian, and Middle Eastern origins composed the remaining 24 percent.

The illness cognition dimensions of self-focus, symptom recognition, and symptom interpretation were measured by instruments developed for this study or adapted from previous work on self-awareness and abnormal illness behaviour. The background and psychometric properties of these measures are described in the following sections.

Self-focus. Chronic awareness of bodily sensations and feelings was measured by the Private Self-Consciousness scale (PSC, Fenigstein et al., 1975) and the Private Body-Consciousness scale (PBC, Miller et al., 1981). These scales identify individuals who are chronically attentive to their inner thoughts and feelings (PSC) and to their bodily sensations (PBC). The PSC is composed of ten true-false items such as "I'm generally attentive to my inner feelings", and "I'm alert to changes in my mood". It has a test-retest correlation of .79 and a correlation of .32 with a physical symptom checklist (Pennebaker and Skelton, 1978). Items were internally consistent (alpha = .69) among our sample of family practice patients.

The PBC includes five true-false questions such as "I am quick to sense the hunger contractions of my stomach", and "I'm very aware of changes in my body temperature". It has a test-retest correlation of .69 among a sample of university students but an alpha of only .32 among our patient sample. The PSC and PBC correlate with each other at .33 among our sample of patients. (See Appendix for intercorrelations of illness cognition measures.) They are used separately and in linear combination to measure intrapsychic versus somatic focus of attention.

Symptom recognition. The tendency for people to conclude that bodily sensations or feelings signify serious disease was measured indirectly. Symptom recognition should be influenced by (a) one's cognitive sense of being vulnerable to illness, (b) the degree of worry or fear about becoming ill, (c) the conviction that one has an illness and, (d) the sense of being more sensitive to symptoms than others. These beliefs might be seen as establishing an expectancy set through which new sensations are more readily experienced as symptoms of a severe illness. Items designed to measure each of these components of somatic symptom recognition were extracted from the Illness Behavior Questionnaire (Pilowsky, Spence, Cobb, and Katsikitis, 1984; items 2, 6, 20, 24, 34, 37, 39). The resulting seven items of the Somatic Symptom Recognition scale (SSR) were internally consistent (alpha = .67).

Items parallel in structure to those of the SSR but modified to have emotional symptom content were designed to measure the tendency to conclude the fluctuations in feelings signify a serious emotional problem. The resulting seven-item Affective Symptom Recognition scale (ASR) includes yes-no questions such as "Do you think there is something seriously wrong with your emotions", and "Do you think you might suddenly lose control of your emotions". The alpha for this scale (.82) suggests adequate internal consistency. Correlation of the ASR with the somatic recognition scale ($r$ = .64) also suggests that the belief that one's emotional symptoms are abnormal often exists together with the belief that one's somatic symptoms are abnormal, and that both beliefs may be traced to a more general feeling of personal vulnerability to illness.

Symptom interpretation. The tendency to interpret symptoms as either somatic, psychological, or environmental (external) in origin was measured by the Symptom Interpretation Questionnaire (SIQ) designed for this study. The SIQ consists of 13 common symptoms such as weakness, dizziness, trouble sleeping, headache and upset stomach. Subjects were asked to imagine that they were experiencing each symptom and hypothesize the predominate cause of each. For example, "If I got dizzy all of a sudden, I would probably think that it is because: (a) there is something wrong with my heart or blood pressure (b) I am not eating enough or I got up too quickly; or (c) I must be under a lot of stress".

A forced-choice response format for each symptom allows for the computation of three scales that are the sum of somatic, affective, and normalizing attributions respectively. The scales measure the tendency to employ one interpretative type (e.g., somatic) in contrast to the other two (e.g., affective or normalizing). The forced-choice design requires that responses to only two of the three scales be used in any multivariate analysis. Response to the third scale is, by design, a perfect linear combination of responses to the other two. (2)

The resulting Affective Symptom Interpretation scale (ASI) is internally

---

2. The Symptom Interpretation Questionnaire and other scales devised for this study are available from the authors.

TABLE 1. CLASSIFICATION OF CLINICAL PRESENTATIONS IN FAMILY MEDICINE

| Clinical Presentation | Inclusion Criteria | Exclusion Criteria | Examples |
|---|---|---|---|
| Psychosocial | Psychosocial complaints with or without additional somatic complaints | None | Depression, mood shifts, feeling stressed because of work tensions, confusion, anxiety attacks |
| Vegetative symptoms of depression (somatic-vegetative) | Complaints of vegetative symptoms of depression as specified by DSM III (APA, 1980) | Psychosocial complaints | Sleeping problems, fatigue, weight gain |
| Somatic symptoms of obscure (somatic-obscure) | Pain not diagnosed as organic in origin or other somatic complaints not diagnosed as organic | Psychosocial complaints, vegetative symptoms of depression, | Shortness of breath, dizziness, weakness in arms and legs, hot flushes, pains in spine, pains in knees, back and shoulder pain, headaches, stomach pains |
| Somatic symptoms of organic origin (somatic-origin) | Somatic complaints, all with organic diagnosis | Psychosocial complaints, vegetative symptoms of depression, somatic symptoms of obscure origin | Chest pain explained by angina, fatigue due to anemia, appetite loss secondary to gastrectomy |
| Health maintenance | Request for check-up, routine test, pregnancy | Complaints or symptoms of any kind | |
| Ineligible | Diagnosed schizophrenic excluded from categorization | | |

consistent (alpha = .82) and reliable over a two-month period among university students (test-retest correlation = .63). (3) The comparison Somatic Symptom Interpretation Scale (SSI) has an alpha of .63 among the patient sample and a test-retest correlation among students of .52. The two scales are negatively correlated at r = -.34 for patients.

Symptom self-report inventories. Affective and somatic symptom reporting was measured by the Center for Epidemiological Studies Depression scale (CES-D; Radloff, 1977) and the somatization subscale of the Symptom Checklist 90 (SCL-90; Derogatis, Lipman, and Covi, 1973). The CES-D consists of 20 items characteristic of clinical depression and, in modified form, was used to measure affective symptom reporting. The CES-D has been shown to be a reliable screening instrument for major depression in community surveys (Radloff, 1977). Items are predominantly affective although somatic and other non-affective symptoms of depression are included. In order to maintain the conceptual distinction between affective and somatic symptom reporting, the CES-D was shortened to include only the 14 purely affective or cognitive depressive symptoms. Deleted were two somatic items (my appetite was poor; my sleep was restless), two ennervation items (everything I did was an effort; I could not get going), and two nonspecific items (I was bothered by things that usually don't bother me; I talked less than usual).

The somatization subscale of the SCL-90 consists of 12 somatic symptoms. (4) The scale was developed as a measure of subjective distress arising from the perception of bodily dysfunction. It has demonstrated high internal consistency (alpha = .86) and correlates highly with MMPI-based scales of bodily symptoms (r = .66) and organic symptoms (r = .62) (Derogatis, Rickels, and Rock, 1976).

Clinical presentation. The classification of patient's clinical presentations has proven to be extraordinarily difficult (McWhinney, 1972; Stewart, McWhinney, and Buck, 1975; Weyrauch, 1984). It is likely that no entirely satisfactory scheme can be devised simply because patients do not present with a single problem and the priority of their problems shifts with information from others. Presentations also must be understood as the result of doctor-patient interaction where the physician assists with language for distress and patients, gauging the receptiveness of their doctors, wait for an appropriate opening to declare their problems. Realizing the limitations of classifying overlapping, heterogeneous and evolving complaints, the categorizations listed below approximate groups of clinical and theoretical significance.

To maintain the distinction between affective and somatic presentations, as well as between somatic complaints of obscure origin and organic somatic complaints, and to arrive at mutually exclusive classifications, presentations have been based on exclusion criteria. Criteria used in classifying presentations and examples of complaints grouped in each category are presented in Table 1. Reading down the table, inclusion criteria for presentations listed higher in order are exclusion criteria for presentations listed lower in order. For example, a patient presenting with psychosocial difficulties and vegatative symptoms of depression is classified as a psychosocial presentation. Similarly, a patient presenting with somatic complaints that receive clear organic diagnoses and at least one somatic complaint of obscure origin is classified as presenting with somatic symptoms

---

3. Robbins and Kirmayer, unpublished data, N = 140.

4. The response format of the somatization subscale was modified slightly to be consistent with the CES-D scale.

TABLE 2. CORRELATIONS OF ILLNESS COGNITION MEASURES WITH SOCIOCULTURAL VARIABLES, LIFE EVENTS, PHYSICIAN VISITS, AND SOCIAL DESIRABILITY

| | Self-focus | | Symptom Recognition | | Symptom Interpretation | |
|---|---|---|---|---|---|---|
| | Body consciousness | Self-consciousness | Somatic recognition | Affective recognition | Somatic interpretation | Affective interpretation |
| Sex (1=female), 0=male) | .20* | .18* | .07 | .26* | -.09 | .21* |
| Age | -.11 | -.28* | -.05 | -.12 | .21* | -.08 |
| Education | -.04 | .14 | -.13 | -.14 | -.11 | -.08 |
| Marital status (1=married, 0=not married) | -.03 | -.27* | -.10 | -.13 | .12 | .05 |
| Jewish | -.13 | -.18* | -.06 | -.16 | .21* | -.21* |
| French Canadian | .09 | .10 | .15 | .07 | .08 | .00 |
| Life events | -.09 | .22* | -.04 | .18 | -.16 | .16 |
| Physician visits, last 12 months | .04 | .07 | .22* | .06 | .17* | -.08 |
| RD16[a] | -.15 | -.62* | -.47* | -.54* | .46 | -.17 |

[a] Correlations based on 100 subjects except for RD16, computed on a subsample of 25

*$p<.05$

TABLE 3. CORRELATIONS AND REGRESSIONS OF AFFECTIVE SYMPTOM REPORTING AND SOMATIC SYMPTOM REPORTING WITH DIMENSIONS OF ILLNESS COGNITION, FAMILY MEDICINE PATIENTS

| | CES-D Affective | | | SCL-90 Somatization | | |
|---|---|---|---|---|---|---|
| | Pearson r | Beta | b | Pearson r | Beta | b |
| Sex (1=female, 0=male) | .12 | -.01 | .23 | .15 | .09 | 1.31 |
| Education | -.19* | -.14 | -1.63 | -.18* | -.11 | -.93 |
| Self-focus | | | | | | |
| Body consciousness | .08 | -.09 | -.68 | .34* | .18 | 1.08* |
| Self-consciousness | .19* | .07 | .28 | .20* | .06 | .16 |
| Symptom Recognition | | | | | | |
| Somatic recognition | .61* | .31 | 1.71* | .41* | .26 | 1.06* |
| Affective recognition | .63* | .29 | 1.27* | .28* | -.03 | -.10 |
| Symptom Interpretation | | | | | | |
| Somatic interpretation | .04 | .08 | .31 | .33* | .35 | 1.03* |
| Affective interpretation | .40* | .25 | .80* | .12 | .15 | .37 |
| Constant | | | 5.48 | | | -3.07 |
| $R^2$ | | .51 | | | .36 | |
| F | | 11.64* | | | 6.29* | |

*p<.05
N=99

of obscure origin. Information used to classify presenting symptoms was collected from three sources: (1) interviews with patients immediately prior to their appointments; (2) a brief questionnaire distributed to physicians two to three months following the patient's visit; and (3) chart reviews conducted two to three months after the patient's visit. Symptoms mentioned in any of these three sources were given equal weight in classifying presentations.

## Sociocultural Measures and Illness Cognition

Data were analyzed to determine sociocultural differences in illness cognition, the relationship between illness cognition and symptom reporting, and the ability of illness cognition to discriminate among types of clinical presentations to family medicine. First, correlations of illness cognition measures with sociocultural variables, life events, physician visits, and social desirability are presented in Table 2. Women in the sample were more body- and self-conscious than were men. They were also more likely to feel emotionally vulnerable and to attribute ambiguous symptoms to emotional causes than were men. Older patients report that they were less focused on their intrapsychic processes than were younger patients but were more apt to see somatic illness as the cause of ambiguous symptoms.

Years of education is unrelated to awareness of oneself and one's bodily sensations, to the conviction that symptoms indicate illness and the tendency to attribute symptoms to somatic or affective causes.

In contrast to other research suggesting that Jews are more introspective and willing to express emotional qualities of illness (Hansell and Mechanic, in press; Zborowski, 1952; Zola, 1966), Jews in this sample tend to attribute ambiguous symptoms to physical causes, are less focused on inner thoughts and feelings, and are less likely to label symptoms as emotional in origin than are non-Jews. These relationships disappear, however, when controlled for age, education and sex and are explained by the fact that Jews in this sample are disproportionately older, less educated men.

The illness cognition of patients of French Canadian background are no different than those without such background, while number of life events within the last three months is related only to the tendency not to be self-reflective. Number of physican visits is positively related to somatic recognition and somatic attributions. Finally, social desirability, measured on a subsample of 25 patients is related strongly and negatively to self-consciousness, somatic recognition and affective recognition, and positively to somatic interpretation.

## The Association of Illness Cognition and Symptom Reports

In studying the relationships between cognitive components of illness and affective and somatic symptom reporting, two outcomes were considered. First, whether there was evidence of a conceptual distinction among components as indicated by their independent association with symptom reports. Second, whether there existed discriminant validity among measures of affective and somatic illness cognitions as indicated by their differential relationships with affective and somatic symptom reports. To do this affective symptom level (CES-D Affective) and somatic symptom level (SCL-90 Somatization) were regressed on illness cognitions. These results are presented in Table 3.

Considering first the bivariate associations between illness cognition and affective symptom reports, it is apparent that all measures except body consciousness and somatic interpretation are related to CES-D Affective. The

TABLE 4. MEANS OF ILLNESS COGNITION MEASURES AND SYMPTOM REPORTS BY TYPE OF CLINICAL PRESENTATION, FAMILY MEDICINE PATIENTS

| | Somatic-organic (n=41) | Psycho-social (n=17) | Somatic-vegetative (n=10) | Somatic-obscure (n=20) | Health Maintenance (n=8) |
|---|---|---|---|---|---|
| Illness Cognitions | | | | | |
| Self-focus | | | | | |
| Private body consciousness | 3.1 | 3.2 | 3.0 | 3.2 | 2.9 |
| Private self-consciousness | 5.1 | 6.1 | 6.2 | 5.3 | 6.3 |
| Symptom Recognition | | | | | |
| Somatic recognition | 1.2 | 2.1 | 2.3 | 1.4 | 1.9 |
| Affective recognition [a] | 1.0 | 3.6 | 3.1 | 1.7 | 2.1 |
| Symptom Interpretation | | | | | |
| Somatic interpretation | 3.4 | 2.6 | 3.0 | 2.9 | 2.8 |
| Affective interpretation [b] | 3.0 | 7.2 | 4.4 | 4.7 | 4.1 |
| Symptom Reports | | | | | |
| SCL-90 | | | | | |
| Somatization | 7.0 | 8.6 | 9.5 | 8.0 | 5.0 |
| CES-D | | | | | |
| (Affective) [c] | 7.4 | 17.4 | 13.8 | 10.5 | 8.1 |

a (F) = 8.37, 4 and 91 degrees of freedom, p<.001; psychosocial significantly different than somatic-obscure; somatic-organic significantly different than somatic-vegetative by Turkey's honestly significant multiple comparison

b (F) = 7.52, 4 and 91 d. f., p<.001; psychosocial significantly different than each other group

c (F) = 4.84, 4 and 90 d. f., p=.001; psychosocial significantly different than somatic-organic strongest relationships are between symptoms and somatic recognition, affective recognition and affective interpretation. These variables remain strong predictors of affective symptoms in the multiple regression model. (5)

While prediction of affective symptoms is dominated by affective cognitions, somatic symptoms are best predicted by somatic cognitions. Heightened awareness of bodily sensations, the conclusion that symptoms represent serious illness, and the tendency to attribute ambiguous symptoms to somatic origin significantly predict level of somatic symptom reporting in the multiple regression model. With the exception that somatic recognition remains strongly predictive of affective symptoms, affective illness cognitions appear more strongly related to affective symptoms while somatic cognitions are predictive of somatic symptoms. These data support the conceptual independence and discriminant validity of affective and somatic illness cognitions and suggest that the model may be useful in understanding symptom reporting.

<u>Discriminating Among Clinical Presentations</u>

An additional test of the clinical utility of the illness cognition model comes with its ability to discriminate among types of clinical presentations in primary care. Though it is likely that presentations to family physicians are biased toward organic illness and communication of distress in somatic terms, patients with psychosocial discomfort are also most likely to complain initially and often exlusively to their family doctor (Katon and Dengerink, 1983). Table 4 presents the results of simple analyses of variance of illness cognition measures by types of clinical presentation.

The most general observation from the table is that patients presenting with psychosocial complaints are unique. Patients who complain of psychosocial distress (most often depression, interpersonal problems or feeling stressed) are distinguished by a greater number of affective symptoms, the belief that their emotional problems represent a serious emotional disorder, and their tendency to trace ambiguous symptoms to emotional origins.

Patients who present with vegetative symptoms of depression (fatigue, weakness, insomnia) in the absence of psychosocial complaints, are generally comparable to those with clear psychosocial complaints, with one major exception. Like psychosocial patients, those with somatic-vegetative symptoms tend to be more focused on their thoughts and feelings and perceive themselves to be more affectively vulnerable than others. They are, however, significantly less likely to see ambiguous symptoms as expressions of affective problems than are patients who acknowledge psychosocial discomfort.

Compared to patients with other somatic symptoms of obscure origin (i.e., pain in limbs, back, chest, or abdomen; headache; dizziness; lump in throat), patients whose somatic symptoms correspond to the vegetative signs of major depression tend to be more self-focused, and to believe that their symptoms represent a serious emotional or physical illness, though the differences between these two groups are not statistically significant. In contrast, the somatic-obscure group, thought by many to represent either non-

---

5. The forced choice format of the Symptom Interpretation Questionnaire will always result in negative correlations beween each pair of the three scales that can be derived from it. This artifactual relationship between the Somatic and Affective Symptom Interpretation scales could influence the strength of regression coefficients when the scales are used together but should not alter their basic relationships with a criterion variable.

TABLE 5. LOGIT REGRESSION ANALYSES OF CLINICAL PRESENTATION BY ILLNESS COGNITIONS, FAMILY MEDICINE PATIENTS

| | A. Psychosocial (1) vs. Somatic-organic (0) | | B. Somatic-vegetative (1) vs. Psychosocial (0) | | C. Somatic-obscure (1) vs. Somatic-vegetative (0) | | D. Somatic-obscure (1) vs. Somatic-organic (0) | |
|---|---|---|---|---|---|---|---|---|
| | (n = 58) | | (n = 27) | | (n = 30) | | (n = 61) | |
| | r | logistic coeff.[a] | r | logistic coeff. | r | logistic coeff. | r | logistic coeff. |
| Sex (1=female), 0=male) | .17 | | .22 | | -.35* | -.89 | .02 | |
| Education | -.08 | | -.27* | -.13 | .72* | .67 | .32* | .11* |
| Body consciousness | .01 | | -.07 | | .05 | | .00 | |
| Self-consciousness | .16 | | .03 | | -.19 | | .00 | |
| Somatic recognition | .22* | -.09 | .06 | | -.31* | -.19 | .03 | |
| Affective recognition | .56* | .25* | -.13 | | -.35* | .12 | .20* | .00 |
| Somatic interpretation | -.17 | | .08 | | -.03 | | .13 | |
| Affective interpretation | .61* | .20* | -.39* | -.13 | .05 | | .34* | .21* |
| Constant | | 3.13 | | 6.82 | | -.76 | | 2.48 |

[a] Unstandardized coefficients are presented
* p <.05

affective presentation of depression (Katon, Kleinman, and Rosen, 1982) or a hypochondriacal concern with the body and illness (Kellner, 1985) appear very similar to those patients for whom the physician has specified an organic origin for all their somatic complaints. They differ only slightly in the tendency for the somatic-obscure group to report more affective symptoms of depression.

To investigate distinctions among presentations with greater precision, logistic regression models were estimated comparing pairs of groups. Four comparisons, selected on the basis of clinical importance, are presented in Table 5. Simple correlations of each illness cognition measure with the presentation dichotomy are presented in the initial column of each panel followed by logistic regression coefficients. Only predictor variables that were significant at the $P < .10$ level in the bivariate case were examined in multivariate models.

Logistic regression is a method of relating a dichotomous dependent variable to one or more independent variables. As in linear regression, the sign and size of coefficients in the model indicate a variable's effect on the dependent variable. In this case, a positive coefficient represents the amount in which a unit change in the independent variable increases the log odds of being in the presentation group coded 1 as opposed to the presentation group coded 0 (Cleary and Angel, 1984).

In the first model, panel A, psychosocial presenations are compared to somatic-organic presentations. Consistent with the ANOVA results, patients who recognize emotional changes as evidence of a serious emotional problem and who apply affective meaning to symptoms are significantly more likely to present psychosocially than somatically.

Panel B compares patients who present with vegetative symptoms of depression to patients who acknowledge psychosocial distress. Correlations confirm that the distinguishing feature of these two groups is that patients in the somatic-vegetative groups are less likely than psychosocial patients to attribute symptoms to a psychosocial cause. In the multivarite model with education controlled the logistic coefficient does not quite reach significance ($p = .07$).

The third model, panel C, compares patients who present with somatic symptoms of obscure origin to the somatic-vegetative group. Based on correlations, patients classified as somatic-obscure tend to be men, higher educated and less likely to believe that they have a serious health problem or emotional problem. In the logistic model, however, only educational differences remain noteable ($p = .06$). Due most likely to the tendency for male and lower educated subjects to score lower on symptom recognition, illness cognition differences between these two groups disappear when sex and education are controlled.

Even with sex and education controlled, somatic-obscure patients remain different than somatic-organic patients in terms of the attribution given ambiguous symptoms (panel D). Somatic-obscure patients are more likely to see stress, tension and emotions as the cause of symptoms than are somatic-organic patients. This suggests that somatic-obscure patients, consistent with the way they are defined, may be more likely to visit the doctor for stress-produced sensations that received neither organic nor psychosocial diagnoses.

To summarize, a model of the cognitive processes involved in symptom reporting and clinical presentation has been proposed. Using individual differences measures designed to reflect these processes, their association with symptom levels and type of presentation (to a family medicine clinic) was examined. Specifically, the hypothesis that expression of distress is mediated by awareness of a change in bodily or feeling state, recognition of such changes as abnormal and thus signifying illness, and interpretation of the symptom as evidence of a physical disease or an emotional problem was examined. A dichotomy between somatic and affective symptom evaluation and expression was advanced not because this is an exhaustive representation of the way people classify their distress but because this distinction fits with popular lay and professional models of illness. The distinction between physical and emotional distress is basic to the social construction of illness experience in the West (Kirmayer, 1984; this volume). Despite efforts to develop an integrated biopsychosocial approach, this duality continues to inform the structure of medical care (Blackwell, 1967; Eisenberg, 1977; Helman, 1985; Kirmayer, in press; Tollefson, Straud, Hughes, and Garvey, 1984).

## Sex, Social Desirability, and Illness Cognition

Initial analyses examined the variation in illness cognition across social categories. If replicated in larger studies, illness cognition variations may be helpful in understanding sociocultural differences in symptom reporting. Group differences in symptomatology may be located in differences in bodily awareness, translation of sensations into symptoms, or objectification of distress in somatic or affective symptoms. For example, clinical and epidemiological studies consistently show that women report more symptoms of depression and more somatic and nonspecific symptoms than do men (Kessler, this volume; Pennebaker, 1982; Weissman and Klerman, 1977). It is unclear, however, whether women experience more morbidity because they are sicker or because they experience their bodies differently or are better able to recognize and label symptoms. Our results have shown that women are more attuned to their bodies and inner thoughts and feelings, perhaps resulting in the experience of sensations and emotions as more intense. They are also more likely to anticipate emotional abnormalities and to consider ambiguous symptoms as rising from affective distress, suggesting that excess female morbidity may also be due to differences in the cognitive appraisal of symptoms. Similarly, unmarried persons have been shown to report greater morbidity (Verbrugge, 1979) but were shown here only to differ from the married in their attentiveness to inner thoughts and feelings, suggesting that emotional sensations may be intensified by introspection among those without a partner.

Illness cognition measures were also shown to be strongly associated with a scale designed to measure social desirability (Schuessler, Hittle, and Cardascia, 1978). Patients who scored higher on the RD16 were significantly less self-conscious, less likely to conclude that something was wrong with their health or emotions, and more likely to select somatic interpretations for ambiguous symptoms. Rather than serving to invalidate these measures as methodologically suspect, it is more useful to consider the substantive meaning of these relationships. McCrae and Costa (1983) have suggested that social desirability scales might best be understood as measures of social adjustment. The authors of the RD16, in fact, have raised the question of whether this scale might be considered a measure of a cheerful or benign temperament (Schuessler et al., 1978). Considering the content of scale items such as "I find that I can help others in many ways", or "The future looks very bleak" (reverse scored), and the fact that the scale is correlated with the CES-D at - .44 among our subsample, it is perhaps best viewed as a measure of social adjustment than of a responding style. It is a substantive finding, not methodological artifact, then, that better adjusted patients report that they are less self-conscious, less physically and emotionally vulnerable and more likely to make somatic attributions than more poorly adjusted patients.

## Cognitive Styles Match Symptoms

In general, measures of somatic illness cognition style were shown to be related to reports of somatic symptoms while affective cognitive style was related to affective symptoms. Heightened awareness of bodily sensations was correlated almost as highly with somatic symptoms as its reliability would allow. Along with somatic recognition and somatic interpretation, these measures remained significant predictors of somatic symptoms in a multiple regression model. Affective awareness, recognition, and interpretation were correlated significantly with affective symptoms, though only recognition and interpretation remained significant in multiple regression. Somatic recognition was also a significant predictor of affective symptoms, suggesting that worry or fear about becoming physically ill may not only increase the recognition and reporting of somatic symptoms but also generate new emotional symptoms consistent with worry.

These findings support the independence of illness cognition styles and the discriminant validity of separate processes of affectively evaluating and somatically evaluating personal distress. In particular, our findings support the work of others (Kleinman, 1980; Robbins and Greenley, 1983; White, 1982) on the importance of causal attributions as an independent factor in illness behaviour and symptom reporting and suggests that the study of introspection (Hansell and Mechanic, in press; this volume; Mechanic, 1980) should be supplemented by measures of symptom recognition and attribution.

## The Importance of Affective Illness Cognition

While differences in affective versus somatic illness cognition succeeded in discriminating affective from somatic symptom reports, only affective illness cognitions successfully discriminated among clinical presentations. Patients who communicated their distress in explicit emotional or interpersonal terms were distinguished from other presentations by reporting greater emotional vulnerability and greater affective interpretations of ambiguous symptoms. Somatic cognitive styles, however, failed to discriminate either somatic presentations from psychosocial presentations or presentations of somatic symptoms of obscure origin from somatic presentations confirmed by organic diagnosis.

Research on abnormal illness behaviour using instruments similar to the somatic illness cognition measures used in this study has tended to emphasize factors that amplify the recognition and expression of somatic concern (Barsky and Klerman, 1983; Pilowsky, 1978; Pilowsky, Murrell, and Gordon, 1979). The present data suggest, however, that a more fruitful approach to the study of a primary care population may be the examination of cognitive mediators of affective symptom expression. It appears that psychologization rather than somatization is a more important contributor to the clinical presentation of these patients.

## Clinical Presentations and Somatization

In understanding the cognitive differences among types of clinical presentations it may prove helpful to trace the correspondence between the use of the term somatization in the literature and the classification of presentations employed in this chapter. Somatization has been used to refer to at least three clinical situations of interest here: (1) somatic presentation of depression; (2) presentation of functional somatic symptoms; and (3) somatic symptoms presented in addition to or accompanying psychosocial distress (Kirmayer, this volume). Each of these situations is addressed in turn.

First, patients with major depressive disorder who present with somatic complaints in the absence of emotional disturbance are said to somatize their depression (Katon, Kleinman, and Rosen, 1982). Without further diagnostic assessment of the participants in this study presenting with vegetative symptoms of depression but without psychosocial complaints, it cannot be concluded they are in fact suffering from affective disorders. This group may include patients with somatic symptoms of obscure origin as well as symptoms caused by psychosocial problems other than affective disorder. This indeterminacy is a general problem with the diagnosis of somatized depression in the absence of affective symptoms. Nevertheless, as done in this study, classification on the basis of symptom presentation suggests that these somatic-vegetative patients appear most similar to patients presenting with psychosocial complaints with the exception that they are less likely to choose affective explantations for ambiguous symptoms. Although they consider themselves just as emotionally vulnerable as patients who present psychosocially, consistent with their non-affective presentation, the somatic-vegetative group avoids affective interpretations of distress. It is difficult to determine whether avoidance of affective interpretations among the somatic-vegetative group presents a defense against the fear of having a psychological problem or is due to the natural history of depression, which may begin with physical symptoms long before emotional complaints or attributions develop (Cadoret, Widmer, and Troughton, 1980).

A second use of the term somatization concerns somatic symptoms of obscure origin. Somatic symptoms that cannot be explained after investigation are often assumed to be functional symptoms. The misattribution of symptoms to organic rather than social or emotional causes is a type of somatization of distress. The present results, however, failed to show that patients with somatic-obscure presentations were different in any respect from patients with somatic symptoms explained organically. Like the somatic-organic group, somatic-obscure patients differ from psychosocial presenters in perceiving themselves as less vulnerable to emotional illness and in making fewer affective attributions for ambiguous symptoms. Contrary to the expectation that unexplained somatic suffering reflects expressions of a somatic bias in evaluation and interpretation of functional symptoms, somatic-obscure patients felt no more vulnerable to physical illness nor were they more somatically focused in symptom attributions than other patients.

Finally, somatization may also refer to patients' emphasis on, or preoccupation with, somatic symptoms that accompany psychosocial distress. Somatic symptoms of obscure origin were common among patients who presented psychosocially. Though they each acknowledged emotional or interpersonal distress, 13 of the 17 patients in this group also complained of somatic symptoms (headache, tiredness, dizziness, numbness, insomnia) that their physicians were unable to explain by organic pathology. Many of their complaints could be considered somatic expressions accompanying psychosocial distress. Functional somatic complaints would appear equally common among patients declaring or revealing psychosocial problems as among those who do not report such difficulties. Thus, the lack of recognition and expression of psychological distress cannot be construed as a cause of functional somatic symptoms in many of these patients.

## CONCLUSIONS

In this chapter a multivariate approach to the cognitive factors of illness behaviour has been presented. Several distinct influences on illness cognition including self- and body focus, somatic and affective symptom recognition and causal attribution were shown to make independent contributions to symptom reports and presentations.

The cross-sectional nature of these data temper the conclusions that can be made. While the conceptualization suggests that cognitive styles should cause symptom experience and reporting, only a consistent relationship between cognitive styles and symptom reporting has been demonstrated. Longitudinal data are required to rule out other, perhaps more parsimonious, explanations of these relationships. It must be considered, for example, that patients with many somatic symptoms become more concerned with their bodily changes and learn to interpret all sensations and feeling states as consistent with the way they feel. A sample of patients are currently being followed over time to determine the prospective utility of illness cognition styles.

Although the use of self-report questionnaires and forced choice items inevitably imposes a conceptual structure on respondents, the present approach complements more open-ended data collection. What the multivariable approach loses in richness it gains in analytic power. This approach may provide useful direction in re-examining the problem of sociocultural factors in illness behaviour. With more precise definitions of patient presentation, such measurement procedures may permit detailed study of the cognitive contributions to somatization and psychologization.

ACKNOWLEDGEMENT

We would like to thank Dr. Sidney Feldman, Dr. Michael Dworkind, Michael Buonvino and Ruth Nabi for their generous assistance. The enthusiasm and hard work of our interviewers made this study possible. This research was supported in part by a grant from the Medical Research Foundation of the Sir Mortimer B. Davis - Jewish General Hospital.

## APPENDIX

### INTERCORRELATIONS OF ILLNESS COGNITION MEASURES, FAMILY MEDICINE PATIENTS

| | Self-focus | | Symptom Recognition | | Symptom Interpretation | |
|---|---|---|---|---|---|---|
| | Body consciousness | Self-consciousness | Somatic recognition | Affective recognition | Somatic interpretation | Affective interpretation |
| Body consciousness | - | | | | | |
| Self-consciousness | .33* | - | | | | |
| Somatic recognition | .23* | .22* | - | | | |
| Affective recognition | .25* | .26* | .64* | - | | |
| Somatic interpretation | .26* | -.03 | .19* | .19* | - | |
| Affective interpretation | -.01 | .19* | .19* | .47* | -.37* | - |
| $\overline{X}$ | 3.08 | 5.53 | 1.56 | 1.01 | 3.05 | 4.32 |
| s.d. | 1.20 | 2.39 | 1.65 | 2.10 | 2.29 | 2.89 |

N = 100
* $p < .05$

REFERENCES


American Psychiatric Association. (1980). Diagnostic and statistical manual, Edition III, Washington: American Psychiatric Association.

Barsky, A. J., & Klerman, G. L. (1983). Overview: Hypochondriasis, bodily complaints, and somatic styles. American Journal of Psychiatry, 140, 273-283.

Blackwell, B. (1967). Upper middle class adult expectations about entering the sick role for physical and psychiatric dysfunctions. Journal of Health and Social Behavior, 8, 83-95.

Cadoret, R., Widmer, R. B., & Troughton, E. P. (1980). Somatic complaints: Harbinger of depression in primary care. Journal of Affective Disorders, 2, 61-70.

Cleary, P. D. & Angel, R. (1984). The analysis of relationships involving dichotomous variables. Journal of Health and Social Behavior, 25, 334-348.

Derogatis, L. R., Lipman, R. S., & Covi, L. (1973). SCL-90: An outpatient psychiatric rating scale: Preliminary report. Psychopharmacology Bulletin, 9, 13-27.

Derogatis, L. R., Rickels, K., & Rock, A. F. (1976). The SCL-90 and the MMPI: A step in the validation of a new self-report scale. British Journal of Psychiatry, 128, 280-289.

Eisenberg, L. (1977). Disease and illness: Distinctions between professional and popular ideas of sickness. Culture, Medicine and Psychiatry, 1, 9-23.

Fava, G. A., Pilowsky, I., Pierfederici, A., et al. (1982). Depressive symptoms and abnormal illness behavior in general hospital patients. General Hospital Psychiatry, 4, 171-178.

Fenigstein, A., Scheier, M. F., & Buss, A. H. (1975). Public and private self-consciousness: Assessment and theory. Journal of Consulting and Clinical Psychology, 43, 522-527.

Hansell, S., & Mechanic, D. (in press). Introspectiveness and adolescent symptom reporting. Journal of Human Stress.

Helman, C. G. (1985). Psyche, soma, and society: The social construction of psychosomatic disorders. Culture, Medicine and Psychiatry, 9, 1-26.

Katon, W., & Dengerink, H. A. (1983). Somatization in primary health care. In J. E. Carr, & H. A. Dengerink (Eds.), Behavioral science in the practice of medicine. New York: Elsevier Biomedical.

Katon, W., Kleinman, A., & Rosen, G. (1982). Depression and somatization: A review. I & II. American Journal of Medicine, 72, 127-135 & 241-247.

Kellner, R. (1985). Functional somatic symptoms and hypochondriasis. Archives of General Psychiatry, 42, 821-833.

Kirmayer, L. J. (1984). Culture, affect and somatization. Transcultural Psychiatric Research Review, 21, 159-188 & 21, 237-262.

Kirmayer, L. J. (in press). Mind and body as metaphors: Hidden values in biomedicine. In M. Lock & D. Gordon (Eds.), Knowledge and practice in medicine. Dordrecht: D. Reidel.

Kleinman, A. (1980). Patients and healers in the context of culture. Berkeley: University of California Press.

Leventhal, H., & Nerenz, D. R. (1985). The assessment of illness cognition. In P. Karoly (Ed.), Measurement strategies in health psychology. New York: John Wiley.

Leventhal, H., Nerenz, D. R., Steele, D. J. (1985). Illness representations and coping with health threats. In A. Baum & J. Singer (Eds.), Handbook of psychology and health. Hillsdale, NJ: Erlbaum.

Leventhal, H., Nerenz, D. R., & Straus, A. (1982). Self-regulation and the mechanisms for symptom appraisal. In D. Mechanic (Ed.), Symptoms, illness behavior and help-seeking. New York: Neale Watson.

McCrae, R. R., & Costa, P. T. (1983). Social desirability scales: More substance than style. Journal of Consulting and Clinical Psychology, 51, 882-888.

McKinlay, J. B. (1973). Social networks, lay consultation, and help-seeking behaviour. Social Forces, 51, 275-292.
McWhinney, I. R. (1972). Beyond diagnosis: An approach to the integration of behavioral science and clinical medicine. New England Journal of Medicine, 287, 384-387.
Mechanic, D. (1980). The experience and reporting of common physical symptoms. Journal of Health and Social Behavior, 21, 146-155.
Meyer, D., Leventhal, H., & Gutmann, M. (1985). Common-sense models of illness: The example of hypertension. Health Psychology, 4, 115-135.
Miller, L. C., Murphy, R., & Buss, A. H. (1981). Consciousness of body: Private and public. Journal of Personality and Social Psychology, 41, 397-406.
Pennebaker, J. W. (1982). The psychology of physical symptoms. New York: Springer.
Pennebaker, J. W., & Skelton, J. A. (1978). Psychological parameters of physical symptoms. Personality and Social Psychology Bulletin, 4, 524-530.
Pilowsky, I. (1967). Dimensions of hypochondriasis. British Journal of Psychiatry, 113, 89-93.
Pilowsky, I. (1969). Abnormal illness behaviour. British Journal of Medical Psychology, 42, 347-351.
Pilowksy, I. (1978). A general classification of abnormal illness behaviours. British Journal of Medical Psychology, 51, 131-137.
Pilowsky, I., Murrell, T. G. C., & Gordon, A. (1979). The development of a screening method for abnormal illness behaviour. Journal of Psychosomatic Research, 23, 203-207.
Pilowsky, I., & Spence, D. (1975). Patterns of illness behaviour in patients with intractable pain. Journal of Psychological Measurement, 1, 385-401.
Pilowsky, I., Spence, N., Cobb, J., & Katsikitis, M. (1984). The illness behavior questionnaire as an aid to clinical assessment. General Hospital Psychiatry, 6, 123-130.
Radloff, L. S. (1977). The CES-D scale: A self-report depression scale for research in the general population. Applied Psychological Measurement, 1, 385-401.
Robbins, J. M., & Greenley, J. R. (1983). Thinking about what's wrong: Attributions of severity, cause, and duration in the problem definition stage of psychiatric help-seeking. In J. R. Greenley (Ed.), Research in Community and Mental Health, Vol. 3, Greenwich, CT: JAI Press.
Schuessler, K., Hittle, D., & Cardascia, J. (1978). Measuring responding desirable with attitude opinion items. Social Psychology, 41, 224-235.
Stewart, M. A., McWhinney, I., & Buck, C. (1975). How illness presents: A study of patient behavior. Journal of Family Practice, 2, 411-414.
Tollefson, G., Straud, L., Hughes, E., & Garvey, M. G. (1984). The functional-organic dichotomy in new patient evaluations by residents in family practice. Comprehensive Psychiatry, 25, 419-425.
Verbrugge, L. M. (1979). Marital status and health. Journal of Marriage and the Family, 41, 267-285.
Weissman, M. M., & Klerman, G. L. (1977). Sex differences and the epidemiology of depression. Archives of General Psychiatry, 34, 98-111.
Weyrauch, K. F. (1984). The decision to see the physician: A clinical investigation. Journal of Family Practice, 18, 265-272.
White, G. M. (1982). The role of cultural explanations in 'somatization' and 'psychologization'. Social Science and Medicine, 16, 1519-1530.
Zborowski, M. (1952). Cultural components in response to pain. Journal of Social Issues, 8, 16-30.
Zola, I. (1966). Culture and symptoms - An analysis of patients' presenting complaints. American Sociological Review, 31, 615-630.

# PART VI COPING: ADAPTATION TO STRESS

# COPING STRATEGIES

Richard Lazarus

Department of Psychology
University of California

This chapter focuses on a metatheory of stress and coping, and advances five main points. Much of what is presented here has been detailed elsewhere (Lazarus and Folkman, 1984; Lazarus, 1966; Lazarus, DeLongis, Folkman and Gruen, 1985). Nonetheless, particularly important new efforts in this area are highlighted.

Based on extensive research, the following points can be made concerning stress. For example, it is not equivalent to life events, no matter what metric is used. Rather, stress is a complex rubric or system of interdependent variables and processes that encompasses emotion as well as other variables.

Table 1 outlines three kinds of variables - antecedents, mediating processes, and adaptational outcomes important in understanding stress. Individual differences in goal hierarchies are illustrative of antecedents. The goals that are most or least important to a given individual are particularly important. A second important antecedent variable involves beliefs about oneself and the world. In addition, there are situational antecedents, for example, demands, constraints, and opportunities or resources. As mediating processes, cognitive appraisal and coping are emphasized and central in the work of Lazarus and associates. Adaptational outcomes are differentiated into those in the short-term and those that occur in the long-term. Among short-term outcomes that occur, the most important is the emotion generated in a particular stressful encounter. Long-term outcome variables include morale or the sense of well-being, health, and social functioning.

The theoretical research task in order to validate such a system is to determine the pathways of influence among the variables. Individual researchers usually concentrate on given segments of the total system and not the interaction between them. This does not mean taking a particular methodological approach, such as path analysis, but examining which variables influence each other and in what ways.

Coping needs to be conceptualized and measured because it is one of the main mediating processes, perhaps the most important one from the point of view of human functioning under conditions of stress. There has been a revolutionary change in the last five to ten years in the way people think about, and do research on, coping. The change is from a top-down search for

TABLE 1 A THEORETICAL SCHEMATIZATION OF STRESS, COPING, AND ADAPTATIION

| CAUSAL ANTECEDENTS | MEDIATING PROCESSES Time 1...T2...T3...Tn Encounter 1...2...3...n | IMMEDIATE EFFECTS | Long-term Effects |
|---|---|---|---|
| Person variables: | Primary appraisal | Physiological changes | Somatic health/ illness |
| values-commitments beliefs: existential sense of control | Secondary appraisal | Positive or negative feelings | Morale (well-being) |
| | Reappraisal | Quality of encounter | Social functioning |
| Environment: | | | |
| | Coping: | | |
| (situational) demands constraints | problem-focused emotion-focused seeking, obtaining and using social support | | |
| resources (e.g., social network) | | | |
| ambiguity of harm | | | |
| | Resolutions of each stressful encounter | | |
| imminence of harm | | | |

*Reprinted (with permission) from Lazarus, R. S., & Folkman, S. (1984). Stress, appraisal, and coping. New York: Springer.

stable traits or styles of coping to a bottom-up focus on the process of coping in specific contexts. In order to understand coping it is essential to describe concretely what people think and do to cope with specific harms and threats in their daily lives.

The essence of a process or transactional approach to coping can be described by three criteria:

(a) There must be a specific context. Coping must be studied in a specific encounter. One must ask not what one might do or would do in that context, or in general, but what is or was actually done or thought. A context can be broad or narrow, and one can get into serious trouble if the context is too broad. An example of a relatively broad context would be having cancer. How the person copes with cancer is an almost meaningless question because so many diverse harms and threats could be involved. Each separate threat may be coped with quite differently by the same individual. For example, the patient does not know for certain whether metastases has occurred and, therefore, whether the cancer is likely to recur. Another threat is the discomfort and pain of treatment or the side effects of chemotherapy or other treatments, such as loss of hair, pain, nausea, loss of energy or the ability to function well. Another potential threat consists of dealing with family or friends. What should one say about one's condition when people ask, and how should it be said? An early-stage cancer is psychologically not the same situation as a late-stage cancer.

Consider also persons who have had cancer surgery and who have to return regularly to the hospital or to the laboratory to get a CAT scan or other tests to see if there have been any metastases. The person may have managed for quite a while without thinking much about the threat. It is on hold and quiescent, not often in consciousness. Then suddenly, the time for the test becomes imminent and now there is a very different psychological situation. What is the test going to reveal? There is a recurrence of apprehension about a problem that had been laid aside but cannot be any longer until the results of the test are known. Each time this occurs the old threat is revived.

The coping process may not be the same in dealing with each of the very different threats associated with an illness like cancer. If all these diverse threats are collapsed into one global but complicated condition (cancer) or are aggregated over time and diverse stages of an illness that does not remain static, one will be confused about exactly what is going on with respect to coping. A clear understanding of the dynamics of coping will be lost. Therefore, what the person thinks and does in a particular context must be examined so that the connection between particular threats and the process of coping is not obscured.

(b) To examine coping as a process means to be in a position to observe changes in coping over time or across occasions. This is what process means. Folkman and Lazarus (1985) did this in a recent study examining the separate temporal stages of a college student examination, which is usually treated as a single unit. In each stage - for example, the warning period, the impact period, and the post-impact period (to use the language of disaster research), coping changes. This is because the relationship that the person has with the environment has, perforce, changed with changes in the psychological situation. Such changes would be obscured if we lumped all stages together as a single encounter or event.

(c) To look at change, one is obliged to use ipsative-normative or longitudinal styles of research. This requires observing the same individual across a variety of encounters or over time.

Two perspectives must be used in the study of the coping process. The first is intra-individual or within the individual and the second is inter-individual. In the intra-individual perspective, the person is compared with himself or herself across diverse contexts or at different stages of an encounter. One can, by doing this, examine how much change or stability there is for the coping process or the person's emotional state. Does the individual do the same thing regardless of the source of stress that he or she is dealing with or, as is consistently found, does the coping process change from one encounter to another (Folkman, Lazarus, Dunkel-Schetter, DeLongis, and Gruen, in press)? One can assess which form of coping is used by a particular person or group to deal with a specific kind of threat, and which mode of coping works best for any given type of person or threat.

Looked at another way, intra-individual analysis permits the examination of an individual's strengths and weaknesses with respect to stress and coping. Most individuals cope well in some situations and badly in others, and from a clinical point of view this provides us with valuable diagnostic information about a person. In a clinical therapeutic interview, one tries to put together a diagnostic picture of the contexts in which the person is in trouble or does well. Attention is often paid, however, only to the pathological side, yet even people who are in trouble manage some things reasonably well. Managing life involves managing many diverse demands, taking into account internal and social constraints, and taking advantage of multiple resources. This complex pattern can only be assessed by employing an intra-individual perspective.

The Ways of Coping Scale contains eight coping factors (Lazarus and Folkman, 1984). Suppose, for example, one wanted to examine the use of distancing, whereby the person tries to be detached from the problem, to cool it, so to speak. Distancing is valuable when nothing can be done except to wait. In other contexts, however, something can be done, in which case the person should mobilize, not cool it, and direct maximum energy toward changing things. The important point here is that it is not sound to assume that one or another process of coping is always good or bad; rather, what works in one context may be counterproductive in another. So we must always examine the effectiveness of coping with respect to its fit with a particular set of demands, constraints and resources, and never disembodied from the context in which it happens.

In contrast, one can compare one person with another with an inter-individual perspective. This is essential for the study of the long-range health consequences of stress and coping because one can consider what is stable about stress and coping in a person over time, and much illness takes a long time to bring about. Lazarus and associates aggregate what a person does over many contexts in an attempt to identify stable stress and coping traits that might affect long-term well-being and functioning, traits that transcend the specific context. It is an unanswered question whether one can locate stable and powerful traits or styles of coping in this way. Previous efforts to identify styles without looking at the coping process in numerous contexts, or over time, have not resulted in fruitful answers.

In a recent effort to aggregate coping across stressful encounters, correlations of the coping process in five specific stressful encounters over a five-month period were obtained (Folkman, Lazarus, Gruen, and DeLongis, in press). The key question was whether the person coped by the same or different thoughts and acts in one encounter compared with another. The obtained correlations were generally low, that is, the coping process varied from one encounter to another. The coping scale with the highest autocorrelations (+.47) across five entirely different stressful encounters was positive reappraisal. A person who used positive reappraisal as a way of dealing with one stressful encounter had a greater probability of doing the same thing in another stressful encounter. The lowest autocorrelation was for the coping scale of seeking social support (+.17); in other words this type of coping was more contextual.

When coping is studied, one should give special attention to certain stresses in a person's life rather than all stresses. In effect, we make a distinction between central and peripheral hassles (Gruen, Folkman, and Lazarus, in press).

Gruen and others asked 150 subjects to choose the one hassle from the ten most frequent hassles they reported over a five-month period which was most central to their lives and another one which was most peripheral. The following were the instructions given the subjects to define central and peripheral hassles:

> Hassles can differ in how much they say about you as a distinctive individual. Some hassles are very central and revealing and others are not. A central hassle is one that expresses what is most important for you. That is, they have to do with enterprises or concerns in which you have a major stake. This kind of hassle might reflect a troubling problem, an ongoing theme in your life such as an unresolved conflict, an unfulfilled need or a personal inadequacy. Other hassles are not central and do not have to do with anything deeply important to you. They deal with matters that are superficial.

Subjects were first asked to rate on Likert-type scales the properties of central and peripheral hassles and, second, to rate the centrality of all the hassles that they had endorsed previously over the four-month period. The findings produced by these procedures have to do with the characteristics of central and peripheral hassles, and with their relationships with health outcomes. The results can be summarized as follows.

Central hassles, more than peripheral ones, reflected problems of emotional control and deficits in coping skills. For example, central hassles were rated as requiring a change in oneself, and were described as caused more by personal needs and expectations than peripheral ones.

What was central for one person was not necessarily so for others, and individual differences in this were enormous. In effect, one cannot rely on normative ratings for stressful events but must identify what is central for each person or like-minded person, which requires ultimately diagnosing each person's distinctive pattern.

Subjects were asked to go back over all 53 hassles on the scale and to rate each one they had endorsed over the previous four months on its degree of centrality. A mean severity score for each subject on his or her central hassles and a mean severity score for peripheral hassles was calculated. These scores were used as a correlate of health status (DeLongis, Coyne, Dakof, Folkman, and Lazarus, 1982) and psychological symptoms (using the Hopkins Symptom Checklist of Derogatis, Lipman, Rickels, Uhlenhuth, and Covi, 1974). Central hassles correlated .58 with psychological symptoms and .18 with somatic health, both statistically significant. In contrast, peripheral hassles correlated only .27, with psychological symptoms, still statistically significant, but only .10 with somatic health, which was not significant. Hassles scores were always negatively associated with these health variables.

When the zero-order relationships involving psychological symptoms were examined by multiple regression analyses, centrality added substantial independent variance to symptoms even when the role of peripheral hassles was statistically eliminated. On the other hand, when the variance contributed by central hassles was statistically eliminated, peripheral hassles contributed little. Peripheral hassles seem to add mainly noise to the stress-symptoms relationship. Somatic health was not analyzed in this way because of its initial marginal relationship to hassles.

Although these data do not prove that centrality is a causal factor in psychological symptoms (there is an unknown degree of confounding between our instructions defining centrality and what subjects reported as characteristics of centrality), these findings are at least consistent with the idea that some hassles (central) are more important in health outcome than others. In all likelihood, they recur because they are problematic for the person and distress probably persists long after the encounter is over, whereas peripheral hassles do not have post-encounter intrusiveness.

Future research must be directed to identify the factors that make different people vulnerable to psychological stress in particular classes of situations and predict the pattern of stress reaction for any given individual. Vulnerability may result from chronic environmental conditions that are destructive, and from person characteristics such as strong commitments that engender threat, problematic generalized beliefs about oneself and the world such as low self-esteem, inflexible coping styles that prove counterproductive in certain types of situations, and neurotic conflicts and/or coping ineptitudes. If vulnerability factors can be identified, then they can be used to predict arenas of living in which a given individual is vulnerable to stress, with the increased likelihood of dysfunction in general or in particular contexts of living.

## REFERENCES


DeLongis, A., Coyne, J. C., Dakof, G., Folkman, S., & Lazarus, R. S. (1982). Relationship of daily hassles, uplifts, and major life events to health status. Health Psychology, 1, 119-136.

Derogatis, L. R., Lipman, R. S., Rickels, K., Uhlenhuth, E. H., & Covi, L. (1974). The Hopkins Symptom Checklist (HSCL): A self-report symptom inventory. Behavioral Science, 19, 1-15.

Folkman, S., & Lazarus, R. S. (1985). If is changes it must be a process: Study of emotion and coping during three stages of a college examination. Journal of Personality and Social Psychology, 48, 150-170.

Folkman, S., Lazarus, R. S., Dunkel-Schetter, C., DeLongis, A., & Gruen, R. (in press). The dynamics of a stressful encounter: Cognitive appraisal, coping, and encounter outcomes. Journal of Personality and Social Psychology.

Folkman, S., Lazarus, R. S., Gruen, R., & DeLongis, A. (in press). Appraisal, coping, health status, and psychological symptoms. Journal of Personality and Social Psychology.

Gruen, R. J., Folkman, S., & Lazarus, R. S. (under review). Are some hassles more equal than others? Manuscript submitted for review.

Lazarus, R. S. (1966). Psychological stress and the coping process. New York: McGraw-Hill.

Lazarus, R. S., DeLongis, A., Folkman, S., & Gruen, R. (1985). Stress and adaptational outcomes: The problem of confounded measures. American Psychologist, 40, 770-779.

Lazarus, R. S., & Folkman, S. (1984). Stress, appraisal, and coping. New York: Springer.

# LIVING WITH CHRONIC DISEASE: THE IMPORTANCE OF COGNITIVE APPRAISAL

Dennis Turk and Thomas Rudy

Departments of Psychiatry and Anesthesiology
University of Pittsburgh School of Medicine

The plight of the chronically ill patient covers a wide array of potential life interruptions and psychological changes as well as illness-related factors such as permanent changes in physical functioning and in physical appearance. Patients with various chronic illnesses may face separation from families, friends, and other sources of gratification, the loss of social and vocational roles, disruption of plans for the future, assaults on self-image and self-esteem, uncertain and unpredictable futures, and distressing emotional reactions (Turk, 1979). Moreover, by nature of the disease, chronic illnesses unlike acute diseases have an extended time course of months or years with repeated demands recurring throughout the adjustment process.

## THE RELATIONSHIP BETWEEN CHRONIC ILLNESS AND DEPRESSION

On the basis of such extensive adjustment demands, it would be no surprise to expect that the presence of a chronic disease would result in significant emotional difficulties. Depending upon how one views the available statistics, the expectancy of psychological distress can be either confirmed or denied. For example, across a heterogeneous set of diseases and disabilities (e.g., chronic pain patients; Romano and Turner, 1985; end-stage renal disease, Devins et al., 1982; cancer patients, Bukberg, Penman, and Holland, 1984; physically disabled, Turner, Noh, and Levin, 1985) there appears to be evidence that between 20 to 50 percent of patients will display some level of depression. As would be expected, severity of the illness does appear to be associated with depressive symptomatology. For example, Moffic and Paykel (1975) reported that 61 percent of patients with severe medical illness were depressed but only 21 percent of those with illnesses classified as only mild to moderately severe were depressed.

These statistics can be taken as providing support for the contention that chronic illnesses are associated with depression or dysphoric mood. However, these incidence rates of depression need to be assessed in comparison to the degree of depression in the general population. Based on two large samples of the general community, 18 to 19 percent of the population show significant signs of depression (Comstock and Helsing, 1976). These percentages are roughly equivalent to those identified by Moffic and Paykel (1975) for those patients with illness of mild to moderate severity. Additionally, in a large study comparing patients with arthritis, diabetes, cancer, renal disease, and dermatological disorders, Cassileth et al. (1984) reported that none of these patient groups were significantly different from each other or the general population in terms of the percentage who revealed signs of dysphoric mood or depressive symptomatology. Schulz and Decker (1985) and Brooks and Matson (1982) reported similar results for spinal cord injured persons and those with multiple sclerosis, respectively. Thus, estimates of the incidence of depression among the chronically ill range from equivalent to two and one-half times the rates reported in the general population. If 20 to 50 percent of chronically ill patients are depressed, that leaves 50 to 80 percent who reveal no significant levels of dysphoric mood despite the presence of illnesses that are clearly disruptive and traumatic.

Measurement Issues

One potential explanation for the variance among incidence rates is that much of the research establishing depression among chronically ill people have employed measures of depression that include symptoms that are as likely to be associated with a major physical problem as they are a sign of depression (Bukberg et al., 1984). For example, among the most common methods used to assess depression are the use of self-report instruments developed for use with psychiatric populations (e.g., Beck Depression Inventory, BDI, Beck, Ward, Mendelsohn, Mock, and Erbaugh, 1961; Hamilton Rating Scale for Depression, HRSD, Hamilton, 1960; and Minnesota Multiphasic Personality Inventory, MMPI, Hathaway and McKinley, 1943). The BDI and HRSD include items concerning sleep dysfunction, changes in appetite and weight, and sexual interest and activity and the MMPI depression scale includes many items concerning somatic functioning. Similarly, the Diagnostic and Statistical Manual of the American Psychiatric Association (DSM-III, American Psychiatric Association, 1980) and the Research Diagnostic Criteria for Major Depression (Feighner et al., 1972) each include items that may be a result of physical illness (e.g., loss or gain of weight, insomnia, reduction in sexual activity). Thus, the application of these assessment procedures to the chronically ill is likely to inflate the estimated prevalence of depression among medical patients.

In considering the incidence and prevalence of depression among people with chronic illnesses, one is reminded of the Thematic Apperception Test (TAT, Murray, 1943) card that shows an acrobat clinging midway on a rope. The question is, is the acrobat half-way up or half-way down? How one responds to the prevalence of depression among the chronically ill may tell more about the observer than the observed. Despite this issue, there is little doubt that although a subset of people with chronic illness are depressed, there is also a substantial number of patients who appear to make satisfactory if not heroic adjustments to their illness with minimal distress (e.g., Binik, 1983; Schulz and Decker, 1985; Tattersall, 1981; Visotsky, Hamburg, Goss, and Lebovits, 1961).

## MEDIATING FACTORS LINKING CHRONIC ILLNESSES AND DEPRESSIVE SYMPTOMATOLOGY

A considerable body of literature has focused on identifying those factors that differentiate patients who show varying degrees of adjustment and dysphoric mood. Three major mediating variables have received the largest degree of attention, (a) predisposing dispositional factors, (b) social supports, and (c) coping strategies or repertoires. Despite historic emphasis and the extensive search for personality factors or styles that differentiate "good" and "poor" adjusters, there is no satisfactory data to support the role of personality dispositions in predicting adjustment to chronic illnesses.

More recently, social support has recieved a great deal of attention (e.g., Kaplan, Cassel, and Gore, 1977). Although social support systems appear to be important, the role of support in the mediation of the illness-depression relationship remains somewhat equivocal. Part of the difficulty with social support relates to confusion and disagreement as to how this construct should be operationalized and the relevant dimensions of support to measure (see recent reviews of this topic presented by Cohen and Wills, 1985 and the special issue of The Journal of Social Issues edited by Brownell and Shumaker, 1984).

As with personality dispositions, the importance of coping styles and coping strategies has also been the focus of much attention. However, there does not appear to be any specific coping style or coping strategy that characterizes those who make satisfactory of unsatisfactory adjustments (Cohen and Lazarus, 1979; Meichenbaum, Turk, and Burstein, 1975). What does appear to be more important than a particular coping style or coping strategy is the ability to respond in a flexible fashion rather than rigidly employing a limited set of coping techniques (Antonovsky, 1979; Turk, Sobel, Follick, and Youkilis, 1980).

## THE ROLE OF COGNITIVE APPRAISAL

As noted earlier, an important characteristic of chronic diseases and disabilities is the temporal dimension. Chronic illnesses extended over time. The individual does not simply cope with a chronic illness but rather the individual is continually called upon to make adjustments. He or she confronts repeated and often new demands over the course of the illness. Throughout this process, the individual continually appraises and reappraises his or her situation, evaluates how well he or she is doing, and continually takes stock of the available resources. These appraisal processes are likely to have an important impact on dysphoric mood, and dysphoric mood, in turn, is likely to influence the appraisal process. Thus, a dynamic transactional process takes place between an individual and his or her environment (Lazarus and Launier, 1978).

To become a source of distress, an event must be judged or appraised as potentially harmful. That is, individuals impose meaning onto their predicament based on their belief systems regarding themselves and the circumstances that confront them. The ongoing appraisal of circumstances, the individual's internal dialogue regarding his or her available coping resources (including social supports), and his/her attitudes and expectancies determine the nature of cognitive, affective, behavioural responses, and subsequently adjustment at any point in time (Lazarus, 1974; Meichenbaum, 1977). It is important to realize, however, that with chronic illness, adjustment should not be viewed as an end-state but rather a continual process. Thus, by means of cognitive appraisal processes, circumstances are repeatedly evaluated and re-evaluated, meaning is ascribed, and the significance of internal as well as external events is established. The reciprocal transaction between the individual with the chronic illness, the illness per se, and the environmental context interact to determine the unique quality of the chronic illness and the adaptive process.

A number of papers (e.g., Devins et al., 1983-1984; Devins, Binik, Hollomby, Barré, and Guttmann, 1981; Schulz and Decker, 1985; Turk, 1979; Turner et al., 1985) have emphasized the importance of the individual patient's appraisal regarding the impact of the disease on his or her life, with particular emphasis on how patients' perceptions of self-control and self-mastery affect adjustment to their illness. Further, these authors have noted that perceptions of self-control and self-mastery may well impact on the individual's mood. Thus, appraisal of the illness, coping resources, and oneself are all important contributors to adjustment and distress at any specific point in time. However, appraisal processes should be viewed as continual and, therefore, patients' levels of distress at any one point in time should not be taken as an indicator of their adjustment to a chronic illness because coping with a chronic condition is a dynamic rather than a static process.

In sum, depression and dysphoric mood might be a readily understandable or even expected secondary reaction to a chronic and incapacitating physical condition. However, the presence of a chronic illness does not appear sufficient or to inevitably cause the subsequent development of depressive symptomatology. Rather, the development of depression may be mediated by personality dispositions, by the absence of or presence of maladaptive social supports, by maladaptive coping styles or inadequate coping repertoires, or more likely, by some combination of these variables. The individual's appraisal of his or her continuing circumstances and resources, however, may play a central mediating role (Linn and Greenfield, 1982; Westbrook and Viney, 1982).

## TOWARD A COGNITIVE-BEHAVIOURAL TRANSACTION MODEL

Rather than assuming a direct link between chronic illness and depression, the authors have proposed a cognitive-behavioural transaction model to explain the apparent association between chronic illness and depression (Turk, Kerns, and Rudy, 1985). This model integrated contemporary behavioural (Ferster, 1973; Lewinsohn, 1974) and cognitive (Beck, 1967; Rehm, 1977; Seligman, 1975) formulations of depression. Specifically, the model hypothesizes that depression is a function of the perception of reduction in instrumental activities and a concomitant decline in important social rewards, as well as a decline in perceptions of control over reinforcement contingencies and self-efficacy. The working hypothesis is that cognitive appraisals rather than actual reductions in instrumental activities, rewards, and control serve as the mediating link between chronic illness and depression.

### A Test of the Cognitive-Behavioural Transaction Model

To provide a preliminary test of the cognitive-behavioural transaction model, a heterogeneous group of chronic pain patients with a diversity of physical conditions was studied. According to the model, the experience of chronic pain is not a sufficient condition for the development of depressive symptomatology. That is, the direct causal link between pain and depression should be small and minimally useful in accounting for the relationship between these two syndromes. Rather, the perception of significant declines in life satisfaction since the onset of pain, the perceived interference of the pain syndrome with various life activities, and lower perceptions of self-control and self-efficacy, are hypothesized to act as necessary mediators or indirect links between the experience of pain and depressive symptoms.

Figure 1 pictorially presents the predictions made by the cognitive-behavioural model. Specifically, as can be seen in Figure 1, this model hypothesizes that increases in pain severity should lead to increases in life interference, which in turn, based on cognitive-behavioural theories of depression, should increase the extent of an individual's depressive symptomatology. Additionally, as also displayed in Figure 1, pain severity is predicted to have an inverse affect on a patient's perceived level of self-control that, as a result of this decline in self-control, should increase a patient's level of depression. Finally, based on the hypothesized effects of interference and self-control and the pain-depression relationship, it is hypothesized that these mediational factors would be sufficient to explain the relationship between pain and depression and that a significant residual indicating a direct connection between pain and depression would not be found. Thus, if the predictions made by the cognitive-behavioural model are plausible, then the following pattern of regression coefficients should be found: (a) the coefficients between pain severity and interference and between interference and depression should both be positive, (b) the coefficients between pain severity and self-control and between self-control and depression should both be negative, and (c) the

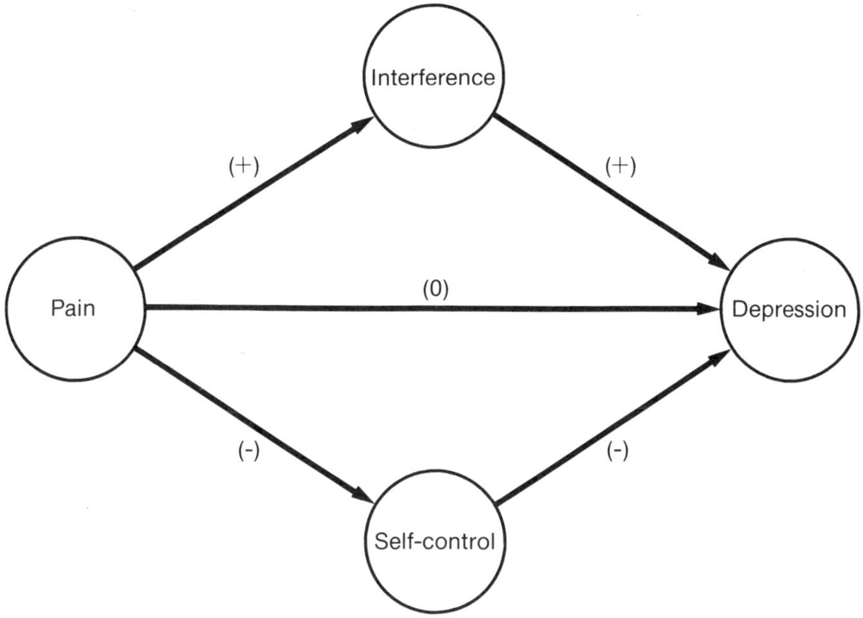


**FIGURE 1.** Hypothesized cognitive-behavioural mediation model of chronic pain and depression

direct link between pain severity and depression should display a nonsignificant coefficient. In this study causal modeling with latent variables was used because it permits a direct test of the degree of congruence between these predictions and the actual relationships observed in data collected from chronic pain patients.

One hundred pain patients who were evaluated at a pain management program (West Haven, Connecticut) served as the subjects for this study. The patients had a diversity of diagnoses and a mean duration of pain of over ten years. A number of measures were employed to assess the relevant constructs, namely, pain intensity, perceived interference, perceived control, and depressive symptomatology. Pain intensity was assessed by pain rating cards (Turk, Meichenbaum, and Genest, 1983), the McGill Pain Questionnaire (MPQ, Melzack, 1975), and the pain severity scale from the West Haven-Yale Multidimensional Pain Inventory (1) (WHYMPI-Pain Severity; Kerns, Turk, and Rudy, 1985).

Depression was measured by the Beck Depression Inventory (BDI; Beck et al., 1961) and the Depression Adjective Checklist (DACL; Lubin, 1965). Perceived interference with life activities attributed by patients to pain was assessed by three scales from the WHYMPI (Kerns et al., 1985), namely

---

1. The West Haven-Yale Multidimensional Inventory is a psychometrically sound instrument developed specifically for chronic pain patients and provides measures on 12 scales related to the impact of pain on the individual's life. Copies of this inventory can be obtained from the authors.

Social, Work, and Family Interference. These interference scales were comprised of items related to how much patients felt pain had affected their ability to participate in social and recreational activities, vocational activities, as well as the amount of satisfaction that they derived from these activities. Finally, perceived control was measured by items from the WHYMPI related to how much control patients felt they had over their lives during the past week (WHYMPI-Life Control), how much they felt they had been able to solve their problems during the past week (WHYMPI-Problem Solving), and the Internal subscale from the Multidimensional Health Locus of Control (MHLC-Internal; Wallston, Wallston, and DeVellis, 1978).

The LISREL-V computer program (Joreskog and Sorbom, 1981) was used to obtain the maximum-likelihood estimates of all model parameters and a chi-square goodness-of-fit statistic. To more fully assess the goodness-of-fit of the model to the obtained data without the potential biasing effects of sample size and departures from a multivariate normal distribution, a normed goodness-of-fit index suggested by Bentler and Bonett, (1980) was also computed. This index, which ranges from 0 to 1 (1 = the model completely explains the observed data), describes the degree to fit of a specific structural model relative to a given baseline. Although several types of baselines may be conceptually appropriate (Bentler and Bonett, 1980), the most frequently used is a null model that postulates no covariation among the variables. In terms of the present study, the null model hypothesis was that depression, pain severity, interference, and self-control were independent. Thus, this index estimated the improvement in variance accounted for by the specific cognitive-behavioural transaction model over a null model that assumed there were no common factors or inter-relationships.

The overall chi-square goodness-of-fit statistic computed by the LISREL-V computer program indicated that this model had a satisfactory level of statistical fit to these data, X(2)(39) = 49.59, p = ns. Additionally, the Bentler-Bonnett (1980) normed index, with the null model employed as the baseline, was computed to be .91. Thus, these goodness-of-fit indices demonstrated that not only did the cognitive-behavioural transaction model statistically fit these data, but also explained a substantial proportion of the total covariation among the observed measures.

The parameter estimates (factor loadings and path coefficients) computed for this analysis are displayed in Figure 2. Examination of this figure indicates that the Pain, Self-Control, Interference, and Depression constructs (latent variables) were adequately operationalized by the measured variables (a) all factor- loading estimates were statistically significant and (b) the correlations between a measured variable with its latent construct were high.

The statistical results for the path-analytic portion of the cognitive-behavioural transaction mediation model are also presented in Figure 2. Significance testing of these regression coefficients indicated that all the regression coefficients hypothesized among the latent variables were found to be statistically significant with the exception of the direct path between pain and depression. Additionally, as can be seen in Figure 2, the paths between pain severity and interference and interference and depression were both computed to be positive, as hypothesized, and the paths between pain severity and self-control and between self-control and depression were both found to be negative, also as predicted by the cogntive-behavioural transaction model.

In sum, the results of this study provide support for the cognitive-behavioural transaction model of depression among chronic pain patients. Specifically, this model predicted that the direct relationship between pain and depression would be nonsignificant and the cognitive appraisal variables of perceived interference and lack of self-control would be significant mediators of the pain-depression relationship. Consistent with

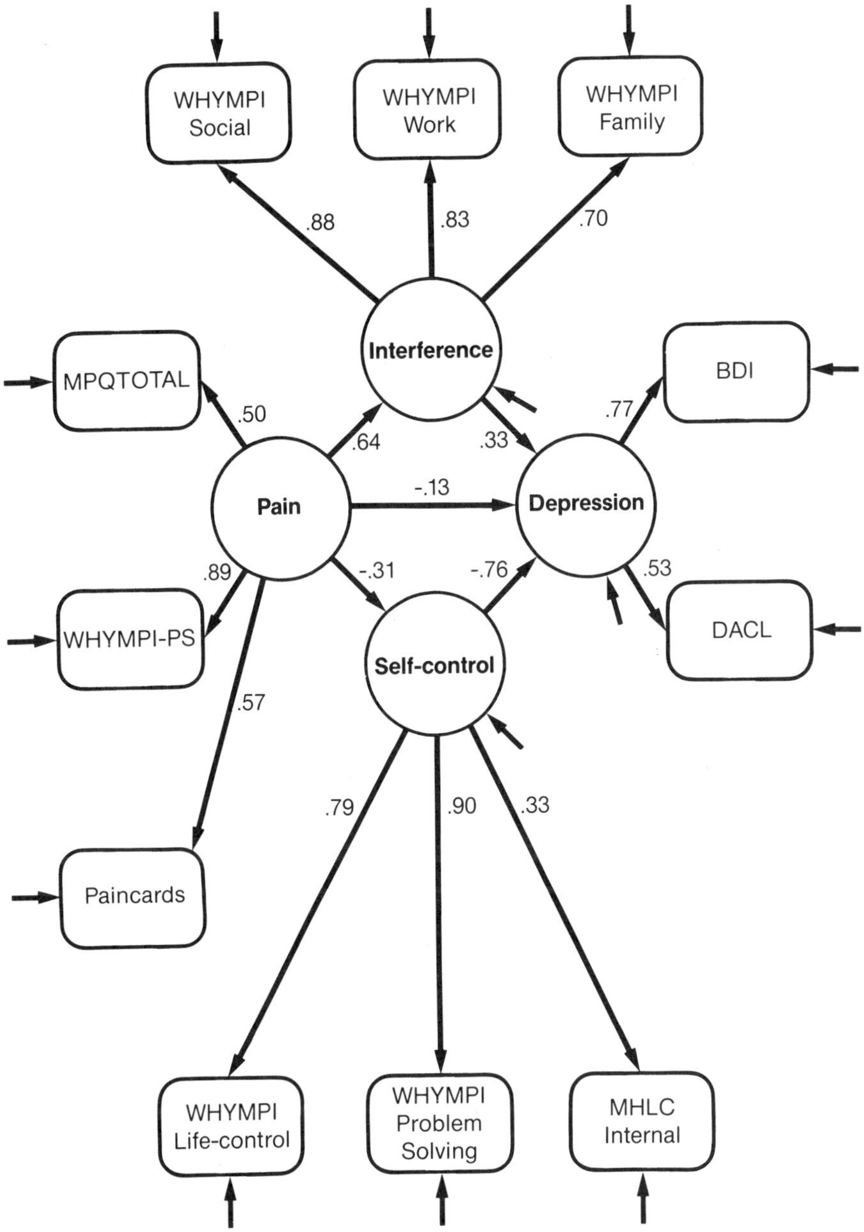


**FIGURE 2.** LISREL parameter estimates for a cognitive-behavioural latent variable model of chronic pain and depression

the general findings of the prevalence of depression among chronic pain patients (see Romano and Turner, 1985), the prevalence of significant levels of depression among the chronic pain patients used in this study was approximately 50 percent. Although a Pearson correlation revealed a modest yet significant association between pain and depression (r = .30), through the use of structural modeling, it was determined that the direct link between pain and depression was not significant. Rather, the association between pain and depression was significantly mediated by perceived interference and lack of self-control. The structural equation that consisted of pain, perceived interference, and perceived lack of self-control accounted for over 68 percent of the variance in depression.

The cognitive-behavioural mediation model suggests that depression among chronic pain patients can be parsimoniously explained by patients' appraisals of the degree to which pain interferes with important areas of functioning and perceptions of self-control. Adapting Lewinsohn's (1974) behavioural model of depression, chronic pain patients may be expected to become depressed as they experience declines in response-contingent reinforcement associated with declines in the frequency and range of instrumental activities. Thus, as patients leave the work place, withdraw social and recreational activities, and limit their activities in the home and with their families, they may be expected to experience declines in the level of contingent rewards in their life.

As attempts at pain relief fail and as efforts to continue or resume activities are unsuccessful, it is understandable that perceptions of helplessness and reduced self-control develop. Cognitive models of depression emphasizing the importance of attributions of helplessness (Abrmason, Seligman, and Teasdale, 1978) and reduced self-control (Rehm, 1977) have been articulated and supported empirically. Results of the present study support the idea that a relatively global perception of lowered self-control and self-efficacy may be an important mediator of the development of depressive symptoms among chronic pain patients. Furthermore, the appraisal of self-control was found to be relatively independent of the appraisal of pain interference (r = -.20), suggesting that each variable should continue to be examined for its theoretical as well as clinical significance. Rehm's (1977) adaptation of Kanfer's (1970) self-control model may prove useful in further understanding the relationshp between self-control and depression. Specifically, to what extent do pain patients manifest deficits in self-monitoring, self-evaluation, or self-reinforcement related to their appraisals of their pain and events in their lives, and to what extent do these specific deficits contribute to the experience of depression?

## Additional Research Support for the Cognitive-Behavioural Mediation Model

The study described above provides some preliminary support for the cognitive-behavioural transaction model of chronic illness and depression. There are several limitations of this study, most notably these analyses are based on cross-sectional data and the use of the BDI that includes items related to somatic symptoms that might be associated with physical illness as well as depression. Future research needs (a) to validate these findings on other populations, (b) employ measures of depressive symptomatology that are influenced by an individual's medical condition, and (c) use longitudinal designs that allow better assessments of the temporal affects of self-appraisals on individuals' mood states. An additional concern might be that the model is specific to chronic pain and would not generalize to other chronic diseases. Recent results from the authors' and other laboratories, however, suggest that the model may be extended beyond chronic pain.

The results reported for chronic pain patients have been replicated in a sample of diabetics (n=225) (Turk and Rudy, 1985). In this study, 31 percent of the sample reported significant levels of dysphoric mood (anxiety, depression, irritability, frustration). Multiple regression analyses revealed that dysphoric mood was significantly predicted ($p < .0001$) by perceived interference with life, perception of diabetes as disabling, and perceptions of limited control over one's life and diabetes. These appraisal factors accounted for 84.4 percent of the variance in dysphoric mood.

Devins et al. (1982) examined the important contribution of perceived control for depression among people with end-stage renal disease. These authors concluded that lower self-efficacy was predictive of depression, subjective feelings of helplessness, and lower self-esteem. In a related study with an end-stage renal disease population, these authors (Devins et al., 1983-1984) established that individuals' perceptions of intrusiveness of their disease and its treatment, as well as their perceptions of having limited control over their lives were significantly and independently associated with negative mood and distress. The importance of perceived control has also recently been demonstrated as an important factor predicting depression and long-term adjustment of spinal cord injured individuals (Schulz and Decker, 1985).

Finally, in a large scale study of depression among physically disabled individuals, Turner et al. (1985) examined the contribution of social support, life stresses and strains, and perceptions of self-mastery. The authors viewed mastery as the extent to which one sees life as being under one's personal control as opposed to being controlled by others or fate. Their sample was divided into different age groups and they reported that across the life span, perceived self-mastery represented the most powerful variable in predicting depression.

## CONCLUSION

The sample of results obtained by the authors and those reported by other investigators provide support for the importance of the subjective appraisals of chronically ill individuals. Future work needs to replicate and extend these findings. The results presented do not exclude the role of coping strategies or social support from contributing to depression among the chronically ill. More likely there is some degree of interaction among these important variables. In viewing adjustment to chronic illness as a process, it is also quite plausible that appraisals of interference and limited control may be the result of a limited coping repertoire or the unavailability of social supports. Future research needs to address this more complex association. However, the results of the studies presented above underscore that significant amounts of variance in depression and dysphoric mood are associated with patient's appraisals.

In the cognitive-behavioural transaction model presented, cognitive appraisal was emphasized. It is worth noting that Lazarus (1966) has distinguished among three types of appraisal: primary, secondary, and reappraisal. Primary appraisal related to evaluation of the situation or circumstances. Secondary appraisal is associated with apraisal of "what can be done" and is associated with the examination of available resources. Reappraisal refers to changed assessment based on new information from the environment and the adequacy of the individual's responses and additional resources. Lazarus (Lazarus and Folkman, 1984) acknowledged the difficulty in establishing what actually comes first and suggests that because coping extends over time, it will simply depend upon how and when we assess different variables. Thus, the utility of classifying three levels of appraisal may be more a function of the timing of assessment than any true "lock-step" sequence. It may be more apropriate to consider the interaction among these variables rather than trying to establish the validity of the specific sequence moving from primary to secondary and finally to reappraisal. Thus, in the cognitive-behavioural transaction model appraisal was identified as a generic construct comprised of individuals' processing information about themselves, circumstances that they confront, and their perception of resources available. The interaction among these appraisals likely mediates the link between chronic illness and depressive symptomatology.

In sum, in studying the chronically ill, greater attention needs to be given to their ongoing appraisals of their circumstances, their ability to maintain some sense of control over their plight, and the resources available to foster adaptive coping. The cognitive-behavioural transaction model presented and the supporting data serve as a useful point of departure. Future research needs to refine the proposed model. It is hoped that the model and the data presented will stimulate further research in this important area.

## ACKNOWLEDGEMENTS

Support for this manuscript was provided by a Veterans Administration Merit Review Grant and a contract from Boehringer Mannheim Diagnostics, Inc.

## REFERENCES

Abramson, L. Y., Seligman, M. E. P., & Teasdale, J. P. (1978). Learned helplessness in humans: Critique and reformulation. Journal of Abnormal Psychology, 97, 49-74.
American Psychiatric Association, Committee on Nomenclature and Statistics. (1980). Diagnostic and statistical manual of mental disorders (3rd ed.). Washington: American Psychiatric Association.
Antonovsky, A. (1979). Health, stress and coping. San Francisco: Jossey-Bass.
Beck, A. T. (1967). Depression: Clinical, experimental, and theoretical aspects. New York: Hoeber.
Beck, A. T., Ward, C. H., Mendelson, M., Mock, J., & Erbaugh, J. (1961). An inventory for measuring depression. Archives of General Psychiatry, 4, 561-571.
Bentler, P. M., & Bonett, D. G. (1980). Significance tests and goodness of fit in the analysis of covariance structures. Psychological Bulletin, 88, 588-606.
Binik, Y. M. (1983). Coping with chronic life-threatening illness: Psychosocial perspectives on end-stage renal disease. Canadian Journal of Behavioural Science, 15, 373-391.
Brooks, N. A., & Matson, R. R. (1982). Social-psychological adjustment to multiple sclerosis. Social Science and Medicine, 16, 2129-2135.
Brownell, A., & Shumaker, S. A. (Eds.). (1984). Social support: New perspectives in theory, research, and intervention. Part 1. Theory and research. Journal of Social Issues, 40, (Whole Issue), 1-138.
Bukberg, J., Penman, D., & Holland J. C. (1984). Depression in hospitalized cancer patients. Psychosomatic Medicine, 46, 199-212.
Cassileth, B. R., Lusk, E. J., Strouse, T. B., Miller, D. S., Brown, L. L., Cross, P. A., & Tenaglia, A. N. (1984). Psychosocial status in chronic illness: A comparative analysis of six diagnostic groups. New England Journal of Medicine, 311, 506-511.
Cohen, R., & Lazarus, R. S. (1979). Coping with the stress of illness. In G. C. Stone, F. Cohen, & N. E. Adler (Eds.), Health psychology - A handbook (pp. 217-254). San Francisco: Jossey-Bass.
Cohen, S., & Wills, T. A. (1985). Stress, social support, and the buffering hypothesis. Psychological Bulletin, 98, 310-357.
Comstock, G. W., & Helsing, K. J. (1976). Symptoms of depression in two communities. Psychological Medicine, 6, 551-563.
Devins, G. M., Binik, Y. M., Gorman, P., Dattel, M., McCloskey, B., Oscar, G., & Briggs, J. (1982). Perceived self-efficacy, outcome expectancies,

and negative mood states in end-stage renal disease. Journal of Abnormal Psychology, 91, 241-244.

Devins, G. M., Binik, Y. M., Hollomby, D. J., Barré, P. E., & Guttmann, R. D. (1981). Helplessness and depression in end-stage renal disease. Journal of Abnormal Psychology, 90, 531-545.

Devins, G. M., Binik, Y. M., Hutchinson, T. A., Hollomby, D. J., Barre, P. E., & Gutmann, R. D. (1983-1984). The emotional impact of end-stage renal disease: Importance of patients' perceptions of intrusiveness and control. International Journal of Psychiatry in Medicine, 13, 327-343.

Feighner, J. P., Robins, E., Guze, S. B., et al. (1972). Diagnostic criteria for use in psychiatric research. Archives of General Psychiatry, 26, 57-63.

Ferster, C. B. (1973). A functional analysis of depression. American Psychologist, 28, 857-870.

Hamilton, M. (1960). A rating scale for depression. Journal of Neurology, Neurosurgery, and Psychiatry, 23, 56-62.

Hathaway, S. R., & McKinley, J. C. (1943). The Minnesota multiphasic personality schedule. Minneapolis: University of Minnesota Press.

Joreskog, K. G., & Sorbom, D. (1981). LISREL-V: Analysis of linear structural relationships by maximum likelihood and least squares methods. Chicago: International Educational Services.

Kanfer, F. H. (1970). Self-regulation: Research issues and speculations. In C. Neuringer, & J. L. Michael (Eds.), Behavior modification in clinical psychology (pp. 178-220). New York: Appleton-Century-Crofts.

Kaplan, B. H., Cassel, J., & Gore, S. (1977). Social support and health. Medical Care, 15, 47-58.

Kerns, R. D., Turk, D. C., & Rudy. T. E. (1985). The West Haven-Yale multidimensional pain inventory. Pain, 23, 345-356.

Lazarus, R. S. (1966). Psychological stress and the coping process. New York: McGraw-Hill.

Lazarus, R. S. (1974). Psychological stress and coping in adaptation and illness. International Journal of Psychiatry in Medicine, 5, 321-333.

Lazarus, R. S., & Folkman, S. (1984). Stress, appraisal, and coping. New York: Springer.

Lazarus, R. S., & Launier, R. (1978). Stress-related transactions between person and environment. In L. A. Pervin & M. Lewis (Eds.), Perspectives in interactional psychology, New York: Plenum.

Lewinsohn, P. M. (1974). Clinical and theoretical aspects of depression. In K. S. Calhoun, H. E. Adams, & K. R. Mitchell (Eds.), Innovative treatment methods in psychopathology. New York: Wiley.

Linn, L. S., & Greenfield, S. (1982). Patients suffering and patient satisfaction among the chronically ill. Medical Care, 20, 425-431.

Lubin, B. (1965). Adjective checklists for measurement of depression. Archives of General Psychiatry, 12, 57-62.

Meichenbaum, D. (1977). Cognitive-behavior modification. New York: Plenum.

Meichenbaum, D., Turk, D. C., & Burstein, S. (1975). The nature of coping with stress. In I. G. Sarason & C. D. Spielberger (Eds.), Stress and anxiety (Vol. 2, pp. 337-360). Washington: Hemisphere.

Melzack, R. (1975). The McGill pain questionnaire: Major properties and scoring methods. Pain, 1, 277-299.

Moffic, H., & Paykel, E. S. (1975). Depression in medical inpatients. British Journal of Psychiatry, 126, 346-353.

Murray, H. A. (1943). Thematic apperception test: Pictures and manual. Cambridge, MA: Harvard University Press.

Rehm, L. P. (1977). A self-control model of depression. Behavior Therapy, 8, 787-804.

Romano, J. M., & Turner, J. A. (1985). Chronic pain and depression: Does the evidence support a relationship? Psychological Bulletin, 97, 18-34.

Schulz, R., & Decker, S. (1985). Long-term adjustment to physical disability: The role of social support, perceived control, and self-blame. Journal of Personality and Social Psychology, 48, 1162-1172.

Seligman, M. E. P. (1975). Helplessness. New York: Freeman.

Tattersall, R. B. (1981). Psychiatric aspects of diabetes - A physician's view. British Journal of Psychiatry, 139, 485-493.

Turk, D. C. (1979). Factors influencing the adaptive process with chronic illness: Implications for intervention. In I. G. Sarson & C. D. Spielberger (Eds.), Stress and anxiety (Vol. 6, pp. 291-311). Washington: Hemisphere.

Turk, D. C., Kerns, R. D., & Rudy, T. E. (1985). Identifying the links between chronic illness and depression. Research in Education, Abstract No. ED 250645.

Turk, D. C., Meichenbaum, D., & Genest, M. (1983). Pain and behavioral medicine: A cognitive-behavioral perspective. New York: Guilford.

Turk, D. C., & Rudy, T. E. (1985). Predictors of dysphoric mood among diabetics. Diabetes Care.

Turk, D. C., Sobel, H. J., Follick, M. J., & Youkilis, H. D. (1980). A sequential criterion analysis for assessing coping with chronic illness. Journal of Human Stress, 6, 35-40.

Turner, R. J., Noh, S., & Levin, D. M. (1985). Depression across the life course - The significance of psychosocial factors among the physically disabled. In A. Dean (Ed.), Depression in multidisciplinary perspective (pp. 32-59). New York: Brunner/Mazel.

Visotsky, H. M., Hamburg, D. A., Goss, M. F., & Lebovits, B. Z. (1961). Coping behavior under extreme stress. Archives of General Psychiatry, 5, 423-448.

Wallston, F. A., Wallston, B. S., & DeVellis, R. (1978). Development of the Multidimensional Health Locus of Control (MHLC) scales. Health Education Monographs, 6, 160-170.

Westbrook, M. T., & Viney, L. L. (1982). Psychological reactions to the onset of chronic illness. Social Science and Medicine, 16, 899-905.

# COPING OVER THE LIFE SPAN

Susan Folkman

Department of Psychology
University of California

It has long been assumed that coping changes over the life span. One point of view is that coping changes normatively as people age. For example, Gutmann (1974) suggests that as people age they move from active mastery, that is, aggressive, controlling modes of coping, to more passive modes, and ultimately to a reliance on magical modes. Vaillant (1977) and Pfeiffer (1977) also suggest that coping changes with age, but in different directions than suggested by Gutmann. Vaillant and Pfeiffer say that people become more effective and realistic in their coping as they age. There is less dependence on immature mechanisms such as projection and acting out, and more use of mature mechanisms such as altruism, humour, and suppression.

Another point of view suggested more recently by McCrae (1982) and Folkman and Lazarus (1980) is that younger and older people cope similarly when they are dealing with similar sources of stress, but that sources of stress change over the life course. Thus, younger adults spend a lot of time coping with the demands associated with establishing careers, marriages, and families, whereas older adults spend a lot of time coping with problems such as declining income and health, and the illness and death of people close to them.

This chapter reports preliminary findings from Folkman and Lazarus (in preparation), comparing the coping of younger and older adults. In this study data were collected about coping and sources of stress from two samples of community residents, one consisting of 75 married couples in which the women were 35-44 years of age and had at least one child still at home and a second sample of 141 individuals aged 65-74 years. The samples were comparable demographically in that they were both white, primarily Protestant or Catholic, above marginal income, and educated beyond high school. The older sample, however, was retired. As might be expected, the somatic health of the older subjects was poorer than the somatic health of the younger subjects. However, the older subjects experienced fewer psychological symptoms than the younger subjects (as measured with the Hopkins Symptom Checklist).

In both samples subjects were interviewed monthly about a recently experienced stressful encounter; the older sample was interviewed four times and the younger sample five times. Subjects then answered a number of questions about each encounter and filled out the Ways of Coping Questionnaire (Lazarus and Folkman, 1984).

The Ways of Coping Questionnaire contains 67 items that describe a broad range of cognitions and actions that people use to manage the demands of the stressful encounters of day-to-day living. Subjects indicated on a Likert scale, the extent to which they used each strategy in a particular situation. Through factor analysis eight forms of coping were identified: (1) confrontive coping, which involves aggressive and somewhat hostile attempts to alter the situtation; (2) distancing, which includes strategies such as "tried to put the problem out of my mind" and "turned to work or other activities"; (3) self-controlling, which includes attempts to keep one's feelings to oneself; (4) seeking social support; (5) escape-avoidance, which includes wishful thinking; (6) accepting responsibility; (7) rational problem-solving; and (8) positive reappraisal, which includes strategies for looking on the bright side of things and seeing opportunities for growth (for a full description of these scales see Folkman, Lazarus, Dunkel-Schetter, DeLongis, and Gruen, in press).

The Ways of Coping Questionnaire reflects a transactional and process-oriented approach, in which coping is conceptualized as a process that is determined by the person's relationship with the environment in a particular transaction (Lazarus and Folkman, 1984). The relationship changes as the encounter unfolds, and from encounter to encounter (Folkman and Lazarus). This approach differs from those in which coping is viewed as a stable personality disposition. It also differs from approaches that ask how the person copes with a general condition such as overload or ill health. Conditions are generally complex and multifaceted. If only general conditions are probed it is unclear what the person is coping with. For example, what does it mean to ask a person how he or she copes with a bad marriage, ambiguity, or with a disease such as cancer?

The question addressed here is whether or not there are differences in the ways younger and older adults cope with similar kinds of situations. The data collected permitted the exploration of this question from two perspectives. First, encounters were grouped according to what they were about; that is, health problems (ranging from minor concerns about weight to major illness), family problems, and maintenance problems (such things as keeping up the house, lawn and car). Second, encounters were grouped along more psychological dimensions according to how they were appraised with respect to what was at stake (primary appraisal) and what the options for coping were (secondary appraisal).

With respect to health, family, and maintenance encounters, older subjects reported more encounters having to do with health than younger subjects, and younger subjects reported more encounters having to do with family problems. The results of a multivariate analysis indicated that older and younger subjects coped in similar ways with stressful encounters that had to do with health and maintenance. Thus, although older subjects reported more health encounters than younger subjects, they coped with these problems in similar ways. However, there was a significant difference in the ways the two groups coped with family problems. The younger subjects used significantly more confrontive coping than the older subjects, and the older subjects used more distancing and positive reappraisal.

Does this mean that age affects the ways people deal with family problems? Or is this difference due to the kinds of family problems that older and younger people face? As part of the interview subjects were asked to report on who was the most important person involved in the situation. In the younger sample, 80 percent of encounters involved spouse or child, whereas in the older sample only 34 percent of the encounters involved spouse or child (presumably an adult child no longer living at home). The age differences in coping with family encounters, therefore, may also be due to differences in what, or with whom, people were coping. The younger subjects were more involved with their immediate family members - namely, spouses and children living at home - whereas the family encounters of the older subjects tended to involve a much higher proportion of family members outside the household. Younger people may use more confrontive coping because they are living in close proximity to the people involved in their stressful encounters. On the other hand, it is also possible that as people age, they become less interested in using confrontive behaviour, regardless of who or what they are coping with.

In these two samples, subjects were asked how they appraised encounters with respect to what was at stake, for example, their self-esteem, their physical well-being, or the well-being of a loved one (primary appraisal). They were also asked what the options for coping were, for example, whether or not the encounter could be changed, or had to be accepted (secondary appraisal). Although the measures of primary and secondary appraisal were not identical in the two samples, they were comparable. Thus, in both studies there were items that assessed threats to the subjects' own self-esteem, and items that assessed threats to a loved one's well-being. There were also items that assessed the extent to which subjects appraised situations as changeable. The issue under investigation is whether the younger and older subjects differed in the ways they coped with encounters that were classified on these psychological dimensions.

With encounters that were classified as high in threat to self-esteem and high in threat to a loved one's well-being, regardless of the nature of the threat, the younger subjects used more confrontive coping than the older subjects, and the older subjects used more distancing and positive reappraisal than the younger subjects. When encounters were classified according to options for coping, the younger subjects again used more confrontive coping and rational problem-solving, and also sought more social support than the older subjects. The older subjects used more distancing and positive reappraisal than the younger subjects. The pattern was very similar in encounters that had to be accepted: the younger subjects sought more social support and used more rational problem-solving than the older subjects, and the older subjects used more distancing and positive reappraisal than the younger subjects.

What is interesting about these findings is that older subjects consistently used more distancing and positive reappraisal than younger subjects, regardless of the appraisal, and younger subjects used more active forms of coping, such as confrontive coping, seeking social support, and problem-solving. Again, it is important to remember that there were differences in sources of stress for the two samples. The younger subjects reported work encounters, which the older subjects, all of whom were retired, did not. In addition, as noted above, the younger subjects were all married and had young children living at home. These differences in the context of living could account for the more active coping pattern displayed by the younger subjects.

It is difficult to know to what to attribute the coping pattern of the older subjects. One possibility is that it is a cohort effect: the older subjects were socialized to cope in these ways. Another possibility is that the older subjects felt more helpless than the younger ones, and thus they coped more passively.

Overall, the results lend some support to both points of view stated earlier. A number of differences in the coping of older and younger subjects seem to be accounted for by differences in their sources of stress. The younger subjects were dealing with their spouses and young children and problems at work, whereas the older subjects were dealing more with health-related problems. On the other hand, there may be some developmental changes in coping that are not associated with changes in sources of stress. Here, the reference is to the greater use of distancing and positive reappraisal among the older subjects. In this light it is interesting to ask if the use of these strategies by older people helps explain why, in the face of declining physical health, they experience fewer psychological symptoms than younger people (Tobin and Lieberman, 1976). If so, the use of these modes of coping by the older subjects, which Gutmann (1974) might label regressive, may in fact be adaptive. This interpretation is consistent with Vaillant's (1977) and Pfeiffer's (1977) hypothesis that people become more effective and realistic in their coping as they age.

Clearly, these issues cannot be addressed satisfactorily with cross-sectional research. What is needed is longitudinal research in which the same person is assessed in diverse domains of living over many years.

REFERENCES

Folkman, S., & Lazarus, R. S. (1980). An analysis of coping in a middle-aged community sample. Journal of Health and Social Behavior, 21, 219-239.

Folkman, S., & Lazarus, R. S. (1985). If it changes it must be a process: Study of emotion and coping during three stages of a college examination. Journal of Personality and Social Psychology, 48, 150-170.

Folkman, S., & Lazarus, R. S. (in preparation). Age differences in stress and coping processes.

Folkman, S., Lazarus, R. S., Dunkel-Schetter, C., DeLongis, A., & Gruen, R. (in press). The dynamics of a stressful encounter: Cognitive appraisal, coping, and encounter outcomes. Journal of Personality and Social Psychology.

Gutmann, D. L. (1974). The country of old men: Cross-cultural studies in the psychology of later life. In R. L. LeVine (Ed.), Culture and personality: Contemporary readings. (pp. 95-121). Chicago: Aldine.

Lazarus, R. S., & Folkman, S. (1984). Coping and adaptation. In W. D. Gentry (Ed.), The handbook of behavioral medicine. (pp. 282-325). New York: Guilford.

McCrae, R. R. (1982). Age differences in the use of coping mechanisms. Journal of Gerontology, 37, 454-560.

Pfeiffer, E. (1977). Psychopathology and social pathology. In J. E. Birren & K. W. Schaie (Eds.), Handbook of the psychology of aging. New York: Van Nostrand Reinhold.

Tobin, S., & Lieberman, M. (1976). Last home for the aged. San Francisco: Jossey-Bass.

Vaillant, G. E. (1977). Adaptation to Life. Boston: Little, Brown.

# ARE THERE COPING STRATEGIES?

Shlomo Breznitz

Ray D. Wolfe Centre for Study of Psychological Stress
University of Haifa

Research on illness behaviour has indicated that the shared images and expectations of people are often determined to a great degree by labels that are used in either describing symptoms or in applying diagnostic labels. For instance, the term "stress", which has become a major topic in both research and clinical practice, owes its popularity to its excess meaning. Today, it is often said that we live in an era of stress. Everything is stress. However, only 20 years ago we were all living in the era of anxiety. There is a psychologically interesting difference between the two words which, perhaps, can account for the transition from anxiety to stress.

Anxiety denotes a very pessimistic condition - one that an individual carries around wherever he/she goes. It is very difficult to get rid of anxiety. The causes are unknown and it is difficult to predict whether treatment will be effective.

Stress, by comparison, is an external condition. It is "something out there", which impinges and, therefore, which is much easier to address. Individuals are submitted or subjected to stressors. Organized actions may be invoked to get rid of some of these stressors, e.g., one can spend a long weekend or a marathon session learning coping skills and relaxation. Our conceptualization of stress implies a sense of control of being able to do something about it, and this may be one reason for our infatuation with the construct in spite of its many theoretical and conceptual shortcomings.

Ever since the concept of stress was introduced, related constructs have been introduced. For instance, shortly after the word "stress" came to be, there was a need for "distress" because stress can sometimes be good. Then "coping" has evolved into "coping strategies" and "social support" has evolved into "social support systems." There is order in this madness which runs like a thread in the evolution of the concepts of the disciplines which are involved in this enterprise. It is the culture that modifies, shapes, and gives survival value to certain concepts which fit the particular biases of the culture involved.

One bias that should be addressed in this area is <u>the optimistic bias</u>. This is the bias of control, of manageability, of being able to do something about problems, as if problems were only opportunities for doing something about them. A good illustration of this particular bias is in the lack of a proper distinction between hopelessness and helplessness.

Helplessness is a major concept in many theories which try to account for disease, for example, Seligman's (1975) theory of learned helplessness. It is as if when there is nothing one can do, there is nothing to be done; whereas hopelessness is a much broader concept. Although one would probably not feel control when one is hopeless, (since there is no reason to even try) <u>one can be hopeful even if one is helpless</u>, as reflected in the following comment: "So, it would not be me that would solve the problem, but that does not mean that from somewhere or somehow a solution cannot come." It is a typical Western, North American bias that help must come from within, from one's resources, one's ability to master his environment, rather than waiting for something good to happen. Unfortunately, it so happens that there tends to be a correlation between the enormity of the stressor and whether it can be controlled or not. Some of the major sources of stress are in fact situations where one can do nothing but learn to live with it. A culture which puts so much emphasis on active coping creates further dilemmas. For example, one Type A characteristic is that whenever there is a problem one immediately has to deal with it. When confronted with a problem that cannot be dealt with in an outright fashion, the Type A individual is more at risk than somebody else for major distress.

The construct of "strategy" needs to be addressed also. Webster's Dictionary gives two definitions of "strategy": first, the science and art of military command employed with the object of meeting the enemy (presumably the stress) under conditions advantageous to one's force; and second, the broader definition, a careful plan or method especially for achieving an end. Therefore, if one uses the of concept coping strategies seriously, there are at least three minimal logical requirements that have to be met.

The first requirement, just on the basis of the denotation of strategy, is <u>planning</u>. It must be demonstrated that there was planning or that there were intentions before the behaviour actually took place, i.e., premeditation in order to consider the behavioural response a "strategy".

The second logical requirement is that there are <u>alternatives</u>. What is the utility of considering strategies if that is the only option facing an individual? Therefore, there must be alternatives. One must demonstrate the availability of alternative modes of coping beyond not only intention, but also choice or preference. Meichenbaum (1985) has stated that the most important thing about a strategy is not what strategy it is, but that it be flexible. This flexibility, in fact, is one of the requirements of the definition of any coping strategy. There must be options available for alternative behavioural responses.

The third minimal logical requirement is that of <u>consistency</u> or pattern in the behaviour. In its absence one might know that something was perhaps planned, but be unable to demonstrate that a strategy was carried out unless expressed in certain consistency patterns. How can one demonstrate coping strategy? This requires planning to permit recognition or introspective analysis prior to action. When one tries to reconstruct coping strategies after the event from an individual's self-report, there is the likelihood of over-estimating the strategical component. This is likely because of the time to put some order into the chaos which is characteristic of a typical stress. After the event, one may find patterns and explanations beyond what is warranted by the actual situation. Ideally, one needs access to thoughts prior to action to prove the presence of a coping strategy.

This raises the issue of how to demonstrate alternatives or choice. The first step was taken by Lazarus and Folkman in their 1985 study of students before and after a mid-term examination (Folkman and Lazarus, 1985). The same students who used more problem-focused strategies before the examination, used more emotion-focused strategies afterwards. This suggested that these students had alternatives. Additionally, it would be useful to demonstrate that in different contexts individuals undertake more than one action.

Consistency, the third requirement, is the only one that is relatively easy to demonstrate by simply observing behaviour. This creates an interesting dilemma because good consistency actually reduces the claim for strategy, because it reduces the probability of alternatives. Ideally, what one would like is to have consistency within which there is embedded inconsistency, so that there is a demonstration that a person can, in fact, do many things, but on the whole does one thing rather than the other. The demonstration of a fully consistent pattern may reflect fixation rather than strategy.

Lazarus and Folkman (1984) empirically find that even in the same situation, most people use six or more different coping acts or thoughts (these will not be labelled as "strategies".) If that is the case, not only is it very difficult to talk about strategies, but perhaps even the consideration of tactics is questionable. People just do things. They muddle through, and if lucky their actions fit well into the requirements of the situation, with very little premeditation, very little planning, and very little choice and volition.

In sum, it appears as though the minimal requirements for a definition (and this is really a weak definition of coping strategy) are very rarely, if ever, met in research. Further, one would not expect them to be able to develop because for some coherent pattern to develop, one would look for situations which allow the opportunity for trial and error, for corrections, and evaluation of consequences. Stressful situations are not ideally suited for this kind of learning. On the contrary, if anything, there is a pull towards stereotypic behaviour, repeating what is most readily available, rather than an opportunity to develop a coherent set of rules which are effective.

Moreover, even if there were strategies, and they could be learned, even then it would probably be nearly impossible to get our subjects to report them properly. Some of the behaviours are just too quick and automatic, and probably do not take the route of premeditation that can be reported. Some are obviously affected by unconscious motivations by which the subjects by definition have no available information. And thirdly, effective coping might be a case where the person has no access to the causes, to the thinking (if there was any) that precedes the actual behaviour. Consider the following, taken from research on artificial intelligence. There is an effort to build data bases of expert systems in various areas so that the data base would be able to fulfill the function of an expert. In order to do that, the researcher who works on this task must be able to extract information from the expert about how he reaches his conclusions. It turns out that experts are very bad in explaining what they do and how they do it. They just know that that is what has to be done. Contrary to what was expected by naive common sense, believing that as long as one is not an expert there is just experience (like in concept formation) and then at some point there is abstraction of rules, so that the expert should be governed by rules, this is not the case. It apparently turns out to be the other way around. Namely, that as long as what should be done is unknown and very little experience is involved, rules are followed. The moment a lot of experience is acquired the answers just pop up. Thus, a person who copes effectively might be the last person who would be able to tell us what were the mediating links that led to a particular kind of behaviour.

If that is the situation, and the conditions for proper usage of "coping strategies" are not met, then there must be other reasons why these concepts are adhered to. It is not because of their utility. It must be something else, which might be the need to prefer concepts that carry with them this excess meaning of controllability, orderliness, responsibility, and so on.

Even the word "coping" itself, not just coping strategies carries this excess meaning. One talks about people who are unable to cope. The adverb "well" is not required. "Unable to cope" is sufficient because the word "coping" already carries this excess meaning. It is positive. It is successful, and therefore it is cherished because it adds to preferences in the larger sense.

One can legitimately ask why this is important. Why are words that important? Kleinman's (this volume) work illustrates the importance of meaning very clearly. There is a real danger that the area of stress is being transformed epistemologically into a challenge, into an opportunity to show one's fortitude, one's coping skills. It is as if the burden was all on the person himself. And that has far-reaching pragmatic and political implications - whether one should invest most of the resources into teaching people to cope or to prevent some of the problems in the first place. It depends on one's orientation and that depends very much on the context of language within which the research is being done.

One can surely make a counterpoint by saying that there is so much positive that one can acquire by being confronted with stress and coping well. One could definitely make the point that if an individual is confronted with a problem and copes with it successfully, it might increase self-esteem with possibly far-reaching implications to health. In several domains of suffering, particularly with chronic problems, or at least problems of long duration, rather than fast, acute stressors, it is not through the mastery of successful coping, but through the misery and the suffering that the main positive lessons are learned. There is so much preoccupation with the conquering of stress that the misery of stress has almost been forgotten.

Finally, consider denial as a way of coping (Breznitz, 1983). Whatever its effectiveness, and whatever its expression, one thing is obvious, namely that <u>denial by definition is without planning and awareness</u>. Try to plan not to see. Try to plan not to hear. Try to plan not to think about something. This very frequent and powerful mode of coping falls totally outside of the scope of what we might legitimately call a coping strategy.

Denial is important for yet another reason. This involves the situation where there is a discrepancy between what the physician reasonably explains to a patient and what the patient maintains even after the explanation. Most frequently the problem is dealt with from one side only; that is when the patient believes there is something wrong, the physician tells him it is all right, and the patient yet maintains that something is wrong. This was called abnormal illness behaviour (Pilowsky, 1969, this volume). But how about the other side of the same coin? How about the physician telling the patient that unless he stops doing this or unless he starts doing that he will be in trouble, and the patient denies the problem, denies the danger and goes on as before? This is yet another type of discrepancy and in line with the importance of words and concepts, it might be appropriate to coin yet another expression, "abnormal health behaviour".

## REFERENCES


Breznitz, S. (1983). The seven kinds of denial. In S. Breznitz (Ed.), The denial of stress. New York: International Universities Press.

Folkman, S., & Lazarus, R. S. (1985). If it changes it must be a process: Study of emotion and coping during three stages of a college examination. Journal of Personality and Social Psychology, 48, 150-170.

Lazarus, R. S., & Folkman, S. (1984). Stress, appraisal and coping. New York: Springer.

Meichenbaum, D. (1985, August). Adaptation to stress. Paper presented at the 2nd International Conference on Illness Behaviour, Toronto, Ontario, Canada.

Pilowsky, I. (1969). Abnormal illness behaviour. British Journal of Medical Psychology, 42, 347-351.

Seligman, M. E. P. (1975). Helplessness. San Francisco: W. H. Freeman.

Webster's Ninth New Collegiate Dictionary. (1983). (p. 1165). Springfield, MA: Merriam-Webster.

# PART VII METHODOLOGY: THEMES AND APPROACHES

# ETIOLOGICAL STUDIES AND ILLNESS BEHAVIOUR

George Brown

Department of Social Policy and Social Sciences
University of London

## General Characteristics of Research on the Etiological Factors in Stress

Four general characteristics of the etiological-stress research will be outlined, and an attempt made to illustrate how these might be incorporated into the study of illness behaviour.

Association between psychosocial etiological factors and clinical variables. Associations between psychosocial and clinical variables, in the particular investigator-based approach to research which will be reviewed, have been considerable. It has, for example, usually been found that some 80 percent of onsets of severe depression in general population samples are preceded by a severely threatening life event, typically involving loss, failure or disappointment or a major long-term difficulty (Brown and Harris, 1978, in press). And with such associations as a basis it has proved possible to develop effective causal models. Four factors, for example, permit prediction in most instances whether or not schizophrenic patients will have a florid relapse: expressed emotion (EE) of relatives, face-to-face contact within the home, use of psychotropic drugs; and life events (Brown and Birley, 1968; Brown, Birley, and Wing, 1972; Vaughn and Leff, 1976). Good models are, of course, not the same as good theory - but such components have usually interrelated together in a way that makes some theoretical sense. For instance, among those schizophrenic patients returning to families with high expressed emotion, life events appear to relate to relapse largely among those taking drugs; the combination of high expressed emotion and no drugs apparently leads too quickly to relapse for events to have much chance of playing a role (Leff and Vaughn, 1985). Events are critical for those with high expressed emotion and drugs, or no drugs and low expressed emotion. Perhaps most surprising of all, findings concerning the etiology and course of schizophrenia and depression have replicated well - even across cultures as disparate as India, California, and Colombia (Leff and Vaughn, 1985; Day, in press; Brown and Harris, in press).

Nature of specific stress-disorder associations. The second point follows from the first: the research appears to begin to show at least some of the hallmarks of successful science - and if this should turn out to be so, it is probably due both to the nature of the phenomena and to the methods used to study them. There appear to be highly specific links between occurrences bearing meaning and psychobiological response patterns. Although there are cultural variations, there is at present more impressive evidence for communality than idiosyncracy of response. For instance, in modern Nairobi, it is still quite common for a man to take a second wife as allowed by traditional culture, although in practice it now can have all the trappings of taking a mistress in Western society and, in a study of out-patient attenders it is of interest that the occurrence of a husband's second marriage was highly related to onset of depression in the first wife (Vadher and Ndetei, 1981). Loss is one of the fundamental human experiences and probably provides the most basic component of clinical depression in any human community.

In this context it is important to take seriously existing diagnostic categories - the etiological agents for depression, anxiety states, schizophrenia and organic brain syndrome, in comparison with functional gastrointestinal disorders are quite different (e.g., Brown and Harris, 1978; Craig and Brown, 1984a, 1984b). In a study of people who underwent an appendicectomy those with a functional disorder had a high rate of events before onset of the kind established to be capable of bringing about a depressive disorder (Creed, 1981). Perhaps most impressive is the observation that mixed depressive and anxiety disorders tend to have life events that are consistent with the different disorders - that is loss for the depressive component and danger for the anxiety component (Finlay-Jones and Brown, 1981). In such affective conditions and in at least some physical states such as gastrointestinal and menstrual disorders, we appear to be dealing with responses that have a marked "automatic" quality. Given a particular biography and current set of circumstances (and doubtless certain constitutional predispositions) the risk of developing fairly quickly a particular disorder is high once a certain kind of stressor bearing a particular meaning or set of meanings, has occurred (Brown and Harris, in press; Craig and Brown, 1984b). Far less than with questions involving "illness behaviour" do we deal in etiological studies with choices and decisions on the part of the subject - at least in the period immediately preceding the onset of the disorder. Indeed, for a number of disorders this kind of automatic role of stressors has now been well enough established for the main research effort to turn to elucidating the role of vulnerability and protective factors in order to explain why only some individuals experiencing such stressors go on to develop a disorder. For example, etiological agents, typically concerning major losses and disappointments only lead to depression in about one in five instances. In the simple model shown in Figure 1, a vulnerability factor, such as lack of a close confiding tie with one's husband, considerably increases risk of depression in the presence of a stressful agent but not without such an agent (see Brown and Harris, 1978).

There is already a tenuous link here with illness behaviour. Such causal models can often be quite close to models that people formulate themselves and <u>their</u> use of the model has a direct bearing on their help-seeking. In a population study in London of women suffering from quite serious depression many said they had doubts about seeking medical help because their suffering was so clearly linked to stressors in their own lives. Many made it clear that the reason they would only present a physical symptom (and not a mental symptom) to their physician was because of this uncertainty of the relevance of their state to medicine (Ginsberg and Brown, 1982). Thus, the women reflect much of the ambivalence and confusion about the implications of etiological research concerning social factors, both in medicine and the social sciences. If depression is produced by adversity should not it be seen as "distress" rather than "disease"? This is an issue still being debated in psychiatric journals in the U.K. (e.g., Bebbington, Tennant, and Hurry, 1981; Brown and Harris, 1982; Brown, Craig, and Harris, 1985; Wing and Bebbington, 1982).

In the case of schizophrenia the question of distress versus disease has not arisen with the same strength and here research has progressed far

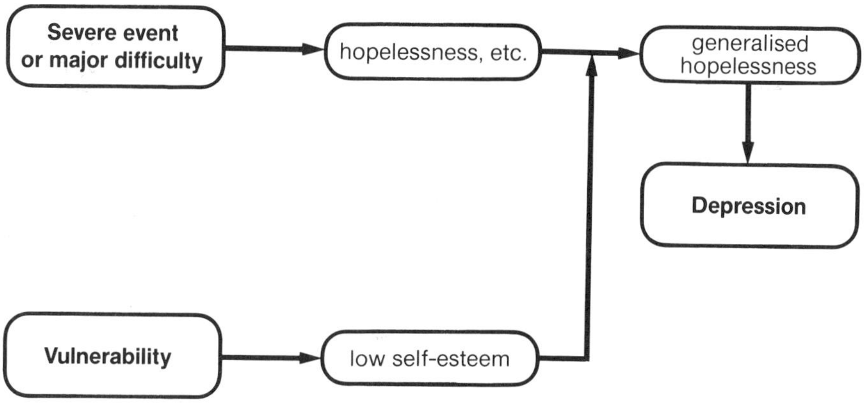


**FIGURE 1**

enough for attempts to be made to bring vulnerability factors under control in terms of intervention with families (Leff, Kuipers, Berkovitz, Eberlein-Vries, and Sturgeon, 1982). However, results from etiological research have been on the whole more ambiguous and uncertain in North America where the bulk of it is carried out. Here it is necessary to recognize that convincing results have tended to emerge most clearly with a particular approach to measurement of both life events and of disorder.

Measurement issues. This leads to the third general point: measurement in the type of work reviewed has been investigator-based. In contrast most research in this field as a whole is respondent-based. The research reviewed has been based on investigator measures in the sense that ratings are made by the investigator after extensive interviews with respondents. Here, the investigator not the respondent is the measuring instrument. Many of these ratings are straightforward - such as the amount of quarrelling in a marital relationship or how often a woman visits her parents. However, two more complex types of judgement have proved to be particularly important. The first concerns making judgements about feelings and attitudes expressed in the interview itself - for example, the Expressed Emotion measure takes account of the tone of voice and facial expression of respondents. The second judgement concerns the likely meaning of a set of circumstances for a person given his or her particular set of biographical and current circumstances. This has been the most important rating of the significance of life events as it allows research to deal with the many potential threats to validity that are present if someone is asked about meaning and yet at the same time it is sufficiently accurate to allow etiological models to be developed (Brown, 1981, 1983). In this way it is possible to deal with highly complex and idiosyncratic material with simple four-point rating scales. Flexible questioning increases accuracy in reporting and various methodological checks can be built into the rating task in which threats to validity are reduced and, in some instances, perhaps ruled out altogether. For instance, in the research on appendicectomy the person who collected the life-event material was blind to whether the condition was organic or functional and those rating the events in terms of threat were blind to whether they were dealing with material collected from a patient or someone from the general population. Given the "double-blind" nature of the ratings it is unlikely that the considerable differences in the nature of events preceding organic and functional conditions could be due to bias on the part of interviewer or rater (Creed, 1981; Craig and Brown, 1984b). Equally important the approach enables the gap between the large-scale epidemiological and the small-scale intensive enquiries to be narrowed. Where reasonably powerful psychosocial effects are present the accuracy of the investigator-based measures allows enquiries to be carried out on quite modest numbers of subjects.

Broadening the scope of research. The fourth and final general point is that, although these enquiries began with the study of a particular disorder, depression and a stressor that had to be closely linked in time to its onset, findings have persistently pointed to the need to push back enquiry to take account of earlier experiences - including childhood and adolescence. One way of viewing such effects is in terms of two strands. The first deals with the outer world and the way it impinges on the indiviudal; the second with the inner world in terms of cognitive sets such as helplessness, hostility and self-esteem (Brown, Harris, and Bifulco, 1986). But while capable of acting independently there are close links between the two strands.

Perhaps the most important principle established by the research is that although the influence of the past can be powerful, there is a good deal of discontinuity. In short, subsequent experience can apparently neutralize the most baleful of earlier experiences. Quinton and Rutter (1984a, 1984b), in a recent prospective study of children in care showed a close link between early adversity and both later poor parenting and affective disorder. However, these effects were almost eliminated if the woman had a satisfactory marriage. Moreover, chances of this effect occurring were quite unrelated to earlier personality disturbance in childhood.

These kind of links are outlined in Figure 2. The top right-hand portion of Figure 2 (involving Strand 1) illustrates the process referred to earlier as an "automatic response". That is, when severe life events and vulnerability factors combine to produce depression. The mid-bottom (Strand 2), moves to the cognitive level and represents critical decisions which often have an impact later on the first, external strand - 'decisions' defined in a broad sense to include, say, a premarital pregnancy (Brown, Harris, and Bifulco, 1986).

It is possible to find parallels between this work and some in the area of illness behaviour. The role of premarital pregnancy, for example, has emerged as a powerful predictive factor in studies of depression and also apparently in a study of the utilization of antenatal services among working-class women in Scotland (McKinlay and McKinlay, 1972). More specifically, the parallel involves the interplay between the cognitive style of planning one's life in a masterful way and the environmental milieu to which a person becomes subject as a result of these plans. A premarital pregnancy seemed in both studies often to land the young couple in a situation where instability in housing and unemployment seemed bound to follow and continue for several years. This frequently leads to depression in London and to under-utilization of antenatal services in Scotland.

It might be argued that a process involving only cognitive factors is involved, that is Strand 2. It is the cognitive set which had originally led to the failure in planning involved in the pre-marital pregnancy and is serving to raise the risk of depression or under-utilization in adult life. In the study of depression, however, it seems that experience earlier in life such as premarital pregnancy, or lack of care in childhood, play an etiological role only if adversity continues in the current period in adulthood. For example, low self-esteem (now known to increase risk of depression once a stressor has occurred, Brown and Bifulco, 1985; Brown et

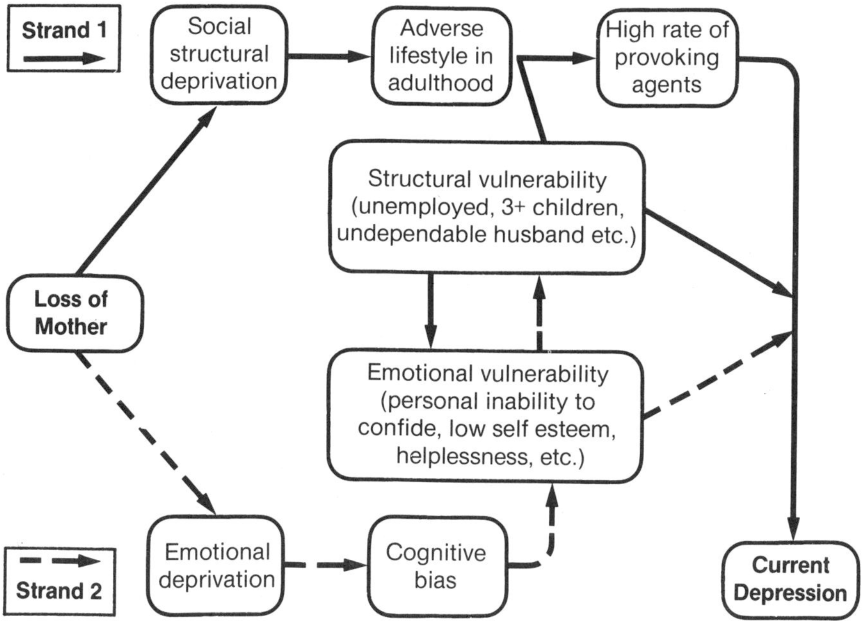


**FIGURE 2.** Speculative casual model showing main lines of impact of loss of mother

al., 1986) is quite highly related to earlier premarital pregnancy and experiences of rejection and indifference in childhood. However, there is evidence that the association between early experience and low self-esteem holds only among women experiencing current difficulties, often within their marriage (Brown and Andrews, 1985). Therefore, the past and present have to be considered together.

Insofar as illness behaviour reflects decisions and choices more than automatic responses, the role of current factors (that is strand 1) may be relatively less important than a continuing cognitive style (that is strand 2) in influencing those decisions and choices. While this may well be so, the parallel is perhaps still worth pursuing; in thinking about illness behaviour there may have been some under-estimation of the role of "automatic" processes. Consider, for example, the process of referral to psychiatrists in a working-class inner city population in North London. Despite using a high threshold to characterize caseness of depression [on average such cases had 19.1 symptoms on the shortened version of the Present State Examination (PSE)], only 13 percent saw a psychiatrist. Yet there was no difference in the severity of depression between those seeing or not seeing a psychiatrist when judged in terms of a count of PSE symptoms. However, those seeing a psychiatrist more often had made a suicidal gesture or had been recorded as having had suicidal plans on the PSE, suggesting that referral was related to uncertainty on the part of the general practitioner in dealing with the condition rather than with the severity of the depression as such.

The finding is of particular interest because of a further result which replicates one in an earlier enquiry in south London. Loss of a mother in childhood by separation (but not by death) was highly associated with such suicidal gestures and plans and thus with referral. This seems best interpreted in terms of symptom-formation and a long-term cognitive set of hostility resulting from the experience of early rejection. These factors determine the expression rather than onset of a depressive disorder (Brown, Craig, and Harris, 1985). Here "choice" may play a modest part in the referral process in contrast to the more "automatic" link between the cognitive set and "acting out".

Methodological Considerations of Possible Importance For the Study of Illness Behaviour

General and introductory points have so far been discussed. There are four specific and more methodological themes that may also be of relevance for the study of illness behaviour.

Need for greater specificity of constructs. Experience suggests that broad concepts such as depression or self-esteem must often be considerably refined if either effective theory is to be developed or statistical associations of any importance to emerge at all. It is not just a matter of differentiating concepts such as depression and anxiety; equally important they usually need to be differentiated internally (Harris and Brown, 1985). For a long time self-esteem has been seen by many as a vital component of any explanation of depression. However, a recent influential prospective enquiry by Lewinsohn and his colleagues (1981) failed to find any link between low self-esteem and subsequent depression. However, once subjects became depressed, their self-esteem tended to decrease. Paralleling this, Brown and others have also found that a measure of self-esteem based on positive comments about the self was totally unrelated to subsequent development of depression following a major loss. On the other hand, negative comments (which were correlated with lack of positive comments) were highly associated with subsequent depression (Brown et al., 1986). A number of recent studies suggest that this differential link of the positive and negative components of self-esteem may be a genuine one (e.g., Warr and Jackson, 1983; Savin-Williams and Jaquish, 1981; Campbell and Teasdale, 1985). An equally clear-cut finding concerns the greatly reduced risk of depression, once a major loss has occurred, if a woman has a confiding and close tie, especially with her husband. Yet there is no hint of such a link among those developing milder depressive conditions (Brown and Harris, 1978; Brown and Prudo, 1981). But it is not just a matter of improving measurement to obtain evidence of etiological processes. Such negative findings can be a valuable source of theoretical insights. For example, it is possible that the lack of a link between inadequacy of support and milder depressive conditions is due to the fact that protected women often develop these milder states rather than avoid depression altogether.

One example of refinement which may have a particular bearing on illness behaviour concerns the position that disorders should be investigated in general, rather than in particular as urged by John Cassel (1974). However, it is now clear that whatever may emerge in the long term, recent progress would have been impossible if this advice had been followed. This surely holds for illness behaviour; it may well be that factors which are relevant for utilization of services for some conditions are irrelevant for others. It is not necessary to dwell on the likely payoff of considering illness behaviour in terms of particular conditions; nor the likely importance of differentiating within diagnostic categories. An obvious need here is to differentiate patients, say receiving an appendicectomy, in terms of whether there is evidence for organic pathology or not (Creed, 1981).

Importance of complex explanatory models. The need for explanatory models to reflect ongoing and complex causal processes has become apparent both for research on illness behaviour and in etiological research. A number of large, prospective studies have recently been carried out to look at affective, and particularly depressive, disorders. But the work has on the whole been deeply disappointing. It is now clear that a prospective design is not sufficient. The potential advantages of such a design are largely nullified without the employment of accurate investigator-based measures to collect data retrospectively. The most glaring shortcoming has been the consistent failure to record life events occurring in the follow-up period (Brown, 1981). Since life events of etiological importance typically occur in the month or so before onset of psychiatric or physical disorders, probably most events of etiological significance have been missed. This problem stems directly from the inability of check-list questionnaires to date events accurately in relation to the onset of a disorder.

Further, it is not only a matter of failing to date events. Henderson (1981) and his colleagues in Canberra have recently concluded that social support plays no protective role in the development of depression. Instead they emphasize that those that are at risk for developing depression have a much greater need for social supports. However, this study was based entirely on reports of feelings of attachment and closeness at one point in time, ignoring the possibility that such reports are not necessarily very good predictors of actual support given in a subsequent crisis. The critical issue of support mobilization was ignored (Gore, 1981, 1985). This information by necessity has to be collected retrospectively. A recent study in London concludes that those who fail to receive support in a crisis, which on the basis of prior reports they might have expected, are particularly likely to develop depression following a major loss. Therefore, it is highly likely that the real link between actual support in a crisis and development of depression can be suppressed in a statistical sense by those who are "let down" in this fashion (Brown et al., 1985). It is essential that prospective studies document by careful retrospective enquiry what happened in the period immediately before the development of disorder.

Quite clearly support in a crisis is unlikely to be restricted to dealing just with the crisis itself. It is likely to have relevance for coping with any distress or psychiatric symptomatology. For women, a husband can be of critical importance in helping to work through distress stemming from puzzling conflicts in her life such as those arising from roles as both wife and mother (Boulton, 1983) and helping to legitimize the translation of affective symptoms into a medical context. While in general women are seen as more nervous and highly strung and subject to psychiatric symptoms, once a particular woman develops serious depression or anxiety there is often great pressure to normalize these as something women must expect and to assume it to be a state that is natural to them (Ginsberg and Brown, 1982).

Addressing the relationship between etiological and "illness behaviour" factors. Following from these points about retrospective enquiry, there is an urgent need to understand more about the complex links between stressor, distress, psychiatric and physical disorder and their relationships to help-seeking. As Mechanic (1976) has noted, most epidemiological studies fail to differentiate the extent to which various independent predictors affect utilization through their influence on the occurrence of symptoms and the extent to which they have an independent effect on help-seeking. Although it is now well-established that many attending general medical and surgical services have diagnosable psychiatric illnesses, little has been established about the nature or role of these disturbances. There may be some surprises here. Murphy, in a study of the onset of new physical illness of the kind commonly seen by general practitioners, found a link between severely threatening events of the kind capable of providing a depressive disorder and the onset of physical disorder, but the event had first to produce at least a minor psychiatric disorder (Murphy and Brown, 1980). Craig (in press) has demonstrated similar findings for gastrointestinal disorders with an organic basis confirmed by laboratory findings. (The events, however, involved for the most part marked goal frustration). Given the claims that have been made for the role of triggers in help-seeking, the issue of dating is critical. Research in illness behaviour has failed to sort out this issue - because of the lack of instruments to date and to juxtapose events and changes in the developing disorder (Rabkin and Struening, 1976). While the technical problems to be overcome are formidable, there is now impressive evidence for the validity of investigator-based methods of interviewing for reconstructing the occurrence of events (e.g., Brown and Harris, 1982).

But such analyses can still leave us with theoretical lacunae. Something occurring at a definite point in time (say support in a crisis) but related to an ongoing variable (say a long history of love and support from the same source) makes it difficult to be sure just what is going on. Support in the crisis may be largely irrelevant given a history of such support and the sense of security and self-esteem that goes with it. In the end it may be only possible to be confident about the effect of some factors by intervening experimentally. Nonetheless, it is far too soon to be despondent about what can be established by traditional theory-based analyses.

Research on the role of triggers or hassles in relation to distress, symptoms and treatment-seeking is puzzling in this context. The most impressive studies have been based on diary-keeping and effects over quite short periods of time, e.g., whether an event on a particular day is associated with distress or treatment-seeking on the same or the following day. The events are typically trivial. Gortmaker, Eckenrode, and Gore (1982) noted that only two percent of daily stresses would alter a family's score on a life-event scale. Given that it is left to the respondent to decide what to count as an event (or for that matter a bad mood, physical malaise or physical symptoms - Verbrugge, 1985), results of such studies are even more likely to be presented with inaccuracy and bias than respondent checklist life-event studies. The results are not without interest, but it is difficult to take seriously assertions about possible causal effects. For this such work would need to be placed in the context of an investigator-based tradition of life-event research and a move made to use more valid methods to record daily events of hassles, physical symptoms and the like. To the degree that essentially trivial phenomena are included this will be difficult and perhaps impossible. The popularity of such research is inexplicable given its general failure to deal adequately with more substantial phenomena. Once this has been achieved there will at least be an established causal framework in which to carry out analyses and develop theoretical insights about the more minor mishaps of daily life.

It may be helpful to note the importance of research that involves less systematic measures. There are superb examples of important insights derived from small samples of people who have been victimized by a particular crisis such as widowhood or rape. Systematic measurement is not an end in itself. We need to avoid measurement that is systematic at the cost of being inaccurate and even trivial. While much of this research is probably best seen as exploratory, it has provided fascinating insights into coping support and for that matter illness behaviour. For example, Weiss illustrates particularly well the strengths of such an approach in a series of studies over a 20-year period dealing with health and marriage (e.g., Weiss, 1973, 1975; Parkes and Weiss, 1983).

Over-reliance on demographic variables. There is an understandable tendency to rely on demographic-type variables. It is easy to overlook the propensity of such variables to represent quite different underlying effects according to their place in a sequence of happenings. The number of children living at home has in a number of studies been shown to relate to an increased chance of a woman developing depression once an important loss or disappointment has occurred. But once depression has developed the number of children at home relates to a decreased chance of receiving treatment from a general practitioner or psychiatrist (Brown and Harris, 1978). What is needed is a theory to interpret such apparently discordant effects. It is also necessary to recognize that the meaning of demographic-type variables may well vary markedly in terms of wider cultural developments. For instance, since the introduction of more effective contraceptive practices in the late 1960's, the presence of three or more young children at home is no longer associated with an increased chance of depression. This probably results from the fact that such children are now more likely to be the product of deliberate planning (Harris, 1986). In this regard "automatic responses" discussed earlier in this chapter, do not devalue the importance of meaning, or for that matter individual choice. Such "automatic" responses occur within an established set of meanings. These meanings can be powerfully influenced by secular changes, not least by those leading to a change in the sense of control.

In these final five points I have discussed (a) the need to refine concepts; (b) the inadequacy of a prospective design on its own to sort out temporal links; (c) the continued need for good retrospective measures; (d) the fact that a satisfactory model may still leave us in the dark theoretically; and finally, (e) the need to reach a satisfactory theoretical understanding of demographic-type measures. These points are enough to suggest that studies integrating both etiology and illness behaviour are in order. The main argument for collaboration between projects on etiology and illness behaviour is the cross-fertilization of ideas and methods that would follow. To be realistic, it must be pointed out that there was a ten-year delay in the investigator-based measures of expressed emotion (EE) reaching North America, and the investigator-based measure of life events (which in its earliest form is over 15 years old) has had little impact on North American research which continues to be largely engaged in the task of trying to improve respondent-based check-lists. Things are much less bleak when it comes to the measurement of psychiatric disorder, but even here there is controversy. The recent history of the Diagnostic Interview Schedule (DIS) illustrates the way of funding research in North America which appears to encourage extravagant hopes that sound data in extremely complex areas can be collected by questionnaire (Klerman, 1985). But here to soften my criticism the superb series of exploratory studies in the tradition of Mechanic (1962) in Students under Stress and Parkes and Weiss (1983) on bereavement promise to provide some of the necessary impetus to sort out the complex effects touched upon in this chapter.

Theoretical advances concerning onset and course may also provide some guidance in coming to terms with the myriad of factors of possible relevance in the study of illness behaviour. For example, recent experimental work aimed to change the level of expressed emotion in the relatives of schizophrenic patients underlines the importance of taking account of what Mechanic refers to as "other's response" to illness (Mechanic, 1968). The degree to which a relative is able to see the patient as ill, appears to be an important factor in lowering the level of critical comments. Given the central role of expressed emotion in determining relapse, there is now good reason to concentrate our effort on the origins of such beliefs and other factors that influence the response of others to a schizophrenic illness (Leff et al., 1982).

It is probable that many readers will consider as exaggerated the possible benefits of the coming together of studies of etiology and illness behaviour given the truly formidable complexities of studying illness behaviour alone. However, as Samuel Johnson noted "there would be few enterprises of great labour or hazard undertaken, if we had not the power of magnifying the advantages which we persuade ourselves to expect from them."

## REFERENCES


Bebbington, P. E., Tennant, C., & Hurry, J. (1981). Adversity and the nature of psychiatric disorder in the community. Journal of Affective Disorders, 3, 345-366.

Boulton, M. G. (1983). On being a mother: A study of women with pre-school children. London: Tavistock Publications.

Brown, G. W. (1981). Contextual measures of life events. In B. S. Dohrenwend & B. P. Dohrenwend (Eds.), Stressful life events and their contexts. New York: Neale Watson Academic Publications.

Brown, G. W. (1983). Accounts, meaning and causality. In G. N. Gilbert & P. Abell (Eds.), Accounts and Action. Gower.

Brown, G. W. & Andrews, B. (1985). Social support and depression. In M. H. Appleby & R. Trumbull (Eds.), Dynamics of stress. New York: Plenum Press.

Brown, G. W., Andrews, B., Bifulco, A., Adler, Z., & Bridge, L. (1986). Social support, self-esteem and depression. Psychological Medicine.

Brown, G. W., & Bifulco, A. (1985). Social support, life events and depression. In I. Sarason (Ed.), Social support: Theory research and applications. Martinus Nijhoff Publishers.

Brown, G. W. & Birley, J. L. T. (1969). Crises and life changes and the onset of schizophrenia. Journal of Health and Social Behaviour, 9, 203.

Brown, G. W., Birley, J. L. T., & Wing, J. K. (1972). The influence of family life on the course of schizophrenic illness: A replication. British Journal of Psychiatry, 121, 241-258.

Brown, G. W., Craig, T. K. J., & Harris, T. (1985). Depression: Disease or distress. British Journal of Psychiatry, 147, 612-622.

Brown, G. W., & Harris, T. O. (1978). Social origins of depression: A study of psychiatric disorder in women. New York: Free Press, London: Tavistock Publications.

Brown, G. S., & Harris, T. O. (1982). Fall-off in the reporting of life events. Social Psychiatry, 17, 23-28.

Brown, G. W., & Harris, T. (1986). Establishing causal links: The Bedford College studies of depression. In H. Katschnig (Ed.), Life events and psychiatric disorders. Cambridge University Press.

Brown, G. W., Harris, T., & Bifulco, A. T. (1986). Long-term effect of early loss of parent. In M. Rutter, C. Izard, & P. Read (Eds.), Depression in childhood: Developmental perspectives. New York: Guildford Press.

Brown, G. W., & Prudo, R. (1981). Psychiatric disorder in a rural and an urban population: 1. Aetiology of depression. Psychological Medicine, 11, 581-599.

Campbell, E., & Teasdale, J. (1985). Self-esteem and depression. (Manuscript).

Cassell, J. (1974). Psychosocial processes and 'stress': Theoretical formulation. International Journal of Health and Services, 4, 471-482.

Craig, T. K. J. (in press). Gastrointestinal disorders. In G. W. Brown & T. Harris (Eds.), Life events and illness. Guilford Press.

Craig, T. K. J., & Brown, G. W. (1984a). Life events, meaning and physical illness: A review. In A. Steptoe, & A. Matthews (Eds.), Health care and human behaviour. London: Academic Press.

Craig, T. K. J., & Brown, G. W. (1984b). Goal frustration and life events in the aetiology of painful gastrointestinal disorder. Journal of Psychosomatic Research, 28, 411-421.

Creed, F. (1981, June). Life events & appendicectomy. Lancet, i, 1381-1385.

Day, R. (in press). Stressful life events and preceding the acute onset of schizophrenia: A cross-national study from the World Health Organization. Culture, Medicine and Society.

Finlay-Jones, R. A., & Brown, G. W. (1981). Types of stressful life event and the onset of anxiety and depressive disorders. Psychological Medicine, 11, 803-815.

Ginsberg, S., & Brown, G. W. (1982). No time for depression: A study of help-seeking among mothers of pre-school children. In D. Mechanic (Ed.), Monographs in Psychosocial epidemiology 3: Symptoms, illness behaviour and help-seeking. New York: Neale Watson Academic Publications Limited.

Gore, S. (1981). Stress-buffering functions of social supports: An appraisal and clarification of research models. In B. S. Dohrenwend, & B. P. Dohrenwend (Eds.), Stressful life events and their contexts. New York: Neale Watson Academic Publications.

Gore, S. (1985). Social support and styles of coping with stress. In S. Cohen, & L. Syme (Eds.), Social support and health. New York: Academic Press.

Gortmaker, S. L., Eckenrode, J., & Gore, S. (1982). Stress and the utilization of health services: A time series and cross-sectional analysis. Journal of Health and Social Behavior, 23, 25-38.

Harris, T., Adler, Z. A., Bridge, L. B., & Brown, G. W. (1986). Instability of indicators in replication studies: Number of children and depression in women.

Harris, T., & Brown, G. W. (1985). Interpreting data in aetiological studies: Pitfalls and ambiguities. British Journal of Psychiatry, 147, 5-15.

Harris, T. O., Brown, G. W., & Eales, M. (1986). Comparing onset of case and borderline case depression: Implications for understanding aetiology. (Manuscript).

Henderson, S., Byrne, D. G., & Duncan-Jones, P. (1981). Neurosis and the social environment. London: Academic Press.

Klerman, G. L. (1985). Diagnosis of psychiatric disorders in epidemiologic field studies. Archives of General Psychiatry, 42, 723-724.

Leff, J., & Vaughn, C. (1985). Expressed emotion in families. London and New York: The Guildford Press.

Leff, J., Kuipers, L., Berkowitz, R., Eberlein-Vries, R., & Sturgeon, D. (1982). A controlled trial of social intervention in the families of schizophrenic patients. British Journal of Psychiatry, 141, 121-134.

Lewinsohn, P. M., Steinmetz, J. L., Larson, D. W., & Franklin, J. (1981). Depression-related cognitions: Antecedent or consequence? Journal of Abnormal Psychology, 90, 213-219.

McKinaly, J. B., & McKinaly, S. M. (1972). Some social characteristics of lower working class utilisers and underutilisers of maternity care services. Journal of Health and Social Behavior, 13, 369-382.

Mechanic, D. (1962). Students under stress: A study in the social psychology of adaptation. New York: Free Press.

Mechanic, D. (1968). Medical sociology - A comprehensive text. (2nd ed.). London: Free Press.

Mechanic, D. (1976). Stress, illness and illness behaviour. Journal of Human Stress, 2, 2-6.

Murphy, E., & Brown, G. W. (1980). Life events, psychiatric disturbance and physical illness. British Journal of Psychiatry, 136, 326-338.

Parkes, C. M., & Weiss, R. S. (1983). Recovery from bereavement. New York: Basic Books.

Quinton, D., & Rutter, M. (1984a). Parents with children in care I. Current circumstances and parenting. Journal of Child Psychology and Psychiatry, 25, 211-229.

Quinton, D., & Rutter, M. (1984b). Parents with children in care II. Intergenerational continuities. Journal of Child Psychology and Psychiatry, 25, 231-250.

Rabkin, J. G., & Struening, E. L. (1976). Life events, stress and illness. Science, 194, 1013-1020.
Savin-Williams, R. C., & Jaquish, G. A. (1981). The assessment of adolescent self-esteem: A comparison of methods. Journal of Personality, 49, 324-336.
Vadher, A., & Ndetei, D. M. (1981). Life events and depression in a Kenyan setting. British Journal of Psychiatry, 139, 134-137.
Vaughn, C. E., & Leff, J. P. (1976). The influence of family and social factors on the course of psychiatric illness: A comparison of schizophrenic and depreseed neurotic patients. British Journal of Psychiatry, 129, 125-137.
Verbrugge, L. M. (1985). Triggers of symptoms and health care. Social Science and Medicine, 20, 855-876.
Warr, P., & Jackson, P. (1983). Self-esteem and unemployment among young workers. Le Travail Humain, 46, 355-366.
Weiss, R. (1973). Loneliness: The experience of emotional and social isolation. Cambridge, MA: M.I.T. Press.
Weiss, R. (1975). Marital separation. New York: Basic Books.
Wing, J. K., & Bebbington, P. (1982). Epidemiology of depressive disorders in the community. Psychological Medicine, 4, 331-345.

# NEW DIRECTIONS IN ILLNESS BEHAVIOUR RESEARCH

Paul Cleary

Department of Social Medicine and Health Policy
Harvard Medical School

Mechanic has defined illness behaviour as "The manner in which persons monitor their bodies, define and interpret their symptoms, take remedial actions, and utilize the health care system." This definition encompasses an immense range of behaviours as well as cognitive and affective processes. The disciplines relevant to the study of illness behaviour, defined in this fashion, include psychology, sociology, economics, education, anthropology, and medicine. It would be presumptuous to attempt to specify what new directions in each of these areas will or should be. Rather, the purpose is to review the major trends in the assumptions, questions, and methodologies of illness behaviour research and the fundamental ways in which future research probably will differ from past work.

Many of the chapters in this volume focus on theoretical issues, and it is important to forge a link between these ideas and research and clinical applications. Several examples of research that illustrate the potential of these new directions in terms of either substantive and/or methodological issues will be cited. Any example is necessarily parochial, and the choice of examples is influenced by research that the author and his colleagues are currently conducting. The translation of theoretical ideas into practical applications is often a difficult process, and it is important to consider the impact that these ideas will have on the study and treatment of clinical problems.

In order to talk about the ways in which new research differs from what has been done in the past, it is necessary to summarize in some way the work that has already been done. Given the breadth of disciplines that study illness behaviour and the complexity of the issues involved, a comprehensive review clearly is beyond the scope of this chapter. However, it is possible to identify major research paradigms which have influenced a substantial amount of research. The majority of illness behaviour research has involved structured interviews or questionnaires administered in a single setting or community that has been cross-sectional in nature. This research has been guided by models that assume rational, conscious behaviour on the part of patients and/or physicians, and is primarily concerned with individual differences. One model that has had an especially prominent role in illness behaviour research is the Health Belief Model. This model and some of the research on it will be reviewed, major limitations will be outlined, and new directions building on this research paradigm will be suggested. It is important to emphasize that the Health Belief Model has been extremely useful and productive. Critical remarks about this model and research on it are not meant to denegrate either the theoretical aspects of the model or the empirical work that researchers have conducted. Rather, it is hoped that critical comment will stimulate thinking about how the work that has already been done can be extended and expanded.

## THE HEALTH BELIEF MODEL

The Health Belief Model (HBM) was developed by Becker (1974), Leventhal, Hochbaum, and Rosenstock (1960), Rosenstock (1960, 1974), Rosenstock and Kirscht (1979). Kasl and Cobb (1966) have also made important contributions to this model of health behaviour, although they have focussed more on the nature of symptoms, pain, and distress. This approach to explaining health behaviours is a synthesis of social psychological theories of value-expectancy and decision-making (Maiman and Becker, 1974). As such, it focuses on behaviours that are under an individual's control and is primarily concerned with conscious decisions about the utility of specific actions (see Garro, this volume, for an illustration of a conscious decision-making model). Variables which are used to predict an individual's behaviour include: 1) perceived susceptibility to a health threat; 2) perceived severity of the consequences of the disease or health threat; 3) the individual's evaluation of the efficaciousness of possible illness actions; 4) the perceived costs of possible illness actions; 5) cues to action such as symptoms or mass media communications; and 6) demographic, structural, and social psychological factors that act as "enabling" factors. A superb summary of the Health Belief Model and other models of health related behaviour has been presented by Becker and Maiman (1983).

The Health Belief Model and models with similar characteristics have received a tremendous amount of attention in the literature. Janz and Becker (1984), for example, recently reviewed 46 empirical studies related to this model. This emphasis on a particular model is surprising, if for no other reason than because it has not consistently given rise to accurate predictions in large scale studies. Furthermore, the reasons the model does not do well in predicting behaviour are not difficult to understand. It is inherently limited in several important ways that have been acknowledged explicitly by Janz and Becker (1984). Perhaps most importantly, it assumes that health behaviour is rational and that people usually attempt to maximize a value expectancy function. Second, it describes only the role of health-relevant variables (e.g. perceived risk, efficacy of action) and ignores the multitude of functions that certain behaviours may serve. Furthermore, it makes no attempt to explicate the processes leading to individual or cultural differences in the independent variables or the specific behaviours under study. Finally, a number of variables that have been shown to be important in different studies are not explicitly incorporated by the Health Belief Model. Although all of these variables can be subsumed under one of the factors described by the model, the complex processes each represents is not described. For example, social and cultural influences are included only to the extent that certain mediators of cultural environments (e.g., barriers to care) are included in the model.

Some authors have argued that the problems with the Health Belief Model have been due to poor measurement, the lack of longitudinal designs, and small sample sizes. Although these observations are accurate to a certain extent, these are relatively minor issues. The research that will be most exciting in the future will not be the research that attempts to refine our knowledge of illness behaviour by including better measures or refining study methodology. Instead the most productive future research will be the work that expands beyond the boundaries of rational, explicit, value-expectancy models and tries to develop an understanding of the psychological, social and organizational factors generating and sustaining particular behaviours.

## AIDS: Behaviour or Contagion?

To demonstrate the limitations of cognitive illness behaviour models and to suggest how a different approach might be useful in developing predictions about health behaviour, the health behaviour of persons who are known to have HTLV-III antibodies in their blood will be considered.

HTLV-III is currently the most likely candidate for the main etiologic agent for Acquired Immune Deficiency Syndrome (AIDS). Recently, screening tests for HTLV-III have been developed and refined so that after a series of tests we can now be relatively certain about whether a person has HTLV-III antibodies in their blood. Blood is currently being screened for HTLV-III and persons are being informed of those test results.

Public health and medical personnel would like to structure the way information is provided and otherwise influence patient behaviour to achieve several goals. First, it is important that information is given in a way that is informative and intelligible. This is a difficult goal to attain in this situation. Persons with HTLV-III antibodies are at high risk for a fatal disease, but the nature of the risk and whether it can be altered is confusing. Second, it is desirable to maximize people's ability and motivation to behave in ways that are functional for both themselves and the public at large. The information about HTLV-III in one's blood and the knowledge that one may develop AIDS can be devastating. Furthermore, the behavioural recommendations for persons with positive results include no unprotected sex, no kissing, not having children, and notification of doctors and dentists. Adhering to these recommendations has a tremendous impact on most peoples' lives, and the factors related to whether people comply or not are extremely complex. Perhaps most importantly, physicians would like to help these people by providing the appropriate support and/or enable people to mobilize support from other sources and potentiate their ability to cope effectively with their new knowledge.

This is one of the most important yet elusive and complicated public health problems in history. Do traditional illness behaviour models provide a theoretical or practical guide on how to address these issues? To a certain extent, yes. Clearly, perceived susceptibility, perceived severity of AIDS, the individual's evaluation of the efficacy of behaviours, the costs of behaviours, cues to action, and enabling factors are important. However, these models fall far short of telling us all of what we need to know in this situation. For example, consider the variable perceived susceptibility. Obviously, this variable will be related to subsequent behaviour. However, what we really need to know is what accounts for the variations in the ways people process information and develop models of susceptibility. For persons with HTLV-III antibodies, the probability of developing AIDS within five years is between five and ten percent, but the factors that discriminate those who will and will not develop the disease are not known. Epidemiologists with the most current information find it difficult to estimate aggregate risk and differentiate persons at high and low risk. A recent Time magazine article compared the situation to playing Russian roulette with one bullet and ten chambers. Imagine how confusing the situation is for someone who has little statistical or medical knowledge, is highly anxious, and perceives a fatal threat associated with the information.

Perception of Risk

In most models dealing with conscious decisions about illness behaviour, perceptions of risk or danger are assumed to be a major determinant of whether the person takes illness action. There is a substantial literature on risk perception. Surprisingly, however, relatively little is known about how the factors affecting such perceptions relate to illness behaviour. Most researchers simply assume that people are aware of the risks they face or that perception of risk is directly related to the information available. Thus, an implicit assumption in much research on illness behaviour is that educating people about their risks will result in more appropriate illness behaviour. There are several problems with this approach. It is clear from the research that has been done that there may be substantial systematic biases in the way people evaluate risk. The estimation of risk is a complex process that depends on the context within which information is presented, the personality of the individual, and cultural factors. For example, a fascinating program of research conducted by Tversky and Kahneman (1981) has demonstrated that seemingly inconsequential changes in the formulation of choice problems causes predictable and significant shifts in preference. The main determinants in such shifts of preference are variations in the framing of acts, contingencies, and outcomes and the characteristic non-linearities of values and decision weights.

It is possible to specify situations in which people are more likely to over-estimate risk and situations in which they will under-estimate risk. For example, a number of studies have shown that there is a general tendency for people to under-estimate risk (Harris and Guten, 1979; Kirscht, Haefner, Kegeles, and Rosenstock, 1966; Larwood, 1978; Robertson, 1977; Weinstein, 1982: Weinstein and Lachendro, 1982). Weinstein (1982) consistently found that college students were generally unbiased about hereditary risk factors and were somewhat pessimistic about environmental risk factors, but they were optimistic about their chances of experiencing health and life-threatening problems. They were also optimistic about their own behaviour patterns; few acknowledged actions or psychological attributes that increased their risk.

Although people tend to under-estimate the frequency of more common causes of death, they over-estimate the frequency of rare causes of death (Slovic, Fischoff, and Lichtenstien, in press). Furthermore, Slovic and colleagues noted that the causes of death that were over-estimated tended to be dramatic and sensational. These data support the importance of available heuristics for the estimation of risk. That is, people tend to judge events as likely or frequent if they are easy to imagine or recall.

The complexities of risk assessment emphasize the inadvisability of adapting a linear, additive model such as the Health Belief Model to predict illness behaviour. Similarly, it is reasonable to expect that individuals who believe in their self-efficacy and in the efficacy of a particular behaviour are more likely to engage in that behaviour to reduce risk. However, Weinstein's (1982) findings suggest that the risks most thought to be preventable by private action are more likely to evoke unrealistic optimism about vulnerability.

Even if more was known about the determinants of risk perception, traditional models of illness behaviour would be inadequate for explaining most types of illness behaviour. Models of cognitive decisions about illness behaviour assume that people consider the barriers to action and the perceived benefits of particular behaviours and act in ways that maximize their outcomes. However, thinking about a person recently informed about HTLV-III emphasized how overly simplistic such an assumption is. For example, it is not clear what behaviours will be most likely to reduce psychological and physical morbidity in patients and what behaviours are directly related to prognosis and transmission of the disease. Given so much ambiguity, patients will undoubtedly develop illness representations or models of their own. Unfortunately, it is unknown how these models will be constructed or how they will influence behaviour. However, one of the implications of the work reviewed in this volume is that it will be critical to develop an understanding of these models before proceeding (Leventhal, 1983; Kleinman, 1980).

## Illness Representations

What are possible models of illness representation in the situation of AIDS? At least two general models have emerged during the short history of AIDS. When AIDS was first being researched, it was reported that there were a number of "risk factors" for AIDS, such as frequent intimate sexual contact, use of amyl nitrate, anal intercourse, etc. The implication was that certain types of behaviour, such as taking intravenous drugs, sniffing amyl nitrate, and engaging in frequent homosexual sex with multiple partners increased one's risk of AIDS because those behaviours make one "vulnerable to AIDS or "caused" AIDS in some way. That is, those behaviours, per se, increase one's risk of developing AIDS. A second, very different, contagion model of AIDS has recently emerged. The most current data suggest that AIDS is caused by an infectious agent that is transmitted by intimate contact or by transfusion of blood products (e.g., see Popovic, Sarngadharan, Read, and Gallo, 1984). In this model, the risk factors mentioned increase one's risk of contacting AIDS to the extent that they bring one into contact with other carriers of the vector that transmits AIDS. This model is supported not only by recent work on AIDS related retroviruses, but also by the striking geographic concentrations of AIDS incidence (Popovic et al., 1984). It is likely that we will eventually confirm both a specific etiologic agent and a number of vulnerability factors.

Depending on which model of risk a person holds, predictions about illness behaviour would be very different. If a person holds the notion that frequent sex increases the risk of AIDS per se, irrespective of whether or not the partner has had occasion to come into contact with the infectious agent, then reducing sexual activity would seem to be an efficacious action. One would have a clear-cut idea about the risk factor, be motivated by both knowledge and fear to reduce risk, assess one's illness action as efficacious, and be likely to take action (in this case inaction).

If, on the other, hand, one holds the apparently correct notion that AIDS clusters among individuals with similar characteristics or behaviours primarily because those indiviudals live in close proximity and have a high probability of coming into contact with one another, then one would make different predictions. People apparently are assuming that the modes of transmission for HTLV-III are much more general than they actually are. In such a situation, since contact with infected individuals may seem inevitable, one might be much less likely to take certain illness actions, such as reducing sexual contacts.

Thus, the risk model that one holds may be a critical determinant of how efficacious one thinks screening is. In addition, there are a number of other variables that are likely to be related to behaviour. Traditional health behaviour models focus on cognitive factors, but consider the potential importance of fear and anxiety. There is a large anxiety component associated with the AIDS risk in the minds of many homosexual men. This fear may inhibit screening if the individual does not see a way of reducing or changing risk and may reduce the probability of adhering to behavioural recommendations if those behaviours simply remind the person of the danger of AIDS. Both Leventhal (1986) and Lazarus (1986) (this volume) have emphasized the complexities of understanding both emotional and problem oriented management. These types of regulation, coping, or processing can occur in parallel and will influence each other. Fear may play a prominent role in how the individual behaves. Leventhal and colleagues (1983) have developed an elegant model of how and when fear will inhibit or facilitate certain types of behaviour.

Individuals both have varying degrees of factual knowledge, and they react differently to this information. Social groups, networks and supports also play critical roles in the way individuals react. Cultural influences must be brought to bear in a careful systematic study of illness behaviour. For example, if one must take into account the fact that persons who are HTLV-III positive are likely to include intravenous drug uses, Haitians, and people who frequently received transfusions, the complexity of the problem can seem overwhelming.

Although the behaviour is complicated, it is possible to derive a number of straightforward hypotheses about illness behaviour in AIDS patients and to test them. Simple multivariate models are not applicable to a large number of situations, but this does not mean that it would be difficult to derive a more appropriate model, given the special characteristics of the risk under consideration. If a better understanding of illness behaviours is to be developed, it is important to focus more on the understanding of how people process cognitive and emotional information, how social context conditions these processes and influence responses, and how culture and ethnicity influence these relationships.

## Illness Behaviour of Older Persons

It is important to take into account the way different subsets of the population vary in terms of the cultural construction of illness. This research tends to focus on groups with different ethnic backgrounds or cultures. However, it is also the case that within a single culture there can be substantial differences in the processes underlying illness behaviour. An interesting example of this is the illness behaviour of persons of different ages.

It might seem that our traditional approaches to studying illness behaviour are perfectly adequate for studying illness behaviour among the elderly, and there is no reason to use new or innovative approaches. However, there is reason to challenge this initial presumption.

A widely held view in social gerontology is that older persons are surprisingly optimistic in their health evaluations (Ferraro, 1980; Shanas, 1962; Fillenbaum, 1979; Linn and Linn, 1980; Maddox and Douglass, 1973). Explanations for this optimism include the idea that older people normalize symptoms of disease because of the belief that old age is necessarily associated with illness (Williamson, 1964). This leads to a broader perspective on the possible range of symptoms and disability and uses a reference group that is relatively sick (Cockerham, Sharp, and Wilcox, 1983). Survey and clinical research suggests that older people under-report certain symptoms, frequently do not seek medical help for relatively important symptoms, and rate their health rather positively (Levkoff, Cleary, and Wetle, 1985).

The research briefly alluded to above at first seems relatively compelling. However, almost none of it is comparative, and very little work has explicitly tried to incorporate the unique social, psychological, and physical characteristics of the aged into their models of health behaviour. There are good theoretical and empirical reasons to suspect that symptom perception, illness models, and the processes leading to and reinforcing help-seeking behaviours are qualitatively different among the aged (Levkoff et al., 1985). Factors that are likely to affect illness behaviour among the aged include increased social isolation, the loss of certain social roles, more loss events, multiple physiological changes, and different symptom and disease experiences. Older persons are more likely to suffer from multiple diseases and the diseases are more likely to be chronic in nature. Further, physical presentations of disease may change with age. For example, symptoms of atherosclerotic heart disease, appendicitis, and pneumonia tend to be less dramatic and noticeable among older persons. One of the consequences of these multiple changes is that elders have qualitatively different patterns of symptom recognition.

There is very suggestive evidence that elders are more likely to somatize psychic dysphoria. Other analyses indicate that the relative importance of different predictors of illness behaviour vary by age group (Levkoff et al., 1985). Peoples' illness representations, and the patterns of introspection are critical to these phenomena. While the Health Belief Model is a reasonable start in analyzing the illness behaviour of the elderly, important differences would be missed unless differences in symptom perception, encoding of sensory information, and differential factors affecting illness behaviour are explored. Not only are the independent variables different among the elderly, but the associations among variables are different. More importantly, the processes giving rise to perceptions and behaviour are different.

## METHODOLOGICAL ISSUES

The preceding examples illustrate some of the substantive issues and processes that will be the focus of illness behaviour research in the future. This volume represents a vast array of approaches to research on clinical problems. Two topics that are represented in a number of chapters in this volume are (1) psychiatric illness in primary care; and (2) coping strategies. There are a number of different ways to research these issues. It is important to reconsider past research and speculate on possible new directions.

### Psychiatric Illness in Primary Care

In primary care settings, there is high prevalence of mental disorders. Patients with these disorders use a large amount of services. Physicians frequently have difficulty either in identifying and treating those disorders or fail to refer patients elsewhere for treatment. Regier and colleagues (1978) have referred to the primary care setting in the United States as an ad hoc mental health care system. A great deal of effort has gone into investigating these phenomena. Issues of illness models, introspection, appraisal, somatization, information processing, and physician attitudes and behaviour are central to developing an understanding of why people go to medical doctors for psychological problems and why physicians respond in the way they do.

The slow growth in the economy recently, the large amount of public budgets accounted for by health spending, questions about the utility of additional care, and second thoughts about a totally egalitarian society have led to an increasing focus on the costs of medical care. There will be some desirable and some undesirable consequences of this revolution. It is clear that social, financial, and organizational factors affecting the cost and efficiency of care are likely to come under increasing scrutiny. There is a growing debate about the desirability of the incursion of the for-profit sector into the provision of health care in the United States. This is an important debate, but the substance of the debate should not blind us to a simple important fact; the medical care system is in flux. If health and illness behaviour are to be understood, the fact is that social factors determine the distribution and characteristics of medical care resources and these in turn determine illness behaviour. Treatment for minor psychological and/or psychosomatic problems is frequently viewed to be of marginal utility. This is especially likely in the study of whether and how patients with psychological and psychiatric disorders receive care. It is expected that in the future an increasing amount of research on the treatment of psychiatric illness in primary care settings will focus on the organization and financing of care. A direction in research that is related to this increasing emphasis on cost and effectiveness is an orientation to a broader range of outcome indicators. Instead of simply examining for the presence of disease, researchers will increasingly focus on physical and social functioning.

## Coping Research

Lazarus and Folkman (1984) have recently detailed an account of the interactive process of stress, appraisal, and coping. They repeatedly emphasize the need to look at stress and adaptation as a transactional process. It is beyond the scope of this chapter to outline what they mean by process and how they apply those ideas to stress and coping. However, they provide an incredibly rich accounting of the factors influencing and influenced by stress and coping. They also differentiate threat appraisal and apprasisal of ability to manage the threat. A similar approach to illness behaviour has been outlined by Leventhal, Safer, and Panagis (1983) and could be expanded to include many of the multitudinous factors discussed by Lazarus and Folkman. Lazarus and Folkman argue that an ipsative-normative approach is necessary to fully understand coping. One extension of these ideas might be that an ipsative-normative approach is necessary to fully delineate the processes underlying illness behaviour. Although such an approach is theoretically elegant, it is not likely to be useful for applied and clinical research. Such a detailed elaboration of the various processes underlying illness behaviour, and an anthropologic approach to illness representations may make the task seem almost unmanageable. If one focuses on such a multiplicity of processes, and intra- and inter- individual differences as well as cultural differences in psychological representations, one might view illness behaviour as ideosyncratic. This would be similar to the situation of personality researchers in the 1960's and 1970's. While one might be convinced that there are regular predictable features to people's behaviour, when one looks at individual characteristics in detail, it is difficult to reliably predict behaviour. For example, Lazarus and Folkman (1984) point out that measures of coping styles or personality traits do not predict how people will cope in a particular situation.

One can find a solution to this dilemma if illness behaviour is not thought of as constant across situations. The complexities described demand that researchers look within homogeneous circumstances to try and develop models for subsets of behaviour. By working to understand the processes underlying specific behaviours, one will be better able to develop models that predict across individuals and situations. One can think of a matrix in which one dimension represents variations in situations and the other represents variations in individual characteristics and dispositions. The predictions of behaviour in each cell would be different. However, if one restricts attention to the same type of situation, then the task of understanding variations in behaviour becomes more manageable. For example, the kinds of illness representations that people can have are infinite. However, it turns out that for particular diseases, a large majority of people tend to choose a limited number. For example, Leventhal and colleagues found that the majority of patients with hypertension have one of a few specific symptoms that they associate with hypertension. Similarly, although people can cope with information about illness in an infinite variety of ways, it appears that patients who are HTLV-III positive develop a relatively small set of illness representations and respond with a limited number of coping strategies. These representations and models may vary across subcultures. For example, the ways gay men and heterosexual women think of AIDS may be qualitatively different. Adoption of some of the research approaches and perspectives discussed in this volume may lead to increased understanding of when and how these differences will affect behaviour. In this way, one can meet the conflicting demands of exploring illness behaviour in more detail while at the same time providing more parsimonious explanations of the complex behaviours under study.

## SUMMARY

Traditional models of illness behaviour have serious limitations in each of the examples discussed. Future research must take into account a broader range of variables and attempt to explicitly model processes underlying the behaviour under investigation.

What are the lessons that should be drawn from this consideration of past research and the examples cited? First, there are certain variables and processes that should receive more attention in the future. These include: a) more detailed and theoretically based investigations of the factors related to the monitoring and interpretation of physical and psychological symptoms; b) studies of how people develop and use intuitive models of the body and illness to regulate their behaviour; c) investigations of how emotional and problem oriented coping processes influence individuals' behaviour; d) new studies of psychological and cultural factors related to somatization; e) research investigating how the organization and financing of health-care affect illness behaviour; f) studies of the way in which both explicit and implicit rationing mechanisms interact with patient characteristics in influencing illness behaviour; and g) more emphasis on functioning and quality of life as outcome indicators. These considerations will lead to the development of a better understanding of health and illness behaviour that will help us to address the important clinical, health service, and epidemiologic issues of a given time period.

## ACKNOWLEDGEMENTS

Thanks extended to S. Levkoff for helpful comments in the preparation of this manuscript.

## REFERENCES

Becker, M. H. (1974). The health belief model and personal health behaviour. Thorofare, NJ: Slack.

Becker, M. H. & Maiman, L. A. (1983). Models of health-related behaviour. In D. Mechanic (Ed.), Handbook of health, health care, and the health professions. (pp. 539-568). New York: The Free Press.

Cockerham, W. C., Sharp, K., & Wilcox, J. (1983). Aging and perceived health. Journal of Gerontology, 38, 349-355.

Ferraro, K. (1980). Self-ratings of health among the old and the old-old. Journal of Health and Social Behavior, 21, 377-383.

Fillenbaum, G. (1979). Social context and self-assessments of health among the elderly. Journal of Health and Social Behavior, 20, 45-51.

Harris, D. M. & Guten, S. (1979). Health-protective behaviour: An exploratory study. Journal of Health and Social Behavior, 20, 17-29.
Janz, N. K. & Becker, M. H. (1984). The health belief model: A decade later. Health Education Quarterly, 11, 1-47.
Kasl, S. V. & Cobb, S. (1966). Health behaviour, illness behaviour and sick role behaviour: I. Health and illness behaviour. Archives of Environmental Health, 12, 246-266.
Kirscht, J. P., Haefner, D. P., Kegeles, S. S., & Rosenstock, I.M. (1966). A national study of health beliefs. Journal of Health and Social Behavior, 7, 248-254.
Kleinman, A. (1980). Patients and healers in the context of culture. An exploration of the borderland between anthropology, medicine, and psychiatry. Berkely: University of California Press.
Larwood, L. (1978). Swine flu: A field study of self-serving biases. Journal of Applied Social Psychology, 8, 283-289.
Lazarus, R. S. & Folkman, S. (1984). Stress, appraisal, and coping. New York: Springer.
Leventhal H. (1983). Behavioral medicine: Psychology in health care. In D. Mechanic (Ed.), Handbook of health, health care, and the health professions. New York: Free Press.
Leventhal, H., Hochbaum, G. M., & Rosenstock, I. M. (1960). Epidemic impact of the general population. In The impact of Asian influenza on community life: A study of five cities. United States Department of Health, Education, and Welfare, Public Health Service, Pub. No. 706, Washington, D.C.
Leventhal, H., Safer, M. A., & Panagis, D. M. (1983). The impact of communications on the self-regulation of health beliefs, decisions, and behavior. Health Education Quarterly, 10, 3-28.
Levkoff, S. E., Cleary, P. D., & Wetle, T. (1985). Differences in the appraisal of health between the aged and middle-aged. Unpublished manuscript, Harvard University.
Linn, B. S., & Linn, M. W. (1980). Objective and self-assessed of health in old and very old. Social Science Medicine, 14, 311-315.
Maddox, G. L., & Douglass, E. B. (1973). Self-assessment of health: A longitudinal study of elderly subjects. Journal of Health and Social Behavior, 14, 87-93.
Maiman, L. A. & Becker, M. H. (1974). The health belief model: Origins and correlates in psychological theory. Health Education Monograph, 2, 236-253.
Popovic, M., Sarngadharan, M. B., Read, E., & Gallo, R. C. (1984). Detection, isolation, and continuous production of cytopathic retroviruses, (HTLV-III) from patients with AIDS and pre-AIDS. Science, 224, 497-500.
Regier, D. A., Goldbert, I. D., & Taube, C. A. (1978). The de facto US mental health services system. A public health perspective. Archives of General Psychiatry, 35, 685-693.
Robertson, L. S. (1977). Car crashes: Perceived vulnerability and willingness to pay for crash protection. Journal of Community Health, 3, 136-141.
Rosenstock, I. M. (1960). What research in motivation suggests for public health. American Journal of Public Health, 50, 295-302.
Rosenstock, I. M. (1974). Historical origins of the Health Belief Model. Health Education Monograph, 2, 409-419.
Rosenstock, I. M., & Kirscht, J. (1979). Why people use health services. In G. Stone, F. Cohen, & N. Adler (Eds.), Health Psychology. San Francisco: Jossey-Bass.
Shanas, E. (1962). The health of older people. Cambridge: Harvard University Press.
Slovic, P., Fischoff, R., & Lichtenstien, S. (in press). Behavioural decision theory perspectives on protective behaviour. In N. Weinstein (Ed.), Taking care: Why people take precautions.

Tversky, A., & Kahneman, D. (1981). The framing of decisions and the psychology of choice. Science, 21, 453-458.
Weinstein, N. D. (1982). Unrealistic optimism about susceptibility to health problems. Journal of Behavioral Medicine, 5, 441-460.
Weinstein, N. D., & Lachendro, E. (1982). Egocentrism as a source of unrealtistic optimism. Personal Social Psychology Bulletin, 8, 195-200.
Williamson, J. (1964). Old people and their unreported needs. Lancet, 1, 1117-1120.

# DEPRESSION: PATTERN OF MEDICAL UTILIZATION AND SOMATIZATION IN PRIMARY CARE

Wayne Katon, Alfred Berg, Anthony Robins and Steven Risse

Department of Psychiatry
University of Washington Medical School

Epidemiologic studies in primary care have documented that between 25 and 75 percent of all patient visits are due to psychosocial stress as opposed to biomedical problems (Stoeckle, Zola, and Davidson, 1964; Manucci, Friedman, and Kaufman, 1961; Garfield, Collen, Feldman, et al., 1976). Studies that have used structured interviews and research diagnostic criteria for psychiatric illness have determined that one in every four primary care patients has a major mental illness. Hoeper and others (1979) in a study of primary care patients utilizing the Schedule for Affective Disorders and Schizophrenia (SADS) and Research Diagnostic Criteria found that 26.7 percent of patients in a primary care clinic suffered from a mental illness. Hoeper, Nyczi, Cleary, et al. (1979) as well as Marsland, Wood and Mayo (1970), have demonstrated that the anxiety and affective disorders are the two most common types of mental disorders afflicting primary care patients.

Epidemiologic studies of depression in primary care have utilized two strategies to study prevalence rates, namely self-rating scales and structured interviews. Multiple studies have used depression self-rating scales to assess prevalence, and these studies have shown that depression occurs in 12 percent to 25 percent of primary care patients (Neilson and Williams, 1980; Hankin and Locke, 1982; Seller, Blaskovich and Lenkei, 1981). However, the depression self-rating scales are more sensitive than specific. These detect virtually all cases of depression, but also select many false positives who do not meet research criteria for major depression. In two recent studies utilizing structured psychiatric interviews and research criteria, Hoeper and Zung found that major depression occurred in six percent to ten percent of primary care patients (Hoeper et al., 1979; Zung, Magill, Moore, et al., 1983). This prevalence rate makes major depression one of the most common clinical problems presenting to primary care physicians (hypertension is the next most frequent diagnosis at 7.0 percent) (Rosenblatt, Cherkin, Schneeweiss, et al., 1982).

Despite the high prevalence rate of major depression, five studies have determined that primary care physicians fail to accurately diagnose 50 to 82 percent of primary care outpatients with major depression (Neilson and Williams, 1980; Hankin and Locke, 1982; Seller et al., 1981; Zung et al., 1983; Moffic and Paykel, 1975). Moreover, two of these studies documented that the primary care physicians were no more accurate in diagnosing depression in the severe depressives than they were in the mild to moderate depressives (Seller et al., 1981; Moffic and Paykel, 1975). This lack of accurate diagnosis can lead to increased morbidity and mortality since untreated depression often results in chronic disability secondary to the social consequences of the illness, i.e., divorce, family problems, vocational loss and self-medication with alcohol and drugs. Moreover, Murphy (1979) documented in a study of 80 patients who had successfully committed suicide that 82 percent had visited a primary care physician in the month prior to their suicide and 55 percent of patients died from an overdose of medication prescribed in that visit.

There have been three problems identified that impede the ability of primary care physicians to diagnose depression. First, many of the patients with depression focus on the somatic symptoms of their illness (such as insomnia, anorexia, fatigue, loss of libido) and minimize the affective and cognitive problems as secondary (Katon, Kleinman, and Rosen, 1982). Second, depression is frequently caused by an acute or chronic medical illness, and that illness tends to mask the depressive problems (Katon, 1984). Many patients with chronic illness who develop major depression simply report worsening of their chronic illness or stop complying with prescribed treatment for their chronic medical illness and relapse. Finally, physicians by nature of their training are somatizers, i.e., they selectively focus on and rule out biomedical illness with psychiatric illness representing a diagnosis of exclusion.

Studies by Brown and Harris (1978), Widmer and Cadoret (1978) and Weissman, Myers and Thompson (1981) have all independently reported increased utilization rates of primary care physicians by patients with major depression. Weissman also found that 50 percent of the patients with major depression were treated in primary care with sedative hypnotics whereas only 17 percent were treated with tricyclic antidepressants (Weissman et al., 1981). Widmer's studies, in particular, suggested that primary care patients with depression presented with nonspecific complaints, pain complaints, tension and anxiety (Widmer and Cadoret, 1978).

This chapter reports on a study designed to investigate whether there are signals of depression that the primary care physician should be attuned to in order to more accurately make the diagnosis of depression. A primary care population with depression was compared to a primary care control group who did not suffer depression over a prospective one-year period after diagnosis and a retrospective two-year period prior to diagnosis. Depressed patients' patterns of medical utilization, i.e., rates of visits, telephone calls and medical evaluations were compared to controls. Also depressed patients' chief complaints on each visit and physician diagnoses were compared to nondepressives.

This study was conducted in the Family Medical Center at the University of Washington. Patients visiting the Medical Center are representative of the general community in terms of sex, ethnicity and insurance status. Subjects were recruited in the following manner. Over a nine-month period individual clinic sessions were randomly selected. Within each session a single physician was identified and a random subgroup of his/her patients (age 18 and over) were approached for participation. Patients completed the Beck Depression Inventory (short form) (Beck and Beck, 1972) and the Zung Self-Rating Depression Scale (Zung and Durham, 1965).

The medical records of study participants were examined for the two years preceding and for the year following the index visit. Data abstracted included; numbers and types of contacts, chief complaints, numbers and types of evaluations (history, physical exam, blood tests, urinalysis, x-rays, microbiologic tests) performed, specific therapies recommended, and diagnoses recorded. A small group of patients with scores on depression rating scales in the moderate to severe depression range was contacted by the investigators and offered further evaluation using the SADS interview (Endicott and Spitzer, 1978). If a patient was found to be severely depressed or suicidal, the personal physician was notified; but in the majority of cases, physicians were not aware of the study's progress or clinical findings unless the patients requested that their physician be so informed.

Chief complaints and diagnoses were initially coded using the International Classification of Primary Care (1984) and ICHPPC (International Classification of Health Problems in Primary Care, 1979) respectively. These classifications were further reduced by the authors to the following 13 clusters of complaints and diagnoses thought more appropriately to reflect the major factors important in this study: (A maximum of six complaints and diagnoses were coded for each time period)

a. Specific diagnosis, infection, objective sign or items not classified, e.g., hypertension, carbuncle, conjunctivitis, diabetes mellitus, pancreatitis, neoplastic disorders;

b. Injury, e.g., lacerations, motor vehicle accident, fractures, head injuries;

c. Headache, e.g., tension or migraine headache;

d. Neck or back pain, e.g., acute or chronic pain, strain;

e. Acute musculoskeletal pain (exclude neck/back), e.g., knee pain, hip pain, general muscle or joint complaints, etc;

f. Chest pain;

g. Abdominal or pelvic pain, e.g., general abdominal pain, stomach-ache, dysuria, menstrual pain;

h. Pain not elsewhere classifed, e.g., generalized pain, eye pain, ear pain, skin pain;

i. Nonspecific or functional complaint, e.g., fatigue, weakness, nausea, change of bowel habits, senility, tinnitus, palpitations, dizziness, itching, weight problems, menstrual problems;

j. Psychiatric symptoms, behaviours, and disorders (exclude depression), e.g., anxiety, sleep disturbances, sexual problems, substance abuse, schizophrenia, obesity, hysterical and hypochondriacal disorders;

k. Depression;

l. Psychophysiologic disorders, e.g., irritable bowel syndrome, premenstrual syndrome, peptic ulcer disease, temporomandibular joint problems;

m. Social problems, e.g., marital problems, unwanted pregnancy, financial or legal problems, death of family member, employment problems.

One hundred forty-seven patients were enrolled as study subjects. Although it proved impossible to keep strict records of refusals to participate, such refusals were very uncommon, and usually due to scheduling difficulties and other factors. The study group was representative of the

TABLE 1 RELATIONSHIP BETWEEN DEPRESSION STATUS AND MEDICAL UTILIZATION INDICES

| | | Medical Utilization States | | | | | | | |
|---|---|---|---|---|---|---|---|---|---|
| | | Office Visits | | Telephone Calls | | Evaluation | | Psychiatric Medications | |
| | | 2 yrs before | 1 yr after | 2 yrs before | 1 yr after | 2 yrs before | 1 yr after | 2 yrs before | 1 yr after |
| Depression Status | None(91) | 6.9 | 3.8 | 0.7 | 0.3 | 4.2 | 1.9 | 0.2 | 0.1 |
| | Mild(29) | 9.0 | 6.6 | 1.2 | 0.6 | 8.4 | 3.6 | 0.2 | 0.3 |
| | Mod(22) | 9.9 | 6.5 | 1.4 | 1.4 | 6.4 | 4.3 | 1.4 | 0.4 |
| | Severe(5) | 12.0 | 15.4 | 3.6 | 0.2 | 9.8 | 3.6 | 2.2 | 0.4 |
| Significance (ANOVA) | | $p=0.14$ | $p<.01$ | $p=0.01$ | $p<.01$ | $p=0.05$ | $p=0.02$ | $p<.01$ | $p=0.07$ |

TABLE 2 NUMBER OF PATIENTS WITH EACH CHIEF COMPLAINT BY DEPRESSION STATUS IN THE TWO YEARS BEFORE AND ONE YEAR AFTER INDEX VISIT

| | Two Years Before Index Visit Depression Status | | | | | One Year After Depression Status | | | | |
|---|---|---|---|---|---|---|---|---|---|---|
| Complaints | None | Mild | Mod | Sev | P value* | None | Mild | Mod | Sev | P value* |
| Specific | 90 | 29 | 22 | 5 | .89 | 90 | 29 | 21 | 5 | .54 |
| Injury | 13 | 6 | 3 | 1 | .84 | 9 | 1 | 4 | 1 | .32 |
| Headache | 11 | 3 | 2 | 0 | .84 | 4 | 0 | 3 | 0 | .14 |
| Back/neck pain | 16 | 2 | 4 | 0 | .39 | 7 | 2 | 5 | 0 | .13 |
| Acute MS pain | 12 | 8 | 2 | 0 | .15 | 7 | 5 | 5 | 1 | .17 |
| Chest pain | 10 | 1 | 1 | 0 | .45 | 2 | 2 | 1 | 0 | .63 |
| Abdominal pain | 15 | 8 | 3 | 1 | .53 | 7 | 6 | 3 | 0 | .20 |
| Pain (other) | 10 | 1 | 2 | 1 | .55 | 6 | 5 | 1 | 0 | .23 |
| Nonspecific | 54 | 15 | 10 | 3 | .65 | 34 | 11 | 9 | 5 | .05 |
| Other Psychiatric | 12 | 2 | 2 | 0 | .65 | 8 | 3 | 3 | 0 | .79 |
| Depression | 4 | 3 | 3 | 1 | .27 | 4 | 2 | 4 | 2 | .05 |
| Psychophysiologic | 7 | 1 | 0 | 0 | .44 | 6 | 1 | 1 | 2 | .02 |
| Social problems | 4 | 3 | 2 | 0 | .57 | 5 | 2 | 2 | 0 | .86 |
| Total: | 258 | 82 | 56 | 12 | | 189 | 89 | 62 | 16 | |

Mod = moderate, Sev = severe
* x(2) statistic

clinic population generally, with the majority women (70 percent) and mean age 33 years.

Each of the 147 individual study subjects was classified by their most depressed Zung or Beck Inventory score into one of four groups: severely depressed (5), moderately depressed (22), mildly depressed (29) and not depressed (91). The 27 patients with moderate to severe depression were contacted and offered a structured psychiatric interview. Eleven of these patients (41 percent) were interviewed with the SADS and eight (73 percent) were found to have major depression by DSM-III criteria. In the one-year period after screening, only ten (37 percent) of the patients with moderate to severe depression on the Beck and Zung Depression Scales were recognized by their physicians as being depressed. Nine (33 percent) of these ten patients were treated with tricyclic antidepressants.

Relationship between depressive status and health care utilization. In the two years before screening, patients with depression made significantly more telephone calls to the physician and were prescribed more psychiatric medications (Table 1). In the one year after the index visit, patients with depression had significantly more office visits, telephone calls and medical evaluations (physical exams, blood tests, X-rays) than controls, and there was a trend toward being prescribed more psychiatric medications.

Relationship between depression status and chief complaints. Patients with depression did not have any more specific complaints in the two-year period before the index visit, but did have significantly more nonspecific complaints, psychophysiologic complaints and depressive complaints in the one year after screening (Table 2).

Relationship between depression status and diagnosis. In the two years prior to the index visit, patients with depression were more likely to be diagnosed as depressed and having a problem with pain (Table 3). In the period of one year after the index visit, patients with depression were more likely to have a specific psychiatric diagnosis, to have a psychophysiologic diagnosis, a diagnosis of acute musculoskeletal pain and a diagnosis of abdominal pain (Table 3).

The results of the prospective portion of this study confirmed results of past retrospective studies in documenting that primary care patients with depression made significantly more visits and more telephone calls to their physicians than nondepressed controls. They also had significantly more medical evaluations (laboratory tests, X-rays, etc.). In the one year after their index visit (at which time their depression was recognized) patients with moderate to severe depression scores were found to have significantly more complaints of depression, nonspecific or vague symptoms (fatigue, weakness, tinnitus, palpitations, dizziness, weight problems) and more psychophysiologic complaints (irritable bowel syndrome, peptic ulcer disease, eczema, temporomandibular joint pain, premenstrual syndrome) than controls. Also during this one-year prospective period, the depressed patients were significantly more likely to receive the diagnosis of depression, acute musculoskeletal pain, abdominal pain, psychophysiologic disorder and other psychiatric disorders than the nondepressed controls.

These findings are important because although past studies have documented that patients with mental illness utilize two to three times as much nonpsychiatric medical care (Widmer and Cadoret, 1978; Weissman et al., 1981), these studies did not specify patients' diagnoses. Studies in primary care have also consistently documented that a small percentage of patients (five to ten percent) utilize a disproportionate share (30 to 50 percent) of medical care. A consistent finding from these studies is that patients with mental illness are over-represented among the high utilization samples

TABLE 3 NUMBER OF PATIENTS WITH GIVEN DIAGNOSIS BY DEPRESSION STATUS IN THE TWO YEARS BEFORE AND ONE YEAR AFTER INDEX VISIT

| | Two Years Before Index Visit Depression Status | | | | | One Year After Depression Status | | | | |
|---|---|---|---|---|---|---|---|---|---|---|
| Complaints | None | Mild | Mod | Sev | P value* | None | Mild | Mod | Sev | P value* |
| Specific | 91 | 29 | 22 | 5 | -- | 91 | 29 | 22 | 5 | -- |
| Injury | 26 | 10 | 5 | 1 | .79 | 14 | 5 | 7 | 2 | .20 |
| Headache | 7 | 3 | 1 | 0 | .79 | 3 | 0 | 2 | 0 | .34 |
| Back/neck pain | 8 | 1 | 1 | 0 | .65 | 3 | 0 | 1 | 1 | .15 |
| Acute MS pain | 2 | 0 | 1 | 0 | .70 | 0 | 1 | 0 | 1 | .001 |
| Chest pain | 2 | 2 | 1 | 0 | .63 | 2 | 0 | 0 | 0 | .74 |
| Abdominal pain | 5 | 4 | 3 | 0 | .33 | 3 | 0 | 3 | 1 | .04 |
| Pain (other) | 0 | 1 | 2 | 0 | .05 | 1 | 2 | 0 | 0 | .22 |
| Nonspecific | 18 | 5 | 5 | 1 | .97 | 10 | 5 | 2 | 1 | .73 |
| Other Psychiatric | 15 | 4 | 6 | 0 | .41 | 7 | 3 | 2 | 3 | .003 |
| Depression | 4 | 4 | 5 | 3 | .001 | 6 | 4 | 4 | 2 | .06 |
| Psychophysiologic | 8 | 4 | 3 | 1 | .74 | 9 | 2 | 1 | 3 | .003 |
| Social problems | 5 | 3 | 1 | 0 | .71 | 4 | 1 | 0 | 0 | .75 |
| Total: | 191 | 70 | 56 | 11 | | 153 | 52 | 44 | 19 | |

Mod = moderate, Sev = severe
* x(2) statistic

(Liptzin, Regier, and Goldberg, 1980; McHugh, Kahn, and Heiman, 1977). The finding that depression is one of the major psychiatric diagnoses associated with high utilization is crucial since it is an illness that is amenable to both psychotherapy and psychopharmacologic treatments.

A second generation of studies should follow from this study to document that treatment of depressive disorders in primary care by a combined psychiatry liaison/primary care physician team would lead to a decrease in depressive symptoms, return of utilization rates to baseline, decreased somatization and decreased iatrogenic injury and financial cost to the patient and medical care system.

Results in the two-year period prior to the diagnosis of depression were less clear in several ways. The depressed patient did make significantly more telephone calls to physicians and had more medical evaluations than controls. However, there were no specific differences noted between depressed and nondepressed patients in patient complaints over the two-year period. Physicians were more likely to diagnose patients with depression as depressed and as suffering from a pain problem, not categorized elsewhere (generalized pain, eye pain, ear pain, skin pain) than controls. It may have been that the two-year retrospective period selected for study was too long since it was unclear when the depressive illness started. Goldberg (1984) has demonstrated that 50 percent of primary care patients with depression had a remission of their symptoms when reinterviewed at six months.

Finally, there was a low rate of accurate diagnosis of depression by the family physicians in the study. Only ten (37 percent) of the patients were accurately diagnosed as depressed. Most likely due to the nonspecific nature of their somatic complaints, the physicians ordered more extensive laboratory and X-ray tests for the patients with depression than the nondepressed controls. The results of this study confirm the tendency of depressed primary care patients to somatize, i.e., selectively focus on somatic symptoms of their illness. This tendency of primary care patients with psychiatric illness to somatize has previously been documented by Goldberg who found that 50 percent of primary care patients with anxiety or depression presented with a somatic symptom (Goldberg, 1984). The recent National Ambulatory Care Survey (in which primary care physicians provided a wide range of information on approximately 90,000 office visits) also demonstrated that 70 percent of patient visits to general medical physicians that result in a psychiatric diagnosis have a physical symptom as the patient's chief complaint (Schurman, Kramer, and Mitchell, 1985).

The study findings suggest that physicians should consider the diagnosis of depression in patients with a pattern of increased clinic utilization (office visits and telephone calls) who present with nonspecific and psychophysiologic symptoms and receive diagnoses such as abdominal pain, acute musculoskeletal pain, a psychophysiologic disorder or another psychiatric illness. The National Ambulatory Care Survey also confirmed that patients with psychiatric diagnoses initially presented with nonspecific symptoms (24 percent complained of chest pain, headaches, dizziness or exhaustion) as well as abdominal or stomach pain or cramps (7.5 percent) or neck, back or leg problems (5.8 percent) (Schurman et al., 1985). It is clear that the patient self-rating depression scales are a sensitive indicator of depression, and the widespread use of these scales in primary care along with adequate psychiatric training of primary care physicians on current effective treatments would increase the accuracy of diagnosis and result in more effective treatment of depression.

SUMMARY

One hundred and forty-seven primary care patients were screened for depression utilizing depression rating scales and psychiatric interview. In the one-year period after screening, the depressed patients visited the physician more frequently, made more telephone calls to their physicians, and had more medical evaluations than the nondepressed patients. The depressed patients were more likely to have nonspecific or vague complaints, psychophysiologic complaints and depressive complaints than the nondepressed patients; their family physicians during this same one-year period were more likely to diagnose the depressed patients as having a psychophysiologic problem, abdominal pain, acute musculoskeletal pain and psychiatric disorders other than depression. In the two years before the screening, depressed patients made more physician telephone calls and had more medical evaluations than controls; they were also more likely during this two-year period to be diagnosed as having a pain problem or as being depressed.

REFERENCES

Beck, A. T., & Beck, R. W. (1972). Screening depressed patients in family practice: A rapid technique. Postgraduate Medicine, 52, 81-85.

Brown, G., & Harris, T. (1978). Social origins of depression: A study of psychiatric disorder in women. New York: The Free Press.

Endicott, J., & Spitzer, R. L. (1978). A diagnostic interview: The schedule for affective disorders and schizophrenia. Archives of General Psychiatry, 35, 837-842.

Garfield, S. R., Collen, M. D., Feldman, R., et al. (1976). Evaluation of an ambulatory medical care delivery system. New England Journal of Medicine, 294, 426-431.

Goldberg, D. (1984). The recognition of psychiatric illness by non-psychiatrists. Australian and New Zealand Journal of Psychiatry, 18, 128-133.

Hankin, J. R., & Locke, B. Z. (1982). The persistence of depressive symptomatology among prepaid group practice enrollees. American Journal of Public Health, 72, 1000-1009.

Hoeper, E. W., Nyczi, G. R., Cleary, P. D., et al. (1979). Estimated prevalence of RDC mental disorder in primary care. International Journal of Mental Health, 8, 30-48.

International Classification of Health Problems in Primary Care. (1979). Oxford: Oxford University.

International Classification of Primary Care. (1984). By North American Primary Care Research Group. Richmond, VA.

Katon, W. (1984). Depression: Relationship to somatization and chronic medical illness. Journal of Clinical Psychiatry, 45, (3, Sec. 2), 4-11.

Katon, W., Kleinman, A., & Rosen, G. (1982). Depression and somatization: A review, part I. American Journal of Medicine, 72, 127-135.

Liptzin, B., Regier, D. A., & Goldberg, I. D. (1980). Utilization of health and mental health services in a large insured population. American Journal of Psychiatry, 137, 553-558.

Manucci, M., Friedman, S. M., & Kaufman, M. R. (1961). Survey of patients who have been seen attending non-psychiatric outpatient department service for ten years or longer. Journal of Mount Sinai Hospital, 28, 32.

Marsland, D. W., Wood, M., & Mayo, F. (1976). Content of family practice: A data bank for patient care, curriculum and research in family practice - 526,196 patient problems. Journal of Family Practice, 3, 25-68.

McHugh, J. P., Kahn, M. W., & Heiman, E. (1977). Relationships between mental health treatment and medical utilization among low income Mexican-American patients: Some preliminary findings. Medical Care, 14, 439-444.

Moffic, H. S., & Paykel, E. S. (1975). Depression in medical inpatients. British Journal of Psychiatry, 126, 346-353.

Murphy, G. L. (1979). The physician's responsibility for suicide. Annals of Internal Medicine, 82, 301-309.

Neilson, A. C., & Williams, T. A. (1980). Depression in ambulatory medical patients. Archives of General Psychiatry, 37, 999-1004.

Rosenblatt, R., Cherkin, D. C., Schneeweiss, R., Hart, L .G., Greenwald, H Kirkwood, and Perkoff, G. T. (1982). The structure and content of family practice: Correct status and future trends. Journal of Family Practice, 15, 681-722.

Schurman, R. A., Kramer, P. D., & Mitchell, J. B. (1985). The hidden mental health network: Treatment of mental illness by nonpsychiatrist physicians. Archives of General Psychiatry, 42, 911-921.

Seller, R. H., Blaskovich, J., & Lenkei, E. (1981). Influence of stereotypes in the diagnosis of depression by family practice residents. Journal of Family Practice, 12, 849-854.

Stoeckle, J. D., Zola, I. K., & Davidson, G. E. (1964). The quantity and significance of psychological distress in medical patients. Journal of Chronic Diseases, 17, 959.

Weissman, M. M., Myers, J. K., & Thompson, W. D. (1981). Depression and its treatment in a US urban community 1975-1976. Archives of General Psychiatry, 39, 417-421.

Widmer, R. B., & Cadoret, R. J. (1978). Depression in primary care: Changes in pattern of patient visits and complaints during a developing depression. Journal of Family Practice, 7, 293-302.

Zung, W. E., & Durham, N. C. (1965). A self-rating depression scale. Archives of General Psychiatry, 12, 63-70.

Zung, W. W. K., Magill, M., Moore, J. T., et al. (1983). Recognition and treatment of depression in a family medicine practice. Journal of Clinical Psychiatry, 44, 3-9.

# MEASURING UTILITIES FOR HEALTH STATES

George Torrance

Management Science, and Clinical Epidemiology and Biostatistics
McMaster University

The paper reviews the history of health state utility measurement; the techniques of health state utility measurement, including rating scales, standard gamble and time trade-off; the performance of health state utility measurement, including acceptability, reliability, validity and cost; the variability in health state utilities across individuals and the relationship to other factors; and the applications of health state utilities, particularly in cost-effectiveness studies.

## Health Utility Measurement

A health state utility index is a cardinal number, usually between 0.0 and 1.0, that is associated with the particular health state. The utility reflects the desirability or preference for the health state as assessed by a rater, who may or may not have had personal experience with the health state being rated. The measure reflects the rater's assessment of the overall impact that the health state would have or does have on the individual's life style - that is, how it affects the individual's overall physical and emotional functioning. The measure is a summary health index that reflects the health-related quality of life associated with the particular health state.

For utility measurement purposes a health state is defined from a performance/behaviour/function point of view. That is, the health state is described in terms of how it affects a person's ability to function, behave or perform. It is not defined in terms of diagnoses, disease labels, or laboratory test results. Within this broad perspective there are many ways in which a health state can be described. Examples of these include: a narrative description in paragraph form; a brief point form description; or video tapes of a person in the particular health state. In a recent study (Cadman, Boyle, Goldsmith and Torrance, 1985) six key attributes have been identified that should be included in a health state description. These are: physical function, emotional function, sensory function, cognitive function, self-care function, and pain. A health state description would describe the level of functioning on each of these six attributes at a particular point in time. Notice that a health state description does not contain explicitly a prognosis. Prognosis is <u>not</u> part of a health state description. Prognosis represents the likely course or change of health states over time. It is important to recognize this distinction and to ensure that prognoses do not creep inadvertently into health state descriptions. Of course, some descriptions imply a particular prognosis and this will be handled in the measurement process to be described later.

The term "utility" is somewhat unfortunate because it can be confusing. It does not refer to the usefulness of the health state or of someone in the health state, but refers to the desirability or preference that individuals exhibit for the health state. In fact, a simple definition of utility is that it is a cardinal measure of the strength of one's preference. To cause further potential confusion there are two kinds of utilities, classical utility and modern utility. Classical utility refers to the concept of utilitarianism and the use of the term utility in this connection prior to the 1950's. Modern utility refers to the use of utilities as based on the work of von Neumann and Morgenstern (1953). These authors founded modern utility theory as a normative approach to decision-making under uncertainty. The theory describes how a decision maker ought to approach a decision problem in which the outcomes are uncertain if he/she wishes to act in a manner defined by the particular set of rational axioms. The axioms have great face validity, and this, in turn, has provided a strong foundation for decision theory.

Table 1 provides some utilities for health states from the literature. Note two states in particular, healthy which has a utility value of 1.00 and dead which has a utility value of 0.00. These two states are reference states and their utility value is defined in order to establish the scale. The utilities for the other health states are determined relative to these two.

Health state utilities are important for several reasons. First, they are important because of a belief in the sovereignty of consumer preferences. That is, the preferences of consumers of health care services should count in health care decisions being made that will affect or potentially affect the consumers. Note that consumers are not being asked for their preferences for therapies or programs, but for their preferences for outcomes or health states. That is, the general public are not asked to express a preference for either a neonatal intensive care unit or a kidney dialysis unit, but they are asked to express their preferences for the different kinds of outcomes (health states) that can occur from each. Second, utilities are a relevant concept because they are based on decision theory under uncertainty, and most health care decisions fall in this domain - that is, the outcomes are uncertain. Third, utilities for health states are important because they support four different kinds of applications: clinical decision analysis, resource allocation using cost-effectiveness analysis or cost-utility analysis, clinical trials, and population health surveys.

The concept of health state utilities originated in the early 1970's. A number of groups have contributed to this development and are noted for further reference, including: Fanshel and Bush, 1970; Kaplan, Bush, and Berry, 1976; Kaplan and Bush, 1982; Torrance, Thomas, and Sackett, 1972; Torrance, 1976a; Torrance, 1976b; Sackett and Torrance, 1978; Torrance, Boyle and Horwood, 1982; Boyle and Torrance, 1984; Torrance and Zipursky, 1984; Churchill, Morgan, and Torrance, 1984; Rosser and Watt, 1971; Rosser and Kind, 1978; Weinstein and Stason, 1977; Weinstein, 1980, 1981; Llewellyn-Thomas et al., 1982; Sutherland, Dunn and Boyd, 1983.

Techniques for Measuring Health State Utility

There are a number of alternative techniques and instruments available for the measurement of health state utilities. The three most common techniques are rating scales, standard gamble, and time trade-off. These three techniques are described in some detail below. In addition, other techniques such as equivalence and ratio scaling are sometimes used. Finally, any of the techniques can be used in conjunction with multi-attribute utility theory in certain circumstances.

TABLE 1

UTILITIES FOR HEALTH STATES

| Health State | Utility |
|---|---|
| Healthy (REF) | 1.00 |
| Life with menopausal symptoms (J) | 0.99 |
| Side effects of hypertension treatment (J) | 0.95 - 0.99 |
| Mild angina (J) | 0.90 |
| Moderate angina (J) | 0.70 |
| Some physical and role limitation with occasional pain (TTO) | 0.67 |
| Hospital dialysis (TTO, Hamilton, dialysis patients) | 0.59 |
| Hospital dialysis (TTO, St. John's, dialysis patients) | 0.57 |
| Hospital dialysis (TTO, general public) | 0.56 |
| Severe angina (J) | 0.50 |
| Anxious/depressed and lonely much of the time (TTO) | 0.45 |
| Being blind or deaf or dumb (TTO) | 0.39 |
| Hospital confinement (TTO) | 0.33 |
| Mechanical aids to walk and learning disabled (TTO) | 0.31 |
| Dead (REF) | 0.00 |
| Quadriplegic, blind and depressed (TTO) | <0.00 |
| Confined to bed with severe pain (RS) | <0.00 |
| Unconscious (RS) | <0.00 |

TTO = time trade off
RS = ratio scaling
J = judgement
REF = reference state

Rating scales. A typical rating scale consists of a line on a page with clearly defined end points. The most preferred health state is placed at one end of the line and the least preferred at the other end. The remaining health states are placed on the line between these two, in order of their preference, and such that the intervals between the placements correspond to the differences in preference as perceived by the subject. Variations on this procedure include category scaling in which a specified number of categories (for example 11 categories) are used. The most preferred health state is placed in category 10, the least preferred in category 0, and the others are placed in the category that seems most appropriate to the subject in order to reflect the strength of the subject's preference, assuming equal change in preference between adjacent categories. Props and visual aids are often helpful in using these techniques. An example of a rating scale prop would be a thermometer with a scale from 0 to 100 on a felt background with foam sticks labelled with the health states. The subject places the foam sticks on the felt background beside the appropriate scale location (Torrance et al., 1982). For category scaling a box with 11 shelves and a deck of cards describing various health states has been developed. The subject places each card on the shelf that represents the appropriate category for that health state (Cadman et al., 1985).

Standard gamble. The standard gamble is the classical method of measuring utilities. It is based directly on the fundamental axioms of utility theory. The method has been used extensively in the field of decision analysis, and good descriptions of the method are available in books from this field (for example, see Holloway, 1979).

The core of the standard gamble method is a paired comparison in which the subject must choose between two alternatives. Alternative '1' is a treatment with two possible outcomes; a good outcome with probability 'p', and a bad outcome with probability '1-p'. Alternative '2' has a certain outcome which is intermediate in desirability between the good and bad outcomes of Alternative '1'. Probability 'p' is varied until the respondent is indifferent between the two alternatives at which point the required utility value for the health state in alternative '2' can be calculated.

Since most subjects cannot readily relate to probabilities, the standard gamble method is often supplemented with the use of visual aids, particularly a probability wheel (Torrance, 1976b). This is an adjustable disk with two sectors, each a different colour and constructed so that the relative size of the two sectors can be readily changed. The alternatives are displayed to the subject on cards, and the two outcomes of the gamble alternative are colour-keyed to the two sectors of the probability wheel. The subject is told that the chance of each outcome is proportional to the similarly coloured area of the disk.

The standard gamble method can be used to measure utilities for chronic health states preferred to death, chronic health states considered worse than death, and temporary health states. Further details of the use of this method are available in Torrance (in press).

Time trade-off (TTO). The time trade-off method was developed specifically for use in health care (Torrance, Thomas and Sackett, 1972). It has been validated against the standard gamble method and has been found to give similar results, although the validation has only been carried out for states preferred to death (Torrance, 1976b). It is an implicit technique like the standard gamble - that is, unlike the rating scale in which the subject provides his preference values explicitly, the time trade-off and the standard gamble methods derive the preference values implicitly based on the subjects responses to decision situations. However, compared to the standard gamble, the time trade-off method has the advantage of being simpler to use. The core of the time trade-off technique is also a paired comparison choice that the subject must make between two alternatives. In the case of a chronic health state, one alternative is to have the health state under consideration for the remainder of life, while the other alternative is to have a shorter but healthy life. The subject is asked to choose between these two alternatives, and the shorter healthy life is varied in length until the subject is indifferent between the two. The less desirable is the health state, the greater is the amount of life that the subject will trade-off in order to be free of the health state. When the indifference point is found, the utility for the health state can be calculated. Again, props and visual aids are generally used with this technique. (e.g., a laminated cardboard time trade-off board with sliders, changeable scales, and changeable health states to facilitate these measurements have been used by the author and his colleagues). Experience shows that the props not only make the task easier for the respondent, but also makes it considerably more enjoyable. With variations on this method, utilities can be measured for chronic health states preferred to death, chronic health states considered worse than death, and temporary health states (Torrance, in press).

Other techniques. In addition to the above, other techniques to measure cardinal preferences for health states include an equivalence technique (Berg, 1973) and ratio scaling (Rosser et al., 1978).

The measurement techniques discussed above have been described in terms of how they are used to measure single health states. However, if the health states are described by a multi-attribute health state classification system, then it is possible to take advantage of multi-attribute utility theory. A multi-attribute classification system would exist if the six key attributes (physical, emotional, sensory, cognitive, self-care, pain) or some subset of these were used to describe each health state (i.e., according to the level of function on each of the attributes). Multi-attribute utility theory can be used to significantly reduce the amount of measurements which must be taken in order to determine a full set of utility values for all possible combinations of attribute levels (for all possible unique health states described by the classification system). This theory does not require any new measurement techniques; instead, any one of the techniques described above can be used. However, additional tests to determine the degree of utility independence are required (see Torrance et al., 1982).

## Performance of Utility Measurement Techniques

Utility measures appear acceptable to subjects, be they members of the general public or patients. Based on six different studies (See Table 2) at least eighty-four percent of subjects were willing to participate in measurement interviews, and at least 96 percent of those who participated, completed the interview. Thus, the methods clearly appear to be acceptable.

The accuracy of utility measures is also an important issue. Accuracy can be assessed by examining reliability, precision and validity. Aggregate data from five studies is shown in Table 3. Internal reliabilities (i.e., consistency) were relatively high. Test-retest reliabilities across the studies (i.e., stability) was satisfactory although reliabilities decreased with greater test-retest time intervals.

The precision of a single measure on a single individual is shown in Table 3. The implication, for example, is that if a single health state utility was measured on a particular individual by the time trade-off instrument and the result was 0.60, the 95 percent confidence interval on this result would be $0.60 \pm 0.26$, a rather wide interval. Thus, although reliability coefficients are satisfactory, the precision of single measurements is only modest.

Two approaches have been taken to examine validity. In one approach, health state utilities are claimed to be utilities obeying the axioms of von Neumann-Morgenstern utility theory for decisions under uncertainty

TABLE 2

ACCEPTABILITY OF UTILITY MEASUREMENT QUESTIONS

| Willingness to Participate | % |
|---|---|
| General Public[1] | 84 |
| University Alumni[1] | 91 |
| Kidney Dialysis Patients[1,2,3] | 94, 88, 88 |
| Kidney Transplant Patients[3] | 88 |
| Cancer Patients[4,5,6] | 100, 91, 83 |
| **Broken Off Interviews** | **%** |
| General Public[1] | 2 |
| University Alumni[1] | 0 |
| Kidney Dialysis Patients[1,2,3] | 3, 4, 3 |
| Kidney Transplant Patients[3] | 3 |
| Cancer Patients[4,5,6] | 0, 0, 0 |

Studies cited

1. Torrance, 1976b
2. Churchill et al., 1984
3. Churchill et al., 1985a
4. Llewellyn-Thomas et al., 1982
5. Sutherland et al., 1983
6. Llewellyn-Thomas et al., 1984

(von Neumann and Morgenstern, 1953). In this case, the standard gamble measurement technique is valid by definition, and the validity of the other techniques can be determined by comparison. In one study, using this approach, the time trade-off technique was found to be relatively valid while the rating scale method was not (Torrance, 1976b). In the other approach to validity, health state utilities are claimed to measure the overall quality of life associated with the health state and thus should be strongly correlated with other trusted measures of health-related quality of life. Using this approach, Churchill and colleagues (1984) determined that patients' measured utilities correlated significantly with nephrologists' ratings of the patients' quality of life. Moreover, groups of patients with different clinical status differed in their measured health state utilities in predictable ways.

Individuals differ greatly in their health state preferences, and the differences cannot be explained by usual demographic characteristics such as age, sex, socioeconomic status, religion, illness, occupation, etc. For example, individual differences among the general public for the same health

TABLE 3

ACCURACY OF UTILITY MEASUREMENTS

| Reliability | Rating Scale | Standard Gamble | Time Trade-off |
|---|---|---|---|
| Internal reliability r[1,2] | 0.86 - 0.94 | 0.77 - 0.92 | 0.77 - 0.88 |
| 1-week test - retest r[3] | 0.77 | 0.80 | 0.87 |
| 4-week test - retest r[4] | | | 0.81 |
| 6-week test - retest r[5] | | | 0.63 - 0.80 |
| **Precision** | | | |
| Standard deviation of measurement error $S_e$[1,2] | 0.09 - 0.15 | 0.13 | 0.13 |
| **Validity** | | | |
| Criterion validity[1] | No | Criterion | Yes |
| Construct validity[5] | | | Yes |

Studies cited

1. Torrance, 1976b
2. Torrance et al., 1982
3. O'Connor et al., 1985
4. Churchill et al., 1985b
5. Churchill et al., 1984

state (on the 0-1 utility scale) result in a standard deviation of scores of approximately 0.30 (Sackett and Torrance, 1978). On the other hand, subjects who are more homogeneous and more knowledgeable about the health state seem to differ less. For example, 29 home dialysis patients rating the home dialysis scenario with the time trade-off method produced a standard deviation of 0.18 compared to 0.28 for the general public (Torrance, 1976b). Fortunately, the imprecision of individual measurements and the considerable differences among individuals can be ameliorated by taking the mean of a large group of subjects. Since the standard error of the mean is $S \sqrt{n}$, the mean utility value for a health state can be made as precise as desired by increasing the group size (n). Moreover, group mean values have been found to be remarkably stable regardless of the makeup of the group (Sackett et al., 1978; Boyd et al., 1982; Wolfson, Sinclair, Bombardier, and McGeer, 1982). These are fortunate findings since group mean utilities are the values required in most applications.

Table 4 summarizes the performance characteristics of the three major measurement techniques (rating scales, standard gamble and time trade-off). Although all are acceptable to subjects they are not equally easy for subjects to use. Two studies have used all three techniques on the same subjects and produced contradictory results regarding ease of use as perceived by the subjects (Torrance, 1976b; McNeil et al., 1986). In one study (Torrance, 1976b) the time trade-off was found to be the easiest to use, while in the other study (McNeil et al., 1986), it was the rating scale. However, in both studies the time trade-off was preferred to the standard gamble. There were no significant differences among the instruments with respect to reliability. Rating scales have shown poor validity when uncorrected, but by applying a power curve correction this can be overcome (Torrance, 1976b; Torrance et al., 1982). Considering the costs of administration, the rating scale is quicker and less expensive. Both the standard gamble and the time trade-off require much more time by the interviewer and the subject. While any of these techniques can be used, it is recommended that the time trade-off technique be used if affordable. If not, a rating scale method is a less expensive but acceptable alternative.

## Applications

Health state utilities are used in four different kinds of applications: clinical decision analysis, resource allocation, clinical trials, and population health surveys. In clinical decision analysis, treatment alternatives for a particular patient are developed in a decision tree format and the patients' utilities for the various outcomes are assessed. The analysis leads to a recommended decision for a particular problem on a particular patient (for examples see Weinstein, 1981, or clinical decision-making rounds in the journal Medical Decision Making).

TABLE 4

PERFORMANCE SUMMARY OF UTILITY MEASUREMENT INSTRUMENTS

| Ease of Use: (Population) | Rating Scale | Standard Gamble | Time Trade-off |
|---|---|---|---|
| General public * (+) | 3 | 2 | 1 |
| Arthritic patients ** (+) | 1 | 3 | 2 |
| **Empirical Evaluation:** | | | |
| Reliability | Acceptable | Acceptable | Acceptable |
| Criterion validity | Unacceptable | Acceptable | Acceptable |
| Construct validity | -- | -- | Acceptable |
| Cost (+) | 1 | 2 | 2 |

* Torrance, 1976b
** McNeil et al., 1985
(+) 1 = best, 2 = 2nd best, 3 = worst

Recently, utility measurement has been incorporated as an outcome measure in some clinical trials (McNeil et al., 1986; Oldridge, Jones, Buyatt, and McKelvie, 1985). In this application the patients assess the utility of the outcomes that they achieve in the trial period. Utilities are generally measured at baseline before the trial and at several follow-up points during the trial for both the experimental and the control groups. Utilities as an outcome are particularly important in clinical trials where mortality is relatively insignificant and where quality of life factors are dominant.

The most recent application of health state utilities is their possible inclusion in population health surveys. A health state utility can be viewed as a global index of health or of health-related quality of life. Population health surveys could be used to ask respondents to assess the utility of their current health state. This would allow cross-sectional comparisons across groups in society and longitudinal comparisons of the same groups over time.

The main use of health state utilities to date has been in the area of resource allocation using cost-effectiveness analysis or cost-utility analysis. The patient outcomes of programs under evaluation are converted by utilities into Quality Adjusted Life-Years (QALY's). In this way the health enhancement created by each program is expressed in comparable units that incorporate both the morbidity improvement and the mortality improvement in the one common measure, Quality Adjusted Life-Years gained. When this is compared to the cost of the program it provides a cost-utility ratio which can be used to compare alternative programs. The advantage of this method is shown by Table 5 taken from Torrance and Zipursky (1984). Here, a number of studies that have used this approach are listed in increasing order of cost per Quality Adusted Life-Years gained. Such comparisons should be used with great caution, but nevertheless can be helpful as one input into resource allocation decision-making.

## CONCLUSIONS

A health state utility is a cardinal number, usually between 0.0 and 1.0 that quantifies the health of an individual or a group, in that state, at a point in time, as an aid to decision-making. The measure reflects the overall impact of the health state on the individual's life style - that is, how it affects her/his overall physical functioning, emotional functioning and social functioning. The measure is a summary health index that reflects health-related quality of life. It is designed to assist in clinical decision analysis, resource allocation decisions using cost-effectiveness analysis, clinical trials, and population health surveys.

Health state utilities can be measured and are particularly relevant when the quality of life of the health outcomes are a significant consideration.

A single measure of health state utility for one individual is relatively imprecise, and such measures should be used with considerable caution and with sensitivity analysis in clinical decision analysis. On the other hand, group means of health state utilities are relatively precise. These can be used with greater confidence in clinical trials, population health surveys, and program evaluation using cost-effectiveness analysis or cost-utility analysis.

Health state utility measurement is not a difficult task. The methodology and the instruments are well-developed and detailed descriptions are available. Researchers interested in the utilities of particular health states are encouraged to incorporate these methods into their work.

TABLE 5

COMPARATIVE COST-UTILITY RESULTS FOR SELECTED PROGRAMS*

| PROGRAM | REPORTED COST/QALY* GAINED IN U.S. DOLLARS (year) | ADJUSTED ‡ COST/QALY + GAINED IN U.S. DOLLARS 1983 |
|---|---|---|
| PKU (phenylketonuria) Screening | <0 (1970) | <0 |
| Prevention of Rh disease of the newborn by postpartum administration of anti-D gamma-globulin | <0 (1977) | <0 |
| Prevention of Rh disease of the newborn by antepartum administration of anti-D gamma-globulin | 1220 (1983) | 1220 |
| Coronary artery bypass surgery for left main coronary artery disease | 3500 (1981) | 4200 |
| Neonatal intensive care, 1000-1499 gm | 2800 (1978) | 4500 |
| T4 (thyroid) screening | 3600 (1977) | 6300 |
| Treatment of severe hypertension (diastolic $\geq$105) in males age 40 | 4850 (1976) | 9400 |
| Treatment of mild hypertension (diastolic 95-104) in males age 40 | 9880 (1976) | 19,100 |
| Estrogen therapy for postmenopausal symptoms in women without a prior hysterectomy | 18,160 (1979) | 27,000 |
| Neonatal intensive care, 500-999 gm | 19,600 (1978) | 31,800 |
| Coronary artery bypass surgery for single vessel disease with moderately severe angina | 30,000 (1981) | 36,300 |
| School tuberculin testing program | 13,000 (1968) | 43,700 |
| Continuous ambulatory peritoneal dialysis | 35,100 (1980) | 47,100 |
| Hospital hemodialysis | 40,200 (1980) | 54,000 |

*These studies use similar, but not identical methods. Generally, costs are net health care costs; however, discount rates and preference weights are not completely consistent. Differences in methods should be considered when comparing the relative cost-utility. For details, see original sources.

+QALY denotes quality-adjusted life-year.

‡Adjusted to 1983 dollars according to the U.S. Consumer Price Index for Medical Care for all urban consumers. Source: U.S. Bureau of Labor Statistics, Monthly Labor Review.

## REFERENCES


Berg, R. L., (1973). Establishing the values of various conditions of life for a health status index. In R. L. Berg (Ed.), Health status indexes (pp. 120-134). Chicago: Hospital Research and Educational Trust.

Boyd, N. F., Sutherland, H. J., Ciampi, A., Tibshirani, R., Till, J. E., & Harwood, A. (1982). A comparison of methods of assessing voice quality in laryngeal cancer. In R. B. Deber & G. G. Thompson (Eds.), Choices in health care: Decision making and evaluation of effectiveness (pp. 141-144). Toronto: Department of Health Administration, University of Toronto .

Boyle, M. H., & Torrance, G. W. (1984). Developing multi-attribute health indexes. Medical Care, 22, 1045-1057.

Cadman, D. T., Boyle, M. H., Goldsmith, C. H., & Torrance, G. W. (1985). Health status index for children in Ontario. (Ontario Ministry of Health Research Grant DM648). McMaster University, Department of Pediatrics.

Churchill, D. N., Morgan, J., & Torrance, G. W. (1984). Quality of life in end-stage renal disease. Peritoneal Dialysis Bulletin, 4, 20-23.

Churchill, D. N., Torrance, G. W., Taylor, D. W., Barnes, C., Ludwin, D., Shimizu, A., & Smith E. K. M. (1985a). Measurement of quality of life in end-state renal disease: The time trade-off approach. McMaster University of Hamilton, Ontario: Working paper.

Churchill, D. N., Torrance, G. W., & Taylor, D. W. (1985b, May 3 - 6). Quality of life in end stage renal disease: Reliability, validity and use of time trade-off method. Abstract. Presented at the 1985 National Meeting of AAP/ASCI/AFCR. Washington, D. C.

Fanshel, S., & Bush, J. W. (1970, November - December). A health-status index and its application to health services outcomes. Operations Research, 18, 1021-1066.

Holloway, C. A. (1979). Decision making under uncertainty: Models and choices. Englewood Cliffs, NJ: Prentice-Hall.

Kaplan, R. M., Bush, J. W., & Berry, C. C. (1976). Health status: Types of validity and the index of well-being. Health Services Research, 4, 478-507).

Kaplan, R. M., & Bush, J. W. (1982). Health related quality of life measurement for evaluation research and policy analysis. Health Psychology, 1, 61-80.

Llewellyn-Thomas, H., Sutherland, H. J., Tibshirani, R., Ciampi, A., Till, J. E., & Boyd, N. F. (1982). The measurement of patients' values in medicine. Medical Decision Making. 2, 449-462.

Llewellyn-Thomas, H., Sutherland, H. J., Tibshirani, R., Ciampi, A., Till, J. E., & Boyd, N. F. (1984). Describing health states: Methodologic issues in obtaining values for health states. Medical Care, 22, 543-552.

McNeil, B. J., Pauker, S. G., & Torrance, G. W. (1986). Measuring health-related quality of life in clinical trials. Working paper.

von Neumann, J., & Morgenstern, O. (1953). Theory of games and economic behavior, (3rd ed.). New York: Wiley.

O'Connor, A. M., Boyd, N. F., & Till, J. E. (1985, April 9 - 11). Influence of elicitation technique. Position order and test-retest error on preferences for alternative cancer drug therapy. Paper presented at the National Nursing Research Conference.

Oldridge, N., Jones, N., Guyatt, G., & McKelvie, R. (1985). Comprehensive early rehabilitation after myocardial infarction. (Clinical trial funded by NHRDP Canada). McMaster University, Department of Medicine.

Rosser, R. M., & Kind, P. (1978). A scale of valuations of states of illness: Is there a social consensus. International Journal of Epidemiology, 7, 347-358.

Rosser, R. M., & Watts, V. (1971, May 5 - 7). The sanative output of a health care system. Paper presented at the Conference of the Operations Research Society of America. Dallas, Texas.

Sackett, D. L., & Torrance, G. W. (1978). The utility of different health states as perceived by the general public. Journal of Chronic Diseases, 31, 697-704.

Sutherland, H. J., Dunn, V., & Boyd, N. F. (1983). Measurement of values for states of health with linear analog scales. Medical Decision Making, 3, 477-487.

Torrance, G. W. (1976a). Health status index models: A unified mathematical view. Management Science, 22, 990-1001.

Torrance, G. W. (1976b). Social preference for health states: An empirical evaluation of three measurement techniques. Socio-Economic Planning Sciences, 10, 128-136.

Torrance G. W. (1984, July 3 - 4). Health status measurement for economic appraisal. Presented at Health Economists' Study Group Meeting. Aberdeen, Scotland.

Torrance, G. W. (in press). Measurement of health state utilities for economic appraisal. Journal of Health Economics.

Torrance, G. W., Boyle, M. H., & Horwood, S. P. (1982). Application of multi-attribute utility theory to measure social preferences for health states. Operations Research, 30, 1043-1069.

Torrance, G. W., Thomas, W. H., & Sackett, D. L. (1972, Summer). A utility maximization model for evaluation of health care programs. Health Services Research, 7, 118-133.

Torrance, G. W., & Zipursky, A. (1984, June). Cost-effectiveness of ante partum prevention of Rh immunization. Clinics of Perinatalogy, 11, 267-281.

Weinstein, M. C. (1980). Estrogen use in postmenopausal women - costs, risks and benefits. New England Journal of Medicine, 30, 308-316.

Weinstein, M. C. (1981). Economic assessments of medical practices and technologies. Medical Decision Making, 1, 309-330.

Weinstein, M. C., & Fineberg, H. E. (1980). Clinical Decision Analysis. Philadelphia: Saunders.

Weinstein, M. C., & Stason, W. B., (1977). Foundations of Cost-effectiveness analysis for health and medical practices. New England Journal of Medicine, 296, 716-721.

Wolfson, A. D., Sinclair, A. J., Bombardier, C., & McGeer, A. (1982). Preference measurement for functional status in stroke patients: Inter-rater and inter-technique comparisons. In Robert Kane & Rosalie Kane (Eds.), Values and Long Term Care (pp. 191-214). Lexington, MA: Lexington Books.

# PART VIII PSYCHIATRY: APPLICATION OF THE MEDICAL MODEL

# THE USE OF ILLNESS BEHAVIOUR CONCEPTS IN PSYCHIATRY

Richard Mayou

Department of Psychiatry
Oxford University

Traditional psychiatric nomenclature developed in mental hospitals is often inappropriate for the much wider variety of common and clinically important psychosocial difficulties encountered in general hospitals and in primary care. These include distress of less than psychiatric severity, social and behavioural problems, and continued medical care-seeking in the absence of disease. Psychiatrists have viewed Mechanic's (1961) description of "illness behaviour" as answering the need for a broader view bringing together the whole variety of psychological and social influence on illness and all the range of psychological and social consequences of being ill.

Although the term "illness behaviour" is increasingly and understandably popular in psychiatry, it is evidently poorly understood since it is used in many different ways. It is often confused with another misused sociological term "sick role". Indeed, the term "illness behaviour" as used by psychiatrists often has only an illusion of meaning. This paper looks at these usages and addresses the utility of the construct.

## Hypochondriasis

Psychiatrists have made particular use of illness behaviour terminology in the discussion of somatic symptoms of psychological origin. The traditional term, hypochondriasis, is an unsatisfactory word for a very wide variety of complaints of which only a highly atypical minority are referred to psychiatrists. Far too little is known of prevalence, but they are undoubtedly very common in the general population, primary care and medical clinics. Most are transient and easily treated by reassurance, but others make considerable demands on medical services (Barsky and Klerman, 1983). The underlying psychological mechanisms are increasingly being referred to under the collective name of somatization and are seen as being much modified by cultural and social factors. Indeed, Kleinman (1982) writes: "somatization sometimes occurs in the absence of psychopathology as a means of coping with social stress and personal distress".

Mechanic's (1961, 1979) definition of illness behaviour refers to undoubted "given" physical symptoms and includes trivial somatic sensations, but has not been concerned with the more dramatic and persistent forms of hypochondriasis. Psychiatrists have extended the concept to similar behaviours by those who have either medically unexplained somatic symptoms or fears of illness (Armstrong, 1984). Recently Mechanic (1979) has placed more emphasis on theory, and he suggests that illness behaviour in response to normal or minor bodily sensations is due to learned patterns of over-preoccupation.

Psychiatrists have used illness behaviour terminology in three ways:

1. Diagnostic Categorgy. The most common usage is in everyday clinical practice where "illness behaviour" is seen as an extra diagnostic category for problems which are not easily put into the standard classifications and where psychopathology is less evident than behavioural difficulty. This usage often seems to imply that illness behaviour is not shown by the ordinary medical patient and is always abnormal.

2. Social Explanation. Illness behaviour is often seen as the social explanation of disturbed behaviour. For example, Kendell (1983) suggests illness behaviour as a mechanism underlying social etiology of hysteria. This view does little justice to the complex social factors that may be involved and assumes that it is always appropriate to refer to dissociative and conversion phenomena as illness (Mayou, 1975). It is essential to recall, as Barsky and Klerman (1983) point out: "The chronic illness behaviour of this sociobehavioural conceptualization is a final common pathway for several distinct entities other than hypochondriasis".

3. Behavioural Category. Although most forms of hypochondriasis can be seen, in part, as problems of illness behaviour, many psychiatrists have tended to reserve this terminology for a psychologically and medically heterogeneous group of chronic problems that are associated with considerable demands on doctors. Pilowsky (1969) has suggested the application of illness behaviour concepts to psychiatry and put forward an idiosyncratic definition. He has worked mainly with chronic pain patients and has exposed the very considerable inadequacies in psychiatric classifications, and writes: "while it is to be expected that patients referred to a pain clinic are a psychologically heterogeneous group, a number of reports suggest that it is "abnormal" illness behaviour of these patients which distinguish them as a group from psychiatric patients and from those with distinct somatic inputs to their pain" (Pilowsky and Bassett, 1982). Pilowsky (1969) defines "abnormal illness behaviour" (AIB) as "the persistence of an inappropriate or maladaptive mode of perceiving, evaluating and acting in relation to one's own state of health, despite the fact that a doctor has offered a reasonably lucid explanation of the nature of the illness and the appropriate course of treatment to be followed". Although, in practice, mainly concerned with intractable hypochondriacal disorder, Pilowsky's (1978) detailed classification of "abnormal illness behaviour" covers many of the subcategories of DSM-III.

There are many ways of defining normality and there are, therefore, considerable difficulties in the use of the word "abnormal". Indeed, psychiatrists are very familiar with the problems in using established terms such as "abnormal personality". Pilowksy's essential criterion of resistance to reasonable medical explanation is entirely arbitrary, excludes important clinical problems, and ignores the patient's own views of his/her symptoms. What is the clinical value of labelling a proportion of those who suffer somatic symptoms as "abnormal" because they do not agree with their doctors?' What is meant by "maladaptive", "reasonably lucid explanation", "appropriate treatment"? Does a reasonable explanation and treatment mean reassurance, which is often ineffective, or does it include psychiatric assessment, full discussion with the patient and behavioural or other treatment? How can one apply the definition to patients who have both permanent and disabling physical illness and hypochondriacal complaints?

Blackwell (1981) and his colleagues find "chronic illness behaviour" a more clinically useful category than psychiatric classification in their work with patients chronically disabled by intractable pain, irritable colon and other predominantly psychologically determined chronic handicaps. Since all patients with chronic physical illness show chronic illness behaviour, Blackwell presumably means problems of chronic illness behaviour when he refers to "the tendency of some patients to become excessively dependent on physicians and to show disability out of proportion to physical findings". His work is of particular interest in that he has developed a theoretical basis in terms of learning theory alongside an impressive and intensive behavioural treatment programme.

The psychiatric usages of illness behaviour as a psychiatric category and as a social explanation are fraught with problems, and other adaptations of illness behaviour terminology use the concept in narrow and idiosyncratic ways. It is undeniably valuable to emphasize the social context and meaning of symptoms and consultation, but the creation of new categories and new names does not necessarily provide any insight into the intricacy of social and psychological mechanisms. Before discussing the application of illness behaviour concepts to major physical disorder, it is convenient to discuss measures.

## Illness Behaviour Measures

In addition to many measures of specific components of illness behaviour, there has been considerable interest in more general measures of illness behaviour. Pilowsky has developed an Illness Behaviour Questionnaire (IBQ) which has been shown to have seven main dimensions when used in a pain clinic population (Pilowsky and Spence, 1975). The IBQ has been used to identify the category of "abnormal illness behaviour" (AIB), but also to establish a dimension of illness behaviour, which extends between AIB and the opposite extreme of denial. This dimension has recently been seen as a possible axis in the multiaxial classification of psychiatric disorder.

The IBQ tells us something about hypochondriacal anxiety and disease conviction, but as with all multivariate techniques, one needs to look at the population studied and the assumptions in the data collection. There are serious problems:

i) Although there are seven dimensions, the questionnaire and interview cover only two aspects (perception of symptoms and mood) of illness behaviour; in the present state of knowledge, it would seem better to assess each aspect of illness behaviour separately (Pilowsky and Spence, 1975; Barnes and Benjamin, 1984).

ii) The research has been based on a very special population of chronic patients, pain clinic attenders. A proportion of such attenders have serious medical problems, but there is also a high prevalence of psychiatric disorder in pain clinic attenders (Edwin, Pearlson and Long, 1984; Tyrer, Capon and Peterson, in press). Responses to questions about disease conviction and bodily preoccupation may reveal unusual attitudes, but they may equally well reflect understandable responses to unpleasant and intractable physical symptoms.

iii) There is no way of knowing how many patients have been given "lucid explanations" by the doctors. It is very difficult to assess the replies to the IBQ without knowledge of patients' physical states. This problem is particularly evident in Pilowsky's preliminary report of an alternative interview procedure, the Illness Assessment Schedule (Pilowksy, Bassett, Barrett, Petrovic, and Minniti, 1983).

iv) Although the instruments have been used in very few other populations, there is some reason to believe that there are considerable differences in responses of various medical groups.

v) It is not surprising that between group differences have been found when the IBQ is used in pain clinics, general practice and rheumatology clinics. However, there is no evidence that the IBQ can discriminate clinically useful sub-groups.

It is claimed that the concept of "abnormal illness behaviour" and the questionnaire (IBQ) and interview all have routine clinical applications. Could these be of help in the diagnosis and treatment of the conditions encountered in clinical practice? There is no evidence that this is so. It is suggested that it would be more appropriate to develop operational definitions of clinically useful sub-categories. These definitions would be dimensional with axes for mental state, physical state and social handicap, as is being proposed for similar problems encountered in primary care. In summary, the present so-called illness behaviour measures are best seen as important but provisional research tools.

Medically Unnecessary Handicaps in Physical Illness

Psychiatrists refer to the problems of medically unnecessary handicap associated with definite physical illness as problems of illness behaviour. This is common in clinical practice both as extra diagnostic category and as the behavioural category, as in Blackwell's definition of chronic illness behaviour.

Although much research describes the psychological and social variables associated with response to acute and chronic physical illness, there have been few attempts to use illness behaviour terminology and concepts. The response to a myocardial infarction is one example. Byrne and his colleagues (1984) have used the IBQ shortly after myocardial infarction. Although there are problems in interpreting replies very early in recovery from a severe illness, and many of the IBQ questions seem inappropriate for those with major medical illness, they believe that the IBQ is useful in examining patterns of psychological and behavioural response to a major acute illness. For instance, they have reported that dimensions of illness behaviour assessed shortly after infarct have a modest predictive value of findings eight months and two years later.

Pritchard (1979) has developed a Response to Illness Questionnaire to examine the meaning to the patient and affective response and used it with dialysis patients and with cardiac patients awaiting surgery (Pilowksy, 1969). Pritchard is rightly cautious in his conclusions, but says that it would be useful to examine the extent to which similar factors are applicable to other chronic illness and suggests the need to examine the value and dimensions of illness behaviour in predicting outcome, and in the management of patients with chronic illness.

Does this sort of research have applications to clinical practice in defining the precise nature of problems and enabling identification of "at risk" patients. Possible predictive factors are best defined and studied separately rather than as statistically derived factors or clusters. It is also essential to consider other equally important illness behaviour variables, the severity of the medical condition, personality and social circumstances, other life events and so on.

It is more sensible to use illness behaviour only as a general term and concentrate specific study of precisely defined components of reactions to major physical illness. It is very doubtful that illness behaviour concepts have any specific applications to the quantitative understanding of the varied individual responses to illness. It is useful to illustrate this with a particular example such as the response to a heart attack. Although impressive how well people cope with myocardial infarcts, a third of these people seem to suffer persistent and medically unnecessary distress and handicaps (Mayou, 1979).

Psychosocial outcome is multidimensional and there are no clear patterns of outcome. It is a much more complex picture than is usually acknowledged and results from the interaction between physical state, personality and social circumstances. Some of the persistent problems might be seen by Blackwell as "chronic illness behaviour", but they are, in fact, a mixture of chronic unchanged problems, worsening of chronic difficulties and a few new problems occurring after the infarct. As time passes, further psychological and social difficulties are sometimes reported, but can usually be attributed to events other than the heart attack. It is misleading to refer to such a variety of behaviours and problems of multiple etiology as illness behaviour. However, it may be convenient to refer collectively to new problems occurring in convalescence, few of which can be diagnosed as psychiatric disorder, as problems of illness behaviour.

## CONCLUSIONS

The sociological concept of illness behaviour has been useful as a corrective to narrow medical and psychiatric views of the impact of illness on patients' everyday lives. It has stimulated research into complex areas of response to illness and exposed the inadequacies in psychiatric nomenclature. The extension of illness behaviour concepts to hypochondriasis has been valuable.

The concept of illness behaviour has been misused and misunderstood within psychiatry so that very often it has no more than the illusion of meaning. Illness behaviour instruments are research tools for examining some aspects of illness behaviour. It is doubtful whether conclusions from the small range of groups so far studied can be generalized to other medical groups. Illness behaviour instruments have not yet been shown to be clinically valuable in diagnosis or in assessing prognosis.

In summary, it is suggested that illness behaviour be used as a general term only in Mechanic's original sense.

## REFERENCES


Armstrong, D. (1984). Illness behaviour revisited. Paper presented at 15th European Conference on Psychosomatic Research, London.

Barnes, D., & Benjamin, S. (1984). The multidimensional assessment of illness behaviour in pain patients. Pain, (Suppl. 2), S40.

Barsky, A. J. & Klerman, G. L. (1983). Overview: Hypochondriasis, bodily complaints and somatic styles. American Journal of Psychiatry, 140(3), 273-283.

Blackwell, B. (1981). Biofeedback in a comprehensive behavioural medicine program. Biofeedback and Self-Regulation, 6, No. 4, 445-472.

Byrne, D. G. (1984). The stability of illness behavior after myocardial infarction. International Journal of Psychiatry in Medicine, 14(4), 285-291.

Edwin, D. H., Pearlson, G. D., & Long, D. M. (1984). Psychiatric symptoms and diagnoses in chronic pain in-patients. Pain, (Suppl. 2), S180.

Kleinman, A. (1982). Neurasthenia and depression: A study of somatization and culture in China. Culture, Medicine and Psychiatry, 6, 117-190.

Kendell, R. E. (1983). Hysteria. In G. F. M. Russell and L. A. Hersov (Eds.), Handbook of Psychiatry 4: The Neuroses and Personality Disorders. Cambridge: Cambridge University Press.

Mayou, R. (1975). The social setting of hysteria. British Journal of Psychiatry, 127, 466-469.

Mayou, R. (1979). The course and determinants of reactions to myocardial infarction. British Journal of Psychiatry, 134, 588-594.

Mechanic, D. (1961). The concept of illness behavior. Journal of Chronic Diseases, 15, 189-194.

Mechanic, D. (1979). Development of psychological distress among young adults. Archives of General Psychiatry, 36, 1233-1239.

Pilowsky, I. (1969). Abnormal illness behaviour. British Journal of Medical Psychology, 42, 347.

Pilowsky, I. (1978). A general classification of abnormal illness behaviours. British Journal of Medical Psychology, 51, 131-137.
Pilowsky, I., & Bassett, L. (1982). Pain and depression. British Journal of Psychiatry, 141, 30-36.
Pilowsky, I., Bassett, D., Barrett, R., Petrovic, L., & Minniti, R. (1983). The illness behaviour assessment schedule: Reliability and validity. International Journal of Psychiatry in Medicine, 13(1), 11-28.
Pilowsky, I, & Spence, N. D. (1975). Patterns of illness behaviour in patients with intractable pain. Journal of Psychosomatic Research, 19, 279-287.
Pritchard, M. J. (1979). Measurement of illness behaviour in patients on haemodialysis and awaiting cardiac surgery. Journal of Psychosomatic Research, 23, 117-130.
Tyrer, S. P., Capon, M. N., & Peterson, D. M. (in press). The detection of psychiatric illness and psychological handicaps in a British pain clinic population. Pain.

# ARE PSYCHIATRIC DISORDERS "REAL"?

Leon Eisenberg

Department of Social Medicine and Health Policy
Harvard Medical School

Psychiatry is dismissed as a medical specialty by some physicians because many of the disorders in its domain have yet to be consistently associated with organ pathology. Critics with a sociologic bent add that psychiatrists misuse medical authority to apply the label "sick" to deviant behaviour which is offensive to community standards. By labelling deviance as a medical disorder, they argue, patients are stripped of the dignity of personal responsibility for their actions and, authorities justify police action by the state to restrict their liberties. Both groups of critics take psychiatric disorders to be less "real" than medical or surgical ones because structural or biochemical defects underlying the pathological behaviour have not yet been demonstrated. The inference is that, were there to be such evidence, the attribution of illness would take on a qualitatively different character.

Thomas Szasz derides mental illness as a "myth" in contrast to brain disease which he takes to be "real" and which he assigns to the neurologist. In his words:

> "The notion of mental symptoms is...inextricably tied to the social (including the ethical) context in which it is made, in much the same way as the notion of bodily symptoms is tied to an anatomical and genetic context." (Szasz, 1960)

He goes on to state:

> "Whereas bodily disease refers to a public, physicochemical occurrence, the notion of mental illness is used to codify relatively more private, sociopsychological happenings of which the observer forms a part...(The psychiatrist) is committed to some picture of what he considers reality -- and to what he thinks society considers reality -- and he observes and judges the patient's behaviour in the light of these considerations." (Szasz, 1960)

In reifying organic illness, Szasz (1960) alleges that bodily symptoms are fully explicable by the "anatomical and genetic context." Yet, this assertion is entirely at variance with clinical experience. The anatomical substrate is insufficient to account for the variability of clinical expression. The insistence that bodily disease is explicable in terms of "public, physicochemical occurrence" disregards the fact that what brings the patient to the doctor is a constellation of behavioural complaints (pain, fatigue, shortness of breath, etc.). Moreover, doctors of every persuasion, no less than their patients, are "committed to some picture of...reality."

Consider an illustrative instance. Few would argue that a compound fracture of the femur is a psychosocial disorder in the usual meaning of that term. Yet when Beecher (1956) compared the extent of pain experienced (as measured by the need for morphine) among soldiers wounded at the Anzio beachhead in World War II and among civilian automobile accident victims, all with comparable anatomical lesions, he found that complaints of pain were significantly less among the soldiers than among the civilians. The social context and the significance of the injury to the victim determined its behavioural consequences even though "the public, physico-chemical occurrence" was the same in the two situations.

Another example is provided by the results of a controlled trial of the treatment of peptic ulcer (Peterson, Sturdevant, and Frankl, 1977). To "confirm" the diagnosis, all patients were endoscoped at the beginning and the end of the trial. To the investigators' surprise, some patients continued to complain of pain despite healing of their endoscopically visualized ulcers, while others whose ulcers were unchanged, became symptom free. The vicissitudes of the clinical condition were not explained in full by the antomical findings. Although ulcer healing was promoted more often by the active agent than by the placebo, relief of pain was the same in both conditions of the therapeutic trial!

While disease concepts are social constructs, it is not implied that diseases would not exist as events in the world if men did not recognize them. Indeed, their existence provides the occasion for their recognition. Nonetheless, the prevalence of a pathological condition in a community is not sufficient in itself to assure its definition as a "disease." For example, the social attitudes over time and space toward persons suffering from pinta have varied considerably. Pinta is a disorder caused by the spirochete treponema carateum, which leads to variegated discolourations of the skin. Among one South American Indian tribe where the pigment disorder is nearly universal, it is the unblemished, disease-free individual, the anomalous variant in <u>their</u> community, who is regarded as abnormal and excluded from marriage (Ackerknecht, 1947). Among the Aztec, those with pinta enjoyed relatively high status; they were selected to bear the litters of the Emperor Montezuma because they set off the multi-coloured displays of his ornaments. In contemporary Mexico, pintados are shunned like lepers (Wood, 1979). Thus, what is and what is not a legitimate "disease" at a given time in the history of a comunity depends on the social organization of knowledge no less than on "a public physicochemical occurrence" and "an anatomical and genetic context." The medical definition of disease is not static, "diseases" come and go.

Until recently, medical students were taught about "chronic brucellosis", a disease which accounted for persistent illness in patients likely to be dismissed as having "neurasthenia" unless a careful history was taken and appropriate laboratory tests performed (Evans, 1947). It had been known since the turn of the century that several species of Brucella micro-organisms can produce an acute infectious illness. Further, some patients, after recovery from an acute episode, go on to display continuing ill health (weakness, fatigue, migratory aches and pains, low grade fever, depression) in the absence of abnormal physical findings. In patients seen long after an initial infection (and even when there was no clear history of an initial infection), the diagnosis was said to be established by a positive serum agglutination test.

There is, however, a serious flaw in this line of reasoning. Agglutins may persist for many years in recovered as well as chronically ill patients. The two groups seem the same in all respects other than complaint pattern. Is it possible that chronic brucellosis is a spurious disease construct which legitimizes (and therefore serves to perpetuate) chronic illness behaviour? Imboden and colleagues (1959) studied 24 patients known to have had acute brucellosis, 16 of whom symptoms had persisted for four to eight years. They were unable to distinguish the recovered from the ill patients by physical or laboratory examination. However, mental status examination revealed clear evidence of emotional disturbance, particularly depression, in those who were symptomatic. Since the chronic patients had been ill for many years, it remained possible that the psychiatric findings were the "result" rather than the "cause" of illness.

To test the hypothesis that prolonged convalescence from an acute infection is a function of pre-existing personality traits, Imboden and others (1961) assessed 600 individuals on the MMPI in order to identify those who were depression-prone. By design, the testing was completed shortly before an epidemic of influenza which had been predicted to strike the area. During the flu season, the rate of infection, as determined by serological testing, was no greater in depression-prone persons than in others (40 percent versus 34 percent). However, the rates of <u>illness</u>, as registered by clinic visits, did differ significantly (17 percent versus 3 percent). Moreover, almost all the patients who exhibited prolonged convalescence from flu (three weeks or more versus two weeks or less) were, as predicted, in the depression-prone group. What is still called by many physicians "chronic brucellosis" appears to be a pattern of illness behaviour fashioned out of the experience of an acute infection in psychologically predisposed individuals, a pattern reinforced by medical responses which sanction complaints by ascribing them to "disease".

Contrast that history with the way the concept of black lung as an occupational disease of miners has developed. Company doctors and public health officials, many of whom identified themselves wholly with mining interests, consistently misinterpreted pulmonary dysfunction among miners. A heavy burden of respiratory morbidity in coal miners had been evident to observers as early as the 19th century. Their disability had been attributed at various times to "miner's asthma," regarded as "ordinary" or "normal" for them, to tuberculosis (although at other times coal dust was said to hinder its progress); to malingering; and as recently as the 1950's (Smith, 1981) to emotional disorder. Three of the author's physician friends were driven out of Kentucky by gunfire because they had diagnosed pneumonconiosis (a compensable disorder) in cases where company doctors, in disregard of medical evidence, diagnosed tuberculosis (an act of God). Ostensibly "objective" medical opinions became ammunition. The legislative outcome was determined by the political coalition built by the union in the fight to win federal benefits for miners who had become respiratory cripples.

Illness among miners was no less real when dismissed as asthma - "normal" for the occupation, than it is today when it has been redefined as black lung. The persistent distress of post-brucella somatization is not mitigated by the redefinition of chronic brucellosis. However, the new conceptions of these disorders have had equally real consequences. In the case of black lung, the change has led to improved, if still inadequate, mine safety standards and to federal benefits for those unable to work because of pulmonary dysfunction. In the case of brucellosis, it has shifted the focus of medical attention.

If medical diagnoses resist strict assignment, it need not surprise us that the same holds true in psychiatry. Is schizophrenia a brain disorder, thus "real" and the proper business of a neurologist, or is the label a "myth" invented by psychiatrists to justify their medical hegemony?

The evidence for brain disease in the schizophrenias rests on studies of familial inheritance (Gottesman and Shields, 1982; McGuffin, Farmer, Gottesman, Murray, and Revely, 1984), neurochemical (Snyder, 1982), circulatory (Gur, Skolnick, and Gur, 1983; Buchsbaum, Ingvar, and Kessler, 1982), and metabolic (Ariel, Golden, and Berg, 1983) abnormalities; and structural defects (Weinberger, Wagner and Wyatt, 1983). Such pathology is present only in some patients and is completely absent in others, but the aggregate evidence is hard to dismiss. Yet, the trajectory of the schizophrenic illness remains exquisitely sensitive to macro and micro cultural differences. In the World Health Organization nine-country study (1979), patients at each of the participating national centers were diagnosed as schizophrenic by common criteria. Yet, at the two year follow-up, there were substantial differences in clinical outcome, with patients in developing countries (Nigeria, India, Colombia) exhibiting a more favorable course than patients in the industrial world (U.S., Czechoslovakia, U.K, and Denmark). The apparent differences may, in part, reflect sampling errors or differences in premorbid factors, but other studies in non-industrialized societies (Murphy and Raman, 1971; Waxler, 1979) report better than expected outcomes.

At the microcultural level, Brown and his colleagues (1962, 1972) in London have shown that the likelihood of relapse in schizophrenic patients discharged from hospital is significantly greater among patients returning to families exhibiting high "expressed emotion", an index which reflects the frequency of critical comments about the patient made by a key family informant in a structured interview (Vaughn and Leff, 1976b). The number of hours of face-to-face contact between the patient and family is decisive; if it is less than 35 hours a week, the likelihood of relapse is half as great. Phenothiazines protect patients in hostile families against relapse, but they offer less benefit to those in more accepting homes, another instance of drug/environment interaction (Vaughn and Leff, 1976a; Leff, Knipers, Berkowitz, Vaughn, and Sturgeon, 1983). When family treatment succeeds in lowering "expressed emotion" in high risk families, the patient relapse rate declines in parallel (Leff, Knipers, Berkowitz, Eberlein-Vries, and Sturgeon, 1982). Randomized controlled trials in the United States have shown that psychosocial interventions directed at patients (Hogarty and Goldberg, 1973) and at families (Falloon et al., 1982) augment the power of neuroleptics to enable chronic schizophrenic patients to maintain themselves in the community. The "problems in living" which accompany presumptive brain disease prove to be responsive to social interventions as well as to medication and to be managed best by combination of both.

The distress and the dysfunction of the schizophrenic patient remains real, whatever name is given to the disorder and whether it is attributed to demonic possession, pathologic rearing, neurotransmitter abnormalities, or dismissed as a "myth". What differs are the ways in which patients and families are regarded by the community and managed by its health practitioners. Definitions of disease have consequences for outcome, sometimes malignant, sometimes benign, but the illnesses themselves cannot be legislated out of existence by changes in terminology.

What of the disorders identified as "psychosomatic"? In the 19th century, eminent physicians contended that there were psychogenic factors in the causation of cholera, typhus, general paresis, and tuberculosis (Ackerknecht, 1982). With the great discoveries of bacteriology in the closing decades of that century, the debate appeared to have been settled, once and for all. The new laboratory medicine with its doctrine of one disease, one cause, emerged triumphant. How well did that paradigm account for even the infectious disease on which it was based?

Consider what might appear to be "open and shut" cases, namely tuberculosis. Throughout the 19th century, controversy raged over the relative contributions of heredity, social circumstance, contagion and psychological predisposition to the pathogenesis of tuberculosis. Koch's brilliant discovery in 1882 established the tubercle bacillus as the necessary condition for the disease in all of its forms. The hereditarians, the social theorists and the psychosomaticists had lost the day. But had they? Secular changes in mortality and the distribution of the disease in the population are not accounted for by identification of the microorganism.

Mortality from tuberculosis fell by half between 1840 and 1880, two years before Koch's discovery. By 1940, it had fallen to one-sixth of its level one hundred years earlier, well before doctors had an effective remedy. The most likely explanations are that improved nutrition had increased host resistance and that better housing and public health control measures had limited the contagion (McKeown, 1976). The introduction of chemotherapy in 1947 sharply accelerated the decline in mortality (McDermott, 1978). But puzzles continue to abound. (1) Why do only five to 15 percent of individuals infected by the tubercle bacillus, as evidenced by a positive tuberculin test, become clinically ill (Glassroth, Robins, and Snider, 1980)? Why does susceptibility in populations continue to vary not only with age, sex, race and place of residence (Center for Disease Control, 1979) but also with HLA phenotype (Al-Arif, Goldstein, and Affronti, 1979) and social class (Feingold, 1975)? The bacillus is a necessary, but not a sufficient condition for the disease. Heredity, personal hygiene and social conditions influence host response. These factors influence the disease equation (Gage, 1935) but have dropped from view in the intellectual excitement generated by the emergence of laboratory science.

There is now a sizeable literature on the extent of the psychopathology to be found among medical patients, whether seen in the dispensary (Editorial, 1979) or on the ward (Moffic and Paykel, 1975). Often major depression goes unrecognized by the internist and the care provided is unresponsive to the patients' problems (Moffic and Paykel, 1975). In a study of 211 women attending a gynecology outpatient clinic, Byrne (1984) found that almost twice as many scored as psychiatric "cases" on a self-administered health questionnaire than among a matched community comparison group (verified by a standardized psychiatric interview conducted on subsamples). The highest rates discovered were among those complaining of pelvic pain. These findings are a striking replication of those reported by Ballinger (1977). In her study of 217 women attending a gynecologic clinic in Dundee, the proportion of attenders who met criteria for psychiatric "caseness" was considerably higher than in the general population, their disorders were more severe, and they had had more contact with local psychiatric services.

How shall we interpret these data? Do the gynecologic complaints "merely" reflect the patient's psychiatric status; that is, are they the somatic expression of psychological symptoms? Or does the psychiatric distress "merely" result from the gynecologic disease? Does the patient have two independent conditions? Or do they interact; that is, are the symptoms arising from each augmented by the presence of the other? If this were a multiple choice question on a National Board examination, the correct answer would be: all of the above! To be a bit more precise, each hypothesis is compatible with a proportion of cases.

---

1. Similar marked secular declines in mortality have been recorded for diphtheria, scarlet fever, pertussis, and measles (Kass, 1971).

At one end of the spectrum are women with Briquet's syndrome (hysteria in the old nomenclature; somatoform disorder in the new) who come to attention with multiple gynecologic complaints and who are hysterectomized to no avail (Martin, Roberts, and Clayton, 1980). At the other end of the spectrum are patients reported by Gath, Cooper, and Day (1982). These women had both menorrhagia and psychiatric disorder, the one eliminated and the other markedly diminished after hysterectomy. Notably, the psychiatric benefit was the same, whether the bleeding was scored as "organic" or "dysfunctional" on the basis of the operative uterine specimen. These authors concluded (Gath, Cooper, Bond, et al., 1982): "psychiatric disorder is more likely to occur in women who have been rendered vulnerable by the discomforts and handicaps resulting from menorrhagia." Selection for surgery may well have been influenced by the co-occurrence of the two disorders but this did not warrant the conclusion that hysterectomy was inappropriate. This evidence, together with other epidemiologic data, highlights the strong association between mental and physical illness in the population, an association which necessitates the integration of mental health into primary health care (Shepherd, 1978).

The task of doctoring is not simply one of diagnosing organic pathology and applying remedies for its correction. It is no less essential to ascertain the events in the patient's life which bring her to the office now rather than at some other time, and to evaluate mental status, cultural background, and what patient and family expect from care (Kleinman, Eisenberg, and Good, 1978). Without that information and a plan of action based on it, medical intervention may well prove both ineffective and irrelevant. It can result in repeated visits, an array of successively more invasive tests, and multiple changes in therapy while the physician pursues a somatic will-o-the-wisp.

Patients are not "either-or" although the practice of medicine would be a great deal simpler if it were so. Under those conditions, physicians could limit themselves to narrowly defined specialties, each justifying its hegemony by technical virtuosity, each boasting itself to be more "scientific" by having excluded uncertainty from its territory. If that sounds familiar, the reader must decide whether this is a caricature or an accurate description of the domains that have been staked out. The only flaw in our scheme is the patients. They stubbornly refuse to come in packages suitable for proper sorting into pre-arranged bins.

## REFERENCES


Ackerknecht, E. H. (1947). The role of medical history in medical education. Bulletin of History and Medicine, 21, 135-145.

Ackerknecht, E. W. (1982). The history of psychosomatic medicine. Psychological Medicine, 12, 17-24.

Al-Arif, L. I., Goldstein, R. A., Affronti, L. F., et al. (1979). HLA-Bw15 and tuberculosis in a North American black population. American Review of Respiratory Disease, 120, 1275-1278.

Ariel, R. N., Golden, C. J., Berg, R. A., et al. (1983). Regional blood flow in schizophrenics. Archives of General Psychiatry, 40, 258-263.

Ballinger, C. B. (1977). Psychiatric morbidity and the menopause: survey of a gynecological outpatient clinic. British Journal of Psychiatry, 131, 83-89.

Beecher, H. (1956). Relationship of significance of wound to the pain experienced. Journal of American Medical Association, 161, 1609-1613.

Brown, G. W., Birley, J. L. T., and Wing, J. K. (1972). Influence of family life on the course of schizophrenic disorders: A replication. British Journal of Psychiatry, 121, 241-258.

Brown, G. W., Monck, E. M., Carstairs, G. M., and Wing, J. K. (1962).

Influence of family life on the course of schizophrenic illness. British Journal of Preventive and Social Medicine, 16, 55-68.
Buchsbaum, M. S., Ingvar, D. H., Kessler, R., et al. (1982). Cerebral glucography with positron tomography. Archives of General Psychiatry, 39, 251-260.
Byrne, P. (1984). Psychiatric morbidity in a gynecology clinic: An epidemiological survey. British Journal of Psychiatry, 114, 28-34.
Center for Disease Control. (1979). Tuberculosis in the United States, 1977. Atlanta: Center for Disease Control (DHEW Publication No. (CDC) 79-8322).
Editorial. (1979). Psychiatric illness among medical patients. Lancet, i, 478-479.
Evans, A. C. (1947). Brucellosis in the United States. American Journal of Public Health, 37, 139-151.
Falloon, I. R. H., Boyd, J. L., McGill, C. W., Razani, J., Moss, H. B., & Gilderman, A. M. (1982). Family management in the prevention of exacerbations of schizophrenia: A controlled study, New England Journal of Medicine, 306, 1437-1440.
Feingold, A. O. (1975). Cost effectiveness of screening for tuberculosis in a general medical clinic. Public Health Reports, 90(6), 544-547.
Gage, S. H. (1935). Theobald Smith 1859-1934, Cornell Veterinarian, 25, 207-228.
Gath, D., Cooper, P., Bond, A., et al. (1982). II. Demographic, psychiatric and physical factors in relation to psychiatric outcome. British Journal of Psychiatry, 140, 343-350.
Gath, D., Cooper, P., and Day, A. (1982). Hysterectomy and psychiatric disorder. I. Levels of psychiatric morbidity before and after hysterectomy. British Journal of Psychiatry, 140, 335-342.
Glassroth, J., Robins, A., and Snider D. (1980). Tuberculosis in the 1980's. New England Journal of Medicine, 302, 1441-1450.
Gottesman, I. I., & Shields, J. (1982). Schizophrenia: The Epigenetic Puzzle. Cambridge University Press, Cambridge.
Gur, R. E., Skolnick, B. E., Gur, R. C., et al. (1983). Brain function in psychiatric disorders, I: Regional cerebral mood flow in medicated schizophrenics, Psychiatry, 40, 1250-1254.
Hogarty, G.E., & Goldberg, S. (1973). Collaborative study group. Drug and sociotherapy in the aftercare of schizophrenic patients. Archives of General Psychiatry, 28, 54-64.
Imboden, J. B., Canter, A., & Cluff, L. E. (1961). Convalescence from influenza. Archives of Internal Medicine, 108, 393-399.
Imboden, J. B., Canter, A., Cluff, L. E., & Trever, R. (1959). Brucellosis: III. Psychologic aspects of delayed recovery. Archives of Internal Medicine, 103, 406-414.
Kass, E. H. (1971). Infectious diseases and social change. Journal of Infectious Diseases, 123, 110-114.
Kleinman, A., Eisenberg, L., & Good, B. (1978). Culture, illness and care. Annals of Internal Medicine, 88, 251-258.
Leff, J. P., Knipers, L., Berkowitz, R., Eberlein-Vries, R., and Sturgeon, D. (1982). A controlled trial of social intervention in the families of schizophrenic patients. British Journal of Psychiatry, 141, 121-134.
Leff, J. P., Knipers, L., Berkowitz, R., Vaughn, C., and Sturgeon, D. (1983). Life events, relatives' expressed emotion and maintenance neuroleptics in schizophrenic relapse. Psychological Medicine, 13, 799-806.
Martin, R. L., Roberts, W. V., and Clayton, P. J. (1980). Psychiatric status after hysterectomy: A one-year prospective follow-up. Journal of American Medical Association, 244, 350-353.
McDermott, W. (1978). Medicine: The public good and one's own. Perspectives in Biology and Medicine, 21, 167-187.
McGuffin, P., Farmer, H. E., Gottesman, I. I., Murray, R. M., and Revely, E.

M. (1984). Twin concordance for operationally defined schizophrenia. Archives of General Psychiatry, 41, 541-545.
McKeown, T. M. (1976). The role of medicine: Dream, mirage or nemesis? London: Nuffield Provincial Hospitals Trust.
Moffic, H., and Paykel, E. S. (1975). Depression in medical inpatients. British Journal of Psychiatry, 126, 346-353.
Murphy, H. B. M., Raman, A. C. (1971). The chronicity of schizophrenia in indigenous tropical peoples: Results of a twelve-year follow-up survey in Maritius. British Journal of Psychiatry, 118, 489-497.
Peterson, W. L., Sturdevant, R. A. L., Frankl, H. D. (1977). Healing of duodenal ulcer with an antacid regimen. New England Journal of Medicine, 297, 341-345.
Shepherd, M. (197). Epidemiologic perspective: Psychosomatic medicine. International Journal of Epidemiology, 7, 201-205.
Smith, B. E. (1981). Black lung: the social production of disease. International Journal of Health Services, 11, 343-359.
Snyder, S.H. (1982). Schizophrenia. Lancet, ii, 970-974.
Szasz, T. S. (1960). The myth of mental illness. American Psychology, 15, 113-118.
Vaughn, C., & Leff, J. P. (1976a). The influence of family and social factors on the course of psychiatric illness. British Journal of Psychiatry, 129, 125-137.
Vaughn, C., & Leff, J. P. (1976b). The measurement of expressed emotion in the families of psychiatric patients. British Journal of Social and Clinical Psychology, 15, 157-165.
Waxler, N. E. (1979). Is outcome for schizophrenia better in non-industrial societies: The case of Sri Lanka. Journal of Nervous and Mental Disease, 167, 144-158.
Weinberger, D. R., Wagner, R. J., and Wyatt, R. J. (1983). Neuropathological studies of schizophrenia: A selective review. Schizophrenia Bulletin, 9, 193-212.
Wood, C. S. (1979). Human sickness and health: A biocultural view. Mayfield, Palo Alto.
World Health Organization. (1979). Schizophrenia: An international follow-up study. New York: John Wiley and Sons.

# ABNORMAL ILLNESS BEHAVIOUR: A REVIEW OF THE CONCEPT AND ITS IMPLICATIONS

Issy Pilowsky

Department of Psychiatry
The University of Adelaide

Patients presenting with illness behaviours which are not congruent with the objective evidence for the presence of illness may be suffering from psychopathologically-based illness behaviour, i.e., "abnormal" illness behaviour. The relevant terms are defined, and the implications for the medical care system are discussed in this chapter.

"Abnormal" illness behaviour is a term coined to refer to a group of psychopathological conditions in which an individual presents with illness behaviour considered out of keeping with the objective evidence for illness. An understanding of this concept is important for the practice of medicine because it has far-reaching implications for the conduct of physicians, who are in one important sense, the only people who can make a definitive decision as to the presence of this condition.

This assertion about the medical role in this diagnosis flows from a consideration of the "sick role" concept as formulated by Parsons (1964). He conceived of this role as a "partially and conditionally legitimated state" which is granted to an individual, provided he accepts that it is undesirable, recognizes his obligation to co-operate with others for the purpose of achieving health, and shows a readiness to utilize the services of those whom society regards as competent to diagnose and treat his/her illness. Having fulfilled these requirements, the individual is exempted from normal obligations and is not held responsible for his/her state, nor expected to be able to recover simply by an act of will. It is suggested that Mechanic and Volkart's (1960) original definition of illness behaviour might be slightly modified. "Illness behaviour" might be referred to as the ways in which individuals perceive, evaluate and respond to aspects of their own functioning which they are predisposed to appraise in terms of "illness" and "health".

What remains ill-defined, however, is the notion of "illness". Writers such as Coe (1970) have emphasized that "illness" and "disease" are not the same thing. "Illness" refers to the individual's subjective experience of a "disease" which, in turn, is essentially a biological concept. The definition of what constitutes "disease" is often difficult. Disease can be construed as a constellation of objectively recognized characteristics of illness. Pilowsky (1978) has suggested that the illness be defined as: "A state of an organism which fulfills the requirements of an appropriate reference group for admission to the sick role." The usefulness of this definition is that it allows the determination, at least operationally, of what "illness" is in any society or culture. It should be noted that the definition of illness in any culture is part of an ongoing process. But at any particular time it should, in theory, be possible to specify what the current criteria are.

When a patient seeks help from a physician the task involves defining the nature of the illness and the appropriate sick role. The consequences of this process have implications for society at large, e.g., determination of sickness benefits and compensation.

The physician's role in this process is clearly pivotal because the physician-patient relationship is not a symmetrical one (Parsons, 1978). A group of patients who are particularly at risk for being regarded as malingerers are those whose illness behaviour strikes doctors as being excessive. This is usually the case when physical symptoms are minor, vague, and not associated with radiopaque lesions and where compensation is involved. Often these patients are labelled hypochondriacs, hysterics and the like.

Because of the problems associated with making these diagnoses it is important to specify as clearly as possible on what basis they should be made. It is suggested (Pilowsky, 1969, 1978) that conditions such as hypochondriasis are best conceptualized as forms of "abnormal" illness behaviour (AIB), defined as:

> The persistence of an inappropriate or maladaptive mode of perceiving, evaluating or acting in relation to one's own state of health, despite the fact that a doctor (or other appropriate social agent) has offered an accurate and reasonably lucid explanation of the nature of the illness and the appropriate course of management to be followed, based on a thorough examination of all parameters of functioning, and taking into account the individual's age, educational and sociocultural background.

This definition places a considerable responsibility on the doctor and has obvious implications for medical education and peer review. It is a definition which emphasizes that the diagnosis of AIB cannot be made definitively unless the doctor has given the patient an "adequate" explanation of what he/she regards the situation to be and that the patient rejects it. As Singh and others (1981) have pointed out, the physician may discharge his/her role in a distinctly abnormal manner. This must be considered along with any notion of "abnormal" illness behaviour.

It may be particularly difficult for a physician to accept that a patient's "illness" is the inability to accept the doctor's view of his/her health status, especially when the patient is hypochondriacal. The same may apply when the patient denies illness or rejects treatment.

It is suggested that "abnormal" illness behaviour can take several forms: (see Table 1)

1. Illness affirming, somatically focused
2. Illness denying, somatically focused
3. Illness affirming, psychologically focused
4. Illness denying, psychologically focused

Since it is the physician's task to assess the patient's illness behaviour, it is reasonable to ask what type of judgement he/she makes. Is it based on his/her own personal experience? Is it based on facts about the

**Table 1.**

**Illness Behaviour**

| | Somatically Focused | Psychologically Focused |
|---|---|---|
| **Illness Affirming** | **Motivation predominantly conscious**<br>1. Malingering<br>2. Chronic factitious syndrome with physical symptoms (Munchausen's Syndrome)<br>3. Factitious disorder with physical symptoms<br>**Motivation predominantly unconscious**<br>1. Neurotic (Somatoform disorders)<br>• Somatization disorder<br>• Conversion disorder<br>• Psychogenic pain disorder<br>• Hypochondriasis<br>2. Psychotic<br>• Hypochondriacal delusions associated with<br>- Major depressive disorder with mood congruent psychotic features<br>- Schizophrenic disorder<br>- Monosymptomatic hypochondriacal psychoses | **Motivation predominantly conscious**<br>1. Malingering<br>2. Factitious disorder with psychological symptoms (Ganser Syndrome)<br>**Motivation predominantly unconscious**<br>1. Neurotic<br>• "Psychic hypochondriasis" (Hunt, 1951)<br>• "Phrenophobia" (Walen, 1982)<br>• Dissociative reactions<br>• Psychogenic amnesia<br>2. Psychotic<br>• Delusions of memory loss or loss of brain function |
| **Illness Denying** | **Motivation predominantly conscious**<br>1. Denial to obtain employment<br>2. Denial to avoid feared therapies<br>3. Denial of illness (e.g. VD) due to shame and guilt<br>**Motivation predominantly unconscious**<br>1. Neurotic<br>• Non-compliance following myocardial infarction<br>• Counterphobic behaviour in hemophilia<br>• Non-compliance with antihypertensive therapy<br>2. Psychotic<br>• Denial of somatic pathology, e.g. as part of hypomanic or schizophrenic disorder<br>**Neuropsychiatric**<br>1. Anosognosia | **Motivation predominantly conscious**<br>1. Denial of psychotic symptomatology to avoid stigma, hospital admission, or to gain discharge from care<br>2. Denial of psychotic illness to avoid perceived discrimination by health care professionals or employers<br>**Motivation predominantly unconscious**<br>1. Neurotic: refusal to accept 'psychological' diagnosis or treatment in the presence of neurotic illness, personality disorder or dependency syndromes (alcohol, opiates, etc.)<br>2. Psychotic: denial of illness ('lack of insight') in psychotic depression, manic states and schizophrenic<br>3. Neuropsychiatric: confabulatory reaction in Korsakoff's psychosis and other organic brain syndromes (Gainotti, 1975) |

**TABLE 2.** Proposed assessment scheme for illness behaviour disturbance

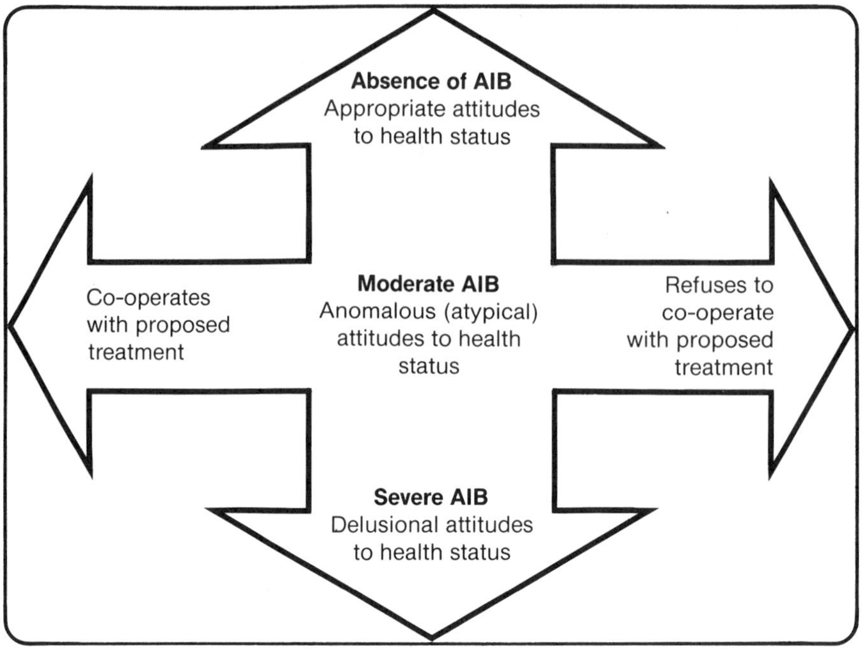


nature and degree of illness behaviour to be expected with specific illnesses?

In an attempt to facilitate the collection of such information, it may be helpful to assess illness behaviour with respect to two variables; severity of the illness behaviour and degree of co-operation with treatment. These two dimensions could be assessed concurrently to yield a framework by which to characterize a given individual. This assessment might even be incorporated into DSM-III forming a sixth axis. Table 2 represents a possible form that this potential axis could take. At the one extreme are severe illness behaviours where attitudes toward health are delusional or quasidelusional. Moderate illness behaviour disturbance would be represented by anomalous but nondelusional attitudes toward health. Finally, minor or absent illness behaviour disturbance would be represented by relatively adaptive attitudes toward health. At each of these levels of severity individuals could co-operate or resist treatment interventions. Co-operation-resistance forms the second dimension of this assessment scheme.

REFERENCES

Coe, R. M. (1970). Sociology of Medicine. London: McGraw Hill.
Gainotti, G. (1975). Confabulation of denial in senile dementia. Psychiatrica Clinica, 8, 99-108.
Hunt, R. C. (1951). The psyche as an object of hypochondriacal preoccupation. Psychiatric Quarterly, 14, 490-495.
Mechanic, D., & Volkart, E. H. (1960). Illness behaviour and medical

diagnosis. Journal of Health and Human Behaviour, 1, 86-96.
Parsons, T. (1964). Social structure and personality. London: Collier MacMillan.
Parsons, T. (1978). Action, theory and the human condition. New York: Free Press.
Pilowsky, I. (1969). Abnormal illness behaviour. British Journal of Medical Psychology, 42, 347-351.
Pilowsky, I. (1978). A general classification of abnormal illness behaviours. British Journal of Medical Psychology, 51, 131-137.
Singh, B., Nunn, D., Martin, J., & Yates, J. (1981). Abnormal treatment behaviour. British Journal of Medical Psychology, 54, 67-73.
Walen, S. R. (1982). Phrenophobia. Cognitive Therapy and Research, 6, 399-408.

# THE TREATMENT OF SOMATIZATION

Robert Kellner

Department of Psychiatry
University of New Mexico School of Medicine

Somatizing patients have been regarded by many authors to have a poor prognosis (Kellner, 1986). In outcome studies of psychotherapy they have been found to respond less well to conventional psychotherapy than patients with emotional symptoms (Rosenberg, 1954; Stone, Frank, Nash, and Imber, 1961) and generally have been judged to be poor candidates for psychotherapy. However, these views are in conflict with good outcomes reported in several uncontrolled studies of patients with functional somatic symptoms. For example, a large proportion of patients with benign chest pain (Cope, 1969) or neurocirculatory asthenia (Cohen and White, 1951), treated only with reassurance and explanation, apparently recovered. In general medical practice a substantial proportion of patients with functional somatic symptoms recover without specific treatments (Thomas, 1978).

Somatizing patients have been generally regarded as poor candidates for psychotherapy for various reasons, such as alexithymia, lack of psychological sophistication and a somatic defense style. Many somatizing patients express the belief that their somatic symptoms are their only burden, which often proves to be false at a later stage. However, even while these individuals have severe somatic symptoms and have not volunteered other concerns, many are willing to express despair in psychological terms when given the opportunity, or are encouraged to do so.

There is evidence, from several controlled studies, that in patients with somatic complaints, psychotherapy leads to improved sense of well-being in comparison to the absence of such treatment. Some of the most successful early controlled studies in psychotherapy were with patients who had psychosomatic diseases or psychophysiologic disorders. Three studies in which psychotherapy was associated with a good outcome are discussed further in the next few paragraphs.

Chappell and Stevenson (1936) carried out the first controlled study of psychotherapy with patients having psychosomatic disorders. This study is not well known, perhaps explaining why the treatment has not been practiced more widely, but it is remarkable for several reasons. Although the study concerns pain caused by physical disease, it is described here because some of the principles of treatment used in this study may be applicable to functional somatic symptoms and persistent pain from other causes. All patients suffered from chronic peptic ulcer and had not responded to previous treatments.

The psychotherapeutic strategies included: 1) Control of worry. The patients who were coached learned to substitute worry with some less unpleasant form of activity. 2) Control of discussion. It was recommended that the patient should seek the co-operation of his family, as well as of close friends, in diverting conversation away from the subject of disease. 3) Explanation and insight. The nature of influence and thought on bodily activity were explained, along with characteristic manners of reacting to common situations. 4) Assurance. The patients were given the assurance of their ability to gain the end they desired. Forty-seven patients were assigned to the experimental group and 20 to the control group. Of these, 15 subjects dropped out early in the experimental treatment and were not followed up. During the first part of the experiment all patients were treated with antacids and an ulcer diet, and were advised to return to a normal diet about half-way through the experiment. All except two could do so in both experimental groups without recurrences of symptoms, whereas in the control group, ten of the 20 subjects had immediate recurrences. The experimental group had lectures seven days a week for six weeks in groups consisting of five to ten subjects, without the usual interaction between patients and therapist. After an eight month follow-up, 30 of 32 patients in the experimental group were in excellent health. At three years follow-up, three patients could not be found; ten remained entirely free of symptoms; five had only minor recurrences; eleven patients had recurrences, but regarded themselves as healthy and were confident of their ability to take care of any symptoms; two subjects had recurrences that were as severe as their previous illness.

The first and so far the largest controlled study of psychotherapy for functional somatic symptoms was conducted by Draspa (1959). One hundred twelve patients with muscular pain for which no organic cause was found were matched with another group with the same complaint. One group had psychotherapy and both groups continued with physical treatments. Psychotherapy was aimed at: 1) teaching both passive and active muscle relaxation; 2) reassuring that pain was only muscular and posed no immediate danger; and 3) "giving insight into the causes of excessive muscular contraction" and so "promoting self-adjustment to change in internal or external environmental situation." In both groups assessment of the degree of recovery was made by the same physician or surgeon who had made the initial diagnosis. Almost twice as many patients in the experimental group as in the control group became free of pain; the mean number of attendances in the experimental group was only half of that of the control group; recovery took twice as long in the control group.

In a recent study, Svedlund and others (1983) compared the outcome of psychotherapy in irritable bowel syndrome with that of routine treatment. A total of 119 patients who fulfilled the criteria of absence of demonstrable organic disease and typical symptoms of an irritable bowel syndrome, were selected. The patients were unaware of the experimental design. One hundred agreed to participate; they were randomly allocated into two groups. In addition, both groups had routine medical treatments, but the psychotherapy group had short-term dynamically oriented individual psychotherapy conducted by psychiatrists. The focus was on means of coping with distress and emotional problems often employing an educative or teaching strategy to illustrate the relationship between stressful life events and abdominal symptoms. Psychotherapy subjects had an average of 7.4 sessions. At the end of treatment, both experimental and control groups were improved, but the improvement in the psychotherapy group was significantly greater in terms of reduced abdominal pain and less bowel dysfunction. On 16 months follow-up this improvement continued in the psychotherapy group, whereas, the control group had deteriorated slightly.

Judging from techniques used in successful controlled studies, and from descriptions of treatments in uncontrolled studies, the strategies of therapy in somatizing subjects should include a thorough physical examination with appropriate laboratory investigations, followed by explanations of the nature of symptoms and reassurance as to their benign nature (Sapira, 1972). These steps may need to be repeated should the individual report new symptoms. They are taught to decrease somatic-focusing tendencies as they often selectively perceive sensations as implying disease. Deliberate suggestion of good health may be used by the therapist when consistent with the known information which suggests absence of physical disease. If the somatizing individual has hypochondriacal beliefs, then special strategies of persuasion may be required (Kellner, 1986). When the somatic symptoms remit, or become less distressing, the patient may need conventional psychotherapy directed to other concerns and conflicts.

There have been numerous contolled studies to show that training in muscular relaxation, or EMG biofeedback, are more effective in the treatment of tension headaches and migraine headaches than control treatments (Jessup, Neufeld, and Merskey, 1979; Editorial - Lancet, 1980; Blanchard, Andrasik, Ahles, Teders, and O'Keefe, 1980). The teaching of coping skills as well as cognitive therapy appear to be effective, at least in the short-term management of pain (Holyroyd, Andrasik, Westbrook, 1977; Rybstein-Blinchik, 1979; Langer, Janis and Wolfer, 1975). These methods may be beneficial in the management of other functional somatic symptoms.

Numerous double-blind controlled studies employing antianxiety or antidepressant drugs have shown that in short-term treatment there is a greater decrease of somatic symptoms with an active drug than with placebo. No adequate long-term studies have been reported.

Group psychotherapy may have advantages over individual psychotherapy. A number of investigations have reported treatment of chronic somatizing patients with group therapy in uncontrolled studies (Mally and Ogston, 1964; Roskin, Mehr, Rabiner, and Rosenberg, 1980-1981; Melson, Rynearson, Dortzbach, Clark, and Snyder, 1982). These authors have expressed the view that group therapy is both effective and economical compared to individual psychotherapy. The emphasis and focus of group therapy differs from that of traditional group therapy in several ways; the patients share persisting and distressing somatic complaints; they all have experienced persistent failure of medical treatment, and were often full of resentment towards their physicians; and, often were unwilling to accept that psychological factors were contributing to their somatic distress. Favourable changes of these attitudes were described by these authors for patients undergoing group psychotherapy.

Individuals who have been ill for a long time with or without a chronic disease are often unresponsive to the methods described in this chapter. Some of these patients appeared to have adapted to their illness or appeared to benefit from assuming the sick role. Additional treatments may be required, aimed at changing the patient's habits and goals as described by Blackwell and Gutmann, (this volume) and Cott (this volume).

## CONCLUSIONS

There is an unmistakable trend for psychological interventions in somatization to be more beneficial than treatments without psychotherapy. The use of inappropriate psychotherapeutic methods may have been one of the reasons that early studies showed poor results. Traditional, non-directive psychotherapy does not address itself to concerns about somatic symptoms and appears to be inadequate when patients are preoccupied with fears and beliefs about disease. More recent research results from the treatment of somatizing individuals do not support the pessimistic conclusions of earlier authors.

## REFERENCES


Blanchard, E. B., Andrasik, F., Ahles, T. A., Teders, S. J., O'Keefe, D. (1980). Migraine and tension headache: A meta-analytic review. Behavioural Therapy, 11, 613-631.

Cope, R. L. (1969). The psychogenic factor in chest pain. Texas Medicine, 65, 78-81.

Cohen, M. E., White, P. D. (1951). Life situations, emotions and neurocirculatory asthenia. Psychsomatic Medicine, 13, 335-357.

Chappell, M. N., Stevenson, T. I. (1936). Group psychological training in some organic conditions. Mental Hygiene, 20, 588-597.

Draspa, L. J. (1959). Psychological factors in muscular pain. British Journal of Medical Psychology, 32, 106-116.

Editorial. (1980). Biofeedback and tension headache. Lancet, pp. 898-899.

Holyrod, K. A. Andrasik, F. & Westbrook, T. (1977). Cognitive control of tension headache. Cognitive Therapy and Research, 1, 121-133.

Jessup, B. A., Neufeld, R. W. J., & Merskey, H. (1979). Biofeedback therapy for headache and other pain: An evaluative review. Pain, 7, 225-270.

Kellner, R. (1986). Somatization and hypochondriasis. New York: Praeger.

Langer, E. J., Janis, I. L., & Wolfer, J. A. (1975). Reduction of psychological stress in surgical patients. Journal of Experimental Social Psychology, 11, 155-165.

Mally, M. A., & Ogston, W. D. (1964). Treatment of the "untreatables". International Journal of Group Psychotherapy, 14, 369-374.

Melson, S. J., Rynearson, E. K., Dortzbach, J., Clark, R. D., & Snyder, A. L. (1982). Short-term intensive group psychotherapy for patients with "functional" complaints. Psychosomatics, 23, 689-695.

Rosenberg, S. (1954). The relationship of certain personality factors to prognosis in psychotherapy. Journal of Clinical Psychology, 10, 341-345.

Roskin, G., Mehr, A., Rabiner, C. J., & Rosenberg, C. (1980-1981). Psychiatric treatment of chronic somatizing patients: A pilot study. International Journal of Psychiatry in Medicine, 10, 181-187.

Rybstein-Blinchik, E. (1979). Effects of different cognitive strategies on chronic pain experience. Journal of Behavioral Medicine, 2, 93-101.

Sapira, J. D. (1972). Reassurance therapy. Annals of Internal Medicine, 77, 603-604.

Stone, A. R., Frank, J. D., Nash, E. H., & Imber, S. D. (1961). An intensive five-year follow-up study of treated psychiatric outpatients. Journal of Nervous and Mental Disorders, 133, 410-422.

Svedlund, J., Ottoson, J., Sjödin, I. & Dotevall, G. (1983, September 10). Controlled study of psychotherapy in irritable bowel syndrome. Lancet, pp. 589-592.

Thomas, K. B. (1978). The consultation and the therapeutic illusion. British Medical Journal, 1, 1327-1328.

# THE MANAGEMENT OF CHRONIC ILLNESS BEHAVIOUR

Barry Blackwell and Mary Gutmann

Department of Psychiatry
University of Wisconsin Medical School

## Introduction

Chronic illness behaviour, of which chronic pain is a subset, can be conceptualized as being composed of seven features. These features are proposed to be broad, in that they apply to the myriad of specific disorders, and useful, in that they lead to specific management principles and interventions.

Earlier research established the characteristics of a syndrome of chronic abnormal illness behaviour seen in patients referred to a psychosomatic inpatient unit (Wooley, Blackwell, and Winget, 1978). These patients suffered from a variety of physical diseases and displayed a range of disabilities including pain, fatigue, breathlessness, depression and obesity.

A somewhat similar conceptualization developed within the chronic pain management field (Pinsky, 1978) and chronic pain can be regarded as the commonest (but by no means only) symptomatic expression of abnormal illness behaviour (Blackwell, Galbraith, and Dahl, 1984).

The purpose of this chapter is twofold. First, to emphasize the common conceptual basis for the treatment of chronic abnormal illness behaviour and chronic pain. To date, these two fields have developed in parallel with little communication. Second, to focus on the underlying principles and strategies of management as opposed to individual treatment methods. The overall objective is to foster a conceptual basis for management that avoids a haphazard eclectism engendered by multimodal treatments applied without an adequate appreciation of etiology.

## CONCEPTUALIZING THE CHRONIC ILLNESS BEHAVIOUR SYNDROME

Rather than resort to the traditional diagnostic labels it is more useful to characterize a chronic illness behaviour syndrome within which individuals display all of the following features, albeit to a varying degree. These are:

Disability Disproportionate to Detectable Disease

This finding is universal whether or not the underlying disease process is trivial or substantive. In the latter instance severe disabling disorders often lay the groundwork for development of superimposed illness behaviour. The discrepancy between the patient's display of suffering and the degree of pathophysiological disease is what triggers the clinician's awareness (and often frustration) about chronic illness behaviour. It is important to train physicians to recognize this perception so that they can rapidly deploy the management strategies discussed below rather than continuing with an exhausting and often expensive pursuit of esoteric diagnoses which inevitably reinforces exaggerated illness behaviour responses.

Search for Disease Validation

Patients often seek to have their worst fears laid to rest, and in the case of chronic illness behaviour, the search may become relentless, reinforced by visits to famous clinics and by the investigative or diagnostic zeal of physicians.

Appeal to Physician Responsibility

Patients who display chronic behaviour readily relinquish control and autonomy to physicians who are often equally ready to accept the burden of diagnosing or curing the patient's condition. This is often established early in history taking when the patient expresses a "well, you're the doctor" attitude while the physician asks leading questions or interrrupts frequently to obtain a sufficient data base to alleviate uncertainty and come to closure. This perpetuates the physician's ignorance of the patient's beliefs and reinforces the patient's dependency on the physician.

Attitudes of Personal Vulnerability and Entitlement

People who readily adopt the sick role are characterized by personal beliefs and attitudes that they are vulnerable to disease and entitled to be cared for by others. In particular, they display a heightened symptom sensitivity, a morbid preoccupation with sickness and a deepseated conviction of ill health. At times the patient's attitudes and beliefs may be shared by the spouse with the intensity of a "folie a deux".

These belief systems are reflected in response to various inventories and questionnaires designed to elicit them. The first three scales on the MMPI (hypochondrias, depression, and hysteria) are almost invariably elevated to give the classical "psychosomatic V". Other rating scales such as the Pilowsky Illness Behaviour Questionnaire (Pilowsky and Spence, 1975), the Kellner Health Attitude Survey (Kellner, Abbott, Pathak, et al., 1983), and the Patient Description Questionnaire (McGashie and Whitenack, 1982) are all reliable measures of such attitudes and beliefs.

The sense of entitlement to care is reflected in interpersonal behaviours by a willingness and skill at soliciting caretaking and reassurance from others as well as by a ready resort to disability, compensation, and litigation to support the sick role.

Avoidance of Healthy Roles Due to Lack of Skills, Excessive Expectations, or Fear of Failure

A useful aphorism is that people do not choose to be sick as long as they are able to be healthy. Adoption of the sick role is invariably associated with some inability to function in a healthy role. This could result from lack of basic intellectual, manual, or social skills to perform adequately, from unrealistic expectations of performance, or from a heightened fear of failure. Adoption of the sick role is facilitated because it reduces or avoids the anxiety associated with the inadequate performance of a healthy role. This avoidance learning becomes self-reinforced not only through the anxiety reduction associated with withdrawal from the healthy role but also by the negative conditions and secondary inertia that results from the sick role.

### Adoption of the Sick Role Due to Environmental Rewards from Family, Friends, Physicians, or Social Entitlement Programs

The sick role position is powerfully maintained by the secondary gain or positive reinforcement derived from a variety of sources including spouse, family, and friends. Patients with sick role tendencies often select physicians with nuturant qualities or lack of limit setting capabilities. Alternatively, they move from one clinic to another exposing themselves to the investigative zeal of inexperienced physicians or those who pride themselves on diagnostic acumen. Finally, such patients validate their sick role either by litigation around accidents or by obtaining disability and compensation through the various social entitlement programs.

### Interpersonal Behaviours to Sustain Sick Role

Patients with psychosomatic disorders or chronic pain have long been recognized to display a range of social and interpersonal behaviours that are designed to sustain the sick role through their effect on the provider. Complaints, demands, threats, and hostility cause the provider to feel guilty; while helplessness and excessive positive compliance invoke caretaking. Patients may also increase the amount of attention by staff splitting or playing off one provider against another.

These various interpersonal behaviours have been characterized as "passive-aggressive" or as "pain games". In the short term they are often effective in obtaining additional attention and sustaining the sick role, but over the longer term they contribute to the development of negative feelings and rejection by the provider.

## GENERAL PRINCIPLES AND SPECIFIC STRATEGIES FOR MANAGEMENT

The above conceptualization of chronic illness behaviour has the major advantage over diagnostic classification in that management intervention follows more directly from the principles themselves. A series of specific management principles are presented in this section. As with the conceptual features presented above, each of these prinicples has relevance for illness behaviour, although they have differential relevance for different individuals.

### Thorough Disease Assessment

This is an essential basis for a rehabilitative approach since it establishes the trust of the patient and the confidence of the provider that nothing has been overlooked. Anything less encourages the patient to doubt the doctor, to criticize the assessment or to allege that the absence of a definitive biomedical diagnosis is either a manifestation of incompetence or an accusation of malingering. It is also important for non-physician team members who may later be called on to ignore the patient's complaints to feel confident that nothing has been overlooked. It is often helpful to ask patients if there is anything they feel has been overlooked or left undone before closing the door to further investigation.

While the assessment needs to be thorough it should not be indiscriminate or adopt a "shotgun" approach. The results of many tests are reported on the basis of statistical probability. If enough tests are done a few are certain to return in the abnormal range creating doubt and ambiguity that may enhance illness behaviour.

## Acceptable Definition of Symptoms That Ends Investigation Without Challenging Their Reality

Since the recognition of abnormal illness behaviour rests on the disparity between the patient's suffering and degree of detectable pathology there is always the risk that patients will perceive the absence of a sufficient biomedical cause as an accusation that they made up the symptoms or imagined them ("you mean it's all in my head?").

In the acute primary care setting it has been shown that vague somatic complaints respond as readily to nonspecific remedies and the absence of a disease label as they do to a specific diagnosis and conventional treatment. This is undoubtedly due to the effects of benign symptom reattribution by the patient (as a result of history taking and examination), to physician reassurance, and to spontaneous remission.

In the case of chronic or recurrent somatic complaints considerable skill may be required to define the patient's symptoms in a manner that ends investigation without challenging their reality. It is important to avoid premature stress attributions but at the same time to begin to establish linkages between the symptoms and the patient's life. This is best done by asking the general question "How do the symptoms interfere with your day to day activities?" followed by specific inquiries about the relationship of symptoms to occupational, social, and parental or sexual activities. This also creates the foundation for a rehabilitative approach based not so much on symptom removal as on strengthening the ability to perform whatever life tasks are interfered with.

Any explanation attempted by the provider is more likely to be acceptable if it takes account of the patient's own attributions and beliefs about the cause, acuity and potential treatment for the symptoms. Patients respond to and cope with their understanding of symptoms. Congruence between patient and provider on illness explanations and expectations facilitates co-operation and an active patient role (Meyer et al., 1985).

Finally, in arriving at an acceptable definition of the symptoms it is important to avoid ambiguity which fosters illness behaviour by feeding into the patient's existing doubts and fears. This is particularly likely to happen if patients are reassured at the same time as further tests are ordered or if they are told nothing serious is wrong but are given a prescription for medication.

## Patient Rather than Physician Responsibility

The reframing of the patient's complaint in an illness behaviour model also requires a subtle but profound change in the locus of control from physician to patient and a switch of expectations from cure to coping or rehabilitation. This is best accomplished by a "good news-bad news" strategy: The "good news" is that based on a thorough examination there is no progressive, malignant, or potentially fatal cause for the symptoms. The "bad news" is that the provider cannot promise to cure them. However, there are many ways in which the sufferer can be helped in learning to cope with disability and to lead a more satisfying life despite it. This message does not challenge the validity or reality of the symptoms, but acknowledges that their final cause or explanation may remain unresolved.

In the case of chronic pain approximately one-third of patients may reject this offer of rehabilitative help and insist on continuing the search for a definitive biomedical answer elsewhere. A useful response is to encourage them to return if they should fail to find a biomedical solution elsewhere. This differs from the kind of hostile disagreement that once characterized the management of psychosomatic patients and which usually led to discharge "against medical advice".

A final strategy in promoting patient responsibility is the avoidance of "first contact" prescribing. This is for two reasons. In acute primary care settings the initiation of drug therapy after the first interview is highly likely to coincide with all the spontaneously occurring curative or restorative factors discussed earlier. For this reason recovery may be mistakenly attributed by both the patient and physician to the medication. (1) The next time that patient experiences the same symptoms (often of minor mood disorder or autonomic arousal) they are likely to return and seek the same medication, thus initiating a cycle of dependency on doctors and drugs. This common, but often overlooked association, accounts for the popularity and prescription of Vitamin B12 shots, thyroid pills, iron tablets, as well as psychotropic drugs in primary care practice. A second reason to avoid this type of prescribing is that in both acute and chronic conditions the contradictory message to the patient is of physician responsibility and authority unless the use of drugs is coupled with the kind of explanation discussed below that emphasizes the role of medication as facilitatory to self-coping strategies.

<u>Symptom Control Strategies That Enhance Self-Esteem and Self-Management</u>

The sequence of strategies offered to assist the illness behaviour patient is highly significant. It consists first of methods to control symptoms, secondly on ways to enhance skills that facilitate healthy behaviour, and lastly on the redeployment of environmental rewards to reinforce healthy responses and minimize illness behaviour. The reason for this sequence is that it places primary emphasis on the patient's complaint and is designed to give the patient new skills and coping strategies <u>before</u> any attempt is made to tamper with or remove the long established and often deeply ingrained secondary gains of the sick role. If this sequence is reversed the patients are likely to panic and to escalate their complaints and illness behaviour.

Specific strategies to facilitate perception of control include the following. First, the role of physical rehabilitation is crucial and is given early emphasis especially in chronic conditions. Disuse atrophy, fatigue and lack of stamina are the natural consequences of fear of disease or injury that accompany sick role behaviour. A progressive stepwise program of physical retraining under skilled medical supervision should be initiated with goals that are set to coincide with whatever activity level is required to restore the individual's independence at work or in the home.

Second, the relationship between increased muscle tension and pain or physical discomfort is usually so self-evident that patients readily accept both the theoretical need and practical value of learning to control their muscle tone either by relaxation training or biofeedback techniques which automatically emphasize self-control.

---

1. (Editors' comment). This is an excellent example of the medicalization process, see McHugh and Vallis, this volume.

Third, a simple but crucial strategy is to teach patients to obtain some cognitive control over their symptoms. Most people readily agree if asked that talking about pain makes it worse. Thus, the way is open to avoid discussing symptoms while at the same time they learn new distraction procedures. This has the dual advantage of both enhancing self-control and eliminating environmental attention to illness statements.

Fourth, many patients with chronic illness behaviour sleep poorly. Although the physician may attribute this to mood disorder the patients usually allege that their symptoms keep them awake. They readily agree, however, that poor sleep impairs coping and magnifies their discomfort so the methods of restoring sleep to normal are acceptable to the patient. This may include sleep hygiene and relaxation strategies or judicious use of low dosage antidepressants.

Once patients have been taught control of their symptoms it is helpful to focus on the relationship between environmental events and the aggravation of symptoms. This can be facilitated either by specific cause and effect questioning, describing situations in which the symptoms arise, or by asking the patient to keep a behavioural diary. Once the symptoms can be linked to environmental events the door is open to looking for new ways that patients can learn to cope with the people or situations that aggravate their complaints. It may be helpful to refer to this as environmental control, although it is traditionally known as stress management.

## Enhancement of Skills or Modification of Expectations to Decrease Anxiety of Healthy Behaviour

A major factor that drives people into chronic illness behaviour is the perceived or real gap between their ability in a healthy role and their expectations or those of others on performance. The negative cognitions or autonomic arousal that accompany this situation amplify or create the physical discomfort.

Perhaps the most common skill deficit in patients with chronic illness behaviour is the ability to get their needs met in a healthy assertive manner. Instead they learn to avoid or control situations by "being sick". Social skills training in general, and assertiveness training in particular, can help patients learn to stick up for themselves without this need. Role playing (often in the doctor's office or with an involved relative or friend) can be a valuable method of reinforcement before an attempt is made to deploy the new skill in actual situations.

The role of more traditional psychotherapy is limited in many patients with chronic illness behaviour because many of them are emotionally illiterate or suffer from what is now called "alexithymia". Inviting them to discuss feelings is like asking a colour blind person to describe the sunset. When the patient and physician are interested or willing to attempt psychotherapy its goals are directed either to lowering the patient's excessive expectations of performance, to the recognition of feelings as determinants of behaviour, and to ways of enhancing self-esteem.

## Redeployment of Environmental Rewards to Reinforce Healthy Behaviour and Ignore Illness Behaviour

Both for short term change as well as long term maintenance it is essential to modify environmental rewards to support the development of new healthy behaviours and to reduce the reinforcement for illness behaviour. Within the patient's immediate social environment this is facilitated by a reduction in talk about symptoms. This is not so difficult as many imagine. Most patients agree that their symptoms worsen when talked about and will accept a suggestion that it would therefore be logical to talk about them less. More specific refocusing can occur as a result of couples or family therapy in which the natural care providers can also learn to alter their response to the patient. Relatives are taught to selectively encourage and reward the patient's attempts to master symptoms and learn new skills but to ignore relapses of pain reporting and displays of pain behaviour. This approach is often a great relief to those who live with the patient since they are eager to help but exhausted by the lack of response to their own indiscriminate nurturance and caretaking behaviours.

In a similar fashion it is vital to ensure consistency and continuity among different members of the health professions who deal with an individual. The patient's tendency to "doctor shop" and to "split" providers in order to sustain the sick role is best dealt with by the identification of a single primary care practitioner whom the patient trusts and who is knowledgeable about chronic illness behaviour management. The fear that psychosomatic patients may develop "symptom substitution" is relatively unfounded but "physician substitution" is quite common, with patient taking the same complaint to a new doctor whenever their sick role needs are not fulfilled.

Finally, attempts to rehabilitate patients or have them return to work are often frustrated by unsettled litigation or the existence of compensation or entitlement benefits. Many disability insurers require either complete invalidism or total return to work. Sometimes it is possible to help patients negotiate a partial or gradual return to work within the realities of the system so that there are no false expectations. In the acute setting the early validation of sick role behaviour by time out often sets the stage for invalidism - rapid return to work is often a better alternative just as early return to the front line is the optimum treatment for battle fatigue.

## Physician Behaviours to Minimize the Sick Role

There is much that the individual physician can do to minimize the adoption of illness behaviour. Application of the principles outlined above requires the avoidance of excessive caretaking or overdirection and the promotion of patient autonomy with attainment of congruence between patient and provider concerning the nature, time course, and treatment of symptoms.

This approach is greatly facilitated if the physician has some knowledge and skill in "pain games" and can tread the middle ground between oversolicitous responses on the one hand and rigid limit setting or patient rejection on the other.

Lastly, there is a definite place for judicious use of psychotropic drugs provided they are presented within a framework that enhances non-drug coping which is time limited and maximizes patient self-control. Such prescribing may often be symptomatic rather than diagnosis related. For example, low dosage tricyclic antidepressants may be used to restore normal sleep patterns as part of enhancing the individual's overall coping capacity. Benzodiazepines may be prescribed not so much to stifle anxiety as to alleviate the socially induced fear that inhibits the expression of normally assertive behaviour. In both instances patients are encouraged to titrate and manage their own medication to maximize the therapeutic benefit.

## REFERENCES

Blackwell, B., Galbraith, J. R., & Dahl, D. S. (1984). Chronic pain management. Hospital and Community Psychiatry, 35, 999.

Kellner, R., Abbott, P., Pathak, D., et al. (1983). Hypochrondriacal beliefs and attitudes in family practice and psychiatric patients. International Journal of Psychiatry in Medicine, 13, 127-137.

Meyer, D., Leventhal, H. & Gutmann, M. (1985). Common-sense models of illness: The example of hypertension. Health Psychology, 4, 115-135.

McGashie, W. C., & Whitenack, D. C. (1982). A scale for measurement of the problem patient labeling process. Journal of Nervous and Mental Disease, 170, 598-604.

Pilowsky, I., & Spence, N. D. (1975). Patterns of illness behaviour in patients with intractable pain. Journal of Psychosomatic Research, 19, 279-287.

Pinsky, J. J. (1978). Chronic intractable benign pain: A syndrome and its treatment with intensive short-term psychotherapy. Journal of Human Stress pp. 17-21.

Wooley, S., Blackwell, B., & Winget, C. (1978). A learning theory model of chronic illness behaviour: Theory, treatment and research. Psychosomatic Medicine, 40, 379-401.

## CONTRIBUTORS

ALFRED BERG, Department of Psychiatry and Behavioural Sciences RP-10, University of Washington Medical School, Seattle, Washington 98195 U.S.A.

MONROE BERKOWITZ, Department of Economics, Rutgers University New Brunswick, New Jersey, 08903 U.S.A.

BARRY BLACKWELL, Department of Psychiatry, Milwaukee Clinical Campus University of Wisconsin Medical School, Milwaukee, Wisconsin 53201 U.S.A.

SHLOMO BREZNITZ, R. D. Wolfe Centre for Study of Psychological Stress University of Haifa, Mt. Carmel, Haifa 31953 Israel

GEORGE BROWN, Department of Social Policy and Social Science Bedford College and Royal Holloway College, University of London 11 Bedford Square, London WC1B 3RA United Kingdom

PAUL CLEARY, Department of Social Medicine and Health Policy, Harvard Medical School, 25 Shattuck Street Boston, Massachusetts 02115 U.S.A.

ARTHUR COTT, Behavioural Medicine Unit, St. Joseph's Hospital 301 James Street South, Hamilton, Ontario L8M 1Y4 Canada

BRUCE CUTHBERT, Department of Clinical Psychology, Box J-165 JHMHC Gainsville, Florida 32610 U.S.A.

LEON EISENBERG, Department of Social Medicine and Health Policy Harvard Medical School, 25 Shattuck Street Boston, Massachusetts 02115 U.S.A.

SUSAN FOLKMAN, Department of Psychology, University of California Berkeley, California 94720 U.S.A.

LINDA GARRO, Department of Social and Preventive Medicine Faculty of Medicine, University of Manitoba 750 Bannatyne Avenue, Winnipeg, Manitoba R3E 0W3 Canada

BYRON GOOD, Department of Social Medicine and Health Policy
Harvard Medical School, 25 Shattuck Street
Boston, Massachusetts 02115 U.S.A.

MARY GUTMANN, Department of Psychiatry, Milwaukee Clinical Campus
University of Wisconsin Medical School,
Milwaukee, Wisconsin 53201 U.S.A.

STEPHEN HANSELL, Institute for Health, Health Care Policy, and Aging Research
Rutgers University, 30 College Avenue
New Brunswick, New Jersey 08903 U.S.A.

WAYNE KATON, Department of Psychiatry and Behavioural Sciences RP-10
University of Washington Medical School
Seattle, Washington 98195 U.S.A.

ROBERT KELLNER, Department of Psychiatry
University of New Mexico School of Medicine
2400 Tucker, N.E., Albuquerque, New Mexico 87131 U.S.A.

RONALD KESSLER, Department of Sociology, University of Michigan
Ann Arbor, Michigan 48109 U.S.A.

LAURENCE KIRMAYER, Department of Psychiatry
Institute of Community and Family Psychiatry, McGill University
4333 Chemin de la Cote Ste-Catherine
Montreal, Quebec H3T 1E2 Canada

ARTHUR KLEINMAN, Department of Anthropology, Harvard University
330 William James Hall, Cambridge, Massachusetts 02138 U.S.A.

DAVID KRANTZ, Department of Medical Psychology
Uniformed Services University of the Health Sciences
4301 Jones Bridge Road, Bethesda, Maryland 20814-4799 U.S.A.

PETER LANG, Department of Clinical Psychology, Box J-165 JHMHC
Gainsville, Florida 32610 U.S.A.

RICHARD LAZARUS, Psychology Department, University of California
Berkeley, California 94720 U.S.A.

JOSEPH LELLA, Department of Humanities and Social Studies in Medicine
McIntyre Medical Sciences Building, 3655 Drummond Street
Montreal, Quebec H3G 1Y6 Canada

VICTORIA LEU, Department of Medical Psychology
Uniformed Services University of the Health Sciences
4301 Jones Bridge Road, Bethesda, Maryland 20814-4799 U.S.A.

HOWARD LEVENTHAL, Department of Psychology
218 Brogden Hall, University of Wisconsin-Madison
1202 West Johnson Street, Madison, Wisconsin 53706 U.S.A.

MARGARET LOCK, Department of Humanities and Social Studies in Medicine
McIntyre Medical Sciences Building, 3655 Drummond Street
Montreal, Quebec H3G 1Y6 Canada

BARBARA MELAMED, Department of Clinical Psychology, Box J-165 JHMHC
Gainsville, Florida 32610 U.S.A.

RICHARD MAYOU, University Department of Psychiatry, Warneford Hospital
University of Oxford, Oxford OX3 7JX United Kingdom

SEAN MCHUGH, GUT Behaviour Unit, Toronto Western Hospital
399 Bathurst Street, Toronto, Ontario M5T 2S8 Canada

DAVID MECHANIC, Institute for Health, Health Care, and Aging Rsearch, Rutgers University, 203 Murray Hall, New Brunswick, New Jersey 08903 U.S.A.

ISSY PILOWSKY, Department of Psychiatry, Royal Adelaide Hospital
The University of Adelaide, Adelaide, South Australia 5001

STEVEN RISSE, Department of Psychiatry and Behavioural Sciences RP-10
University of Washington Medical School, Seattle, Washington 98195 U.S.A.

JAMES ROBBINS, Department of Sociology
Institute of Community and Family Psychiatry, McGill University
4333 Chemin de la Cote Ste-Catherine, Montreal, Quebec H3T 1E2 Canada

ANTHONY ROBINS, Department of Psychiatry and Behaviorual Sciences RP-10
University of Washington medical School, Seattle, Washington 98195 U.S.A.

THOMAS RUDY, Center for Pain Evaluation and Treatment
University of Pittsburgh School of Medicine, 230 Lothrop Street
Pittsburgh, Pennsylvania 15213 U.S.A.

ZINDEL SEGAL, Clarke Institute of Psychiatry
250 College Street, Toronto, Ontario M5T 1R8 Canada

BRIAN SHAW, Clarke Institute of Psychiatry
250 College Street, Toronto, Ontario M5T 1R8 Canada

GEORGE TORRANCE, Faculty of Business, McMaster University
1280 Main Street West, Hamilton, Ontario L8S 4M4 Canada

DENNIS TURK, Center for Pain Evaluation and Treatment
University of Pittsburgh School of Medicine
230 Lothrop Street, Pittsburgh, Pennsylvania 15213 U.S.A.

MICHAEL VALLIS, Clarke Institute of Psychiatry
250 College Street, Toronto, Ontario M5T 1R8 Canada

STANLEY WALLACK, Health Policy Center, Heller Graduate Center
Brandeis University, 415 South Street
Waltham, Massachusetts 02254 U.S.A.

IRVING ZOLA, Department of Sociology, Brandeis University
Waltham, Massachusetts 02254 U.S.A.

INDEX